T0195201

Endoscopic Surgery

Editors

JOHN H. RODRIGUEZ
JEFFREY L. PONSKY

SURGICAL CLINICS OF NORTH AMERICA

www.surgical.theclinics.com

Consulting Editor
RONALD F. MARTIN

December 2020 • Volume 100 • Number 6

ELSEVIER

1600 John F. Kennedy Boulevard • Suite 1800 • Philadelphia, Pennsylvania, 19103-2899

http://www.surgical.theclinics.com

SURGICAL CLINICS OF NORTH AMERICA Volume 100, Number 6
December 2020 ISSN 0039–6109, ISBN-13: 978-0-323-76310-3

Editor: John Vassallo, j.vassallo@elsevier.com

Developmental Editor: Nicole Congleton

Surgical Clinics of North America (ISSN 0039–6109) is published bimonthly by Elsevier Inc., 360 Park Avenue South, New York, NY 10010-1710. Months of publication are February, April, June, August, October, and December. Business and Editorial Offices: 1600 John F. Kennedy Blvd., Suite 1800, Philadelphia, PA 19103-2899. Periodicals postage paid at New York, NY and additional mailing offices. Subscription prices are $430.00 per year for US individuals, $891.00 per year for US institutions, $100.00 per year for US & Canadian students and residents, $507.00 per year for Canadian individuals, $1130.00 per year for Canadian institutions, $536.00 for international individuals, $1130.00 per year for international institutions and $250.00 per year for foreign students/residents. To receive student/resident rate, orders must be accompanied by name of affiliated institution, date of term, and the *signature* of program/residency coordinator on institution letterhead. Orders will be billed at individual rate until proof of status is received. Foreign air speed delivery is included in all *Clinics* subscription prices. All prices are subject to change without notice. POSTMASTER: Send address changes to *Surgical Clinics*, Elsevier Health Sciences Division, Subscription Customer Service, 3251 Riverport Lane, Maryland Heights, MO 63043. **Customer Service (orders, claims, online, change of address): Telephone: 1-800-654-2452 (U.S. and Canada); 314-447-8871 (outside U.S. and Canada). Fax: 314-447-8029. E-mail: journalscustomerservice-usa@elsevier.com (for print support); journalsonlinesupport-usa@elsevier.com (for online support).**

Reprints. For copies of 100 or more, of articles in this publication, please contact the Commercial Reprints Department, Elsevier Inc., 360 Park Avenue South, New York, New York 10010-1710. Tel. 212-633-3874, Fax: 212-633-3820, E-mail: reprints@elsevier.com.

The Surgical Clinics of North America is also published in Spanish by McGraw-Hill Interamericana Editores S.A., P.O. Box 5-237 06500 Mexico D.F. Mexico; and in Portuguese by Interlivros Edicoes Ltda., Rua Comandante Coelho 1085, CEP 21250, Rio de Janeiro, Brazil; and in Greek by Paschalidis Medical Publications, Athens Greece.

The Surgical Clinics of North America is covered in *MEDLINE/PubMed (Index Medicus), EMBASE/Excerpta Medica, Current Contents/Clinical Medicine, Current Contents/Life Sciences, Science Citation Index,* and *ISI/BIOMED.*

Printed in the United States of America.

Contributors

CONSULTING EDITOR

RONALD F. MARTIN, MD, FACS
Colonel (Retired), United States Army Reserve, York, Maine, USA

EDITORS

JOHN H. RODRIGUEZ, MD, FACS
Director of Surgical Endoscopy, General Surgery, Digestive Disease Institute, Cleveland Clinic, Cleveland, Ohio, USA

JEFFREY L. PONSKY, MD, FACS
Professor of Surgery, Cleveland Clinic Lerner College of Medicine, Lynda and Marlin Younker Chair in Developmental Endoscopy, Case Western Reserve University, Cleveland, Ohio, USA

AUTHORS

AMAN ALI, MD
Resident, General Surgery, Department of Surgery, Houston Methodist Hospital, Houston, Texas, USA

JUAN S. BARAJAS-GAMBOA, MD
Research Fellow, Digestive Disease Institute, Cleveland Clinic Abu Dhabi, Abu Dhabi, United Arab Emirates

STACY BRETHAUER, MD
Professor of Surgery, Vice Chair of Surgery for Quality and Patient Safety, Department of Surgery, The Ohio State University, Columbus, Ohio, USA

PRABHLEEN CHAHAL, MD, FACG, FASGE
Program Director, Advanced Endoscopy Fellowship, Advanced Endoscopist, Department of Gastroenterology, Hepatology and Nutrition, Cleveland Clinic Foundation, Cleveland, Ohio, USA

CHEN CHEN, MD
Resident, General Surgery, Department of Surgery, Houston Methodist Hospital, Houston, Texas, USA

SARAH CHOI, MD
Resident, Department of General Surgery, Cleveland Clinic, Cleveland, Ohio, USA

SABRINA DREXEL, MD
Fellow, Minimally Invasive Surgery and Flexible Endoscopy, University Hospitals, Cleveland Medical Center, Cleveland, Ohio, USA

KEVIN EL-HAYEK, MD, FACS
Section Head, Endoscopic Surgery, Division of General Surgery, Section Head, Hepato-Pancreato-Biliary Surgery, Division of Surgical Oncology, MetroHealth System, Associate Professor of Surgery, Case Western Reserve University, Cleveland, Ohio, USA

TOLGA ERIM, DO
Department of Gastroenterology and Hepatology, Digestive Disease Institute, Chair, Department of Gastroenterology, Director of Endoscopy, Cleveland Clinic Florida, Weston, Florida, USA

FRANCISCO X. FRANCO, MD
Department of Gastroenterology and Hepatology, Digestive Disease Institute, Cleveland Clinic Florida, Weston, Florida, USA

ELEANOR FUNG, MD
Associate Professor, Department of Surgery, University at Buffalo, Buffalo, New York, USA

EMRE GORGUN, MD, FACS, FASCRS
Section Head, Surgical Colorectal Oncology, Department of Colorectal Surgery, Digestive Disease and Surgery institute, Cleveland Clinic, Cleveland, Ohio, USA

A. DANIEL GUERRÓN, MD, FACS, FASMBS
Assistant Professor of Surgery, Director, Research Fellowship, Division of Metabolic and Bariatric Surgery, Duke University, Durham, North Carolina, USA

SAMI KISHAWI, MD
Resident, Department of General Surgery, University Hospitals, Cleveland Medical Center, Cleveland, Ohio, USA

MATTHEW KROH, MD
Chairman, Digestive Disease Institute, Cleveland Clinic Abu Dhabi, Abu Dhabi, United Arab Emirates; Associate Professor of Surgery, Cleveland Clinic Lerner College of Medicine

MacKENZIE D. LANDIN, MD
Minimally Invasive and Bariatric Surgery Fellow, Division of Metabolic and Bariatric Surgery, Duke University, Durham, North Carolina, USA

MEGAN LUNDGREN, MD
Advanced Laparoscopic and Endoscopic Fellow, General Surgery, Digestive Disease Institute, Cleveland Clinic, Cleveland, Ohio, USA

JEFFREY MARKS, MD, FACS, FASGE
Professor of Surgery, Department of General Surgery, Director, Surgical Endoscopy, Jeffrey L. Ponsky, M.D. Professor of Surgical Education, Cleveland, Ohio, USA

ERIC M. PAULI, MD, FACS, FASGE
Director of Endoscopic Surgery, Chief, Division of Minimally Invasive and Bariatric Surgery, Department of Surgery, Penn State Health, Hershey, Pennsylvania, USA

JEFFREY L. PONSKY, MD, FACS
Professor of Surgery, Cleveland Clinic Lerner College of Medicine, Lynda and Marlin Younker Chair in Developmental Endoscopy, Case Western Reserve University, Cleveland, Ohio, USA

JOHN H. RODRIGUEZ, MD, FACS
Director of Surgical Endoscopy, General Surgery, Digestive Disease Institute, Cleveland Clinic, Cleveland, Ohio, USA

MADHUSUDHAN R. SANAKA, MD
Director of Third Space Endoscopy, Department of Gastroenterology, Cleveland Clinic, Cleveland, Ohio, USA

IPEK SAPCI, MD
Department of Colorectal Surgery, Digestive Disease and Surgery Institute, Cleveland Clinic, Cleveland, Ohio, USA

STEVE R. SIEGAL, MD
Fellow, Division of Minimally Invasive and Bariatric Surgery, Department of Surgery, Penn State Health, Hershey, Pennsylvania, USA

SHELINI SOOKLAL, MD
Advanced Endoscopy Fellow, Department of Gastroenterology, Hepatology and Nutrition, Cleveland Clinic Foundation, Cleveland, Ohio, USA

ANDREW T. STRONG, MD
Department of General Surgery, Cleveland Clinic, Cleveland, Ohio, USA

NABIL TARIQ, MD, FACS, FASMBS
Associate Program Director, General Surgery Residency, Weill Cornell Medical College, Assistant Professor, Department of Surgery, Houston Methodist Hospital, Houston, Texas, USA

CHRISTINE TAT, MD
Research Fellow, Digestive Disease Institute, Cleveland Clinic Abu Dhabi, Abu Dhabi, United Arab Emirates

MICHAEL B. UJIKI, MD, FACS
Department of Surgery, NorthShore University HealthSystem, Evanston, Illinois, USA

CHAITANYA VADLAMUDI, MD, MBA
Assistant Professor, Department of Surgery, Georgetown University, Washington DC, USA

CATHERINE F. VOZZO, DO
Gastroenterology Fellow, Department of Gastroenterology, Cleveland Clinic, Cleveland, Ohio, USA

VAIBHAV WADHWA, MD
Department of Gastroenterology and Hepatology, Digestive Disease Institute, Cleveland Clinic Florida, Weston, Florida, USA

KELLY T. WAGNER, MD
Surgical Resident, Department of Surgery, University at Buffalo, Buffalo, New York, USA

HARRY J. WONG, MD
Department of Surgery, University of Chicago Medicine, Chicago, Illinois, USA;
Department of Surgery, NorthShore University HealthSystem, Evanston, Illinois, USA

Contents

> Surgeons have played a central role in the development of endoscopy from its primitive origins to the development of modern high definition flexible endoscopes. In addition to creating new devices, they have been instrumental in developing new techniques and expanding therapeutic applications. Surgeons will continue to innovate new applications for existing technology and develop innovative new tools to expand therapeutic capabilities.

> Flexible endoscopic procedures, such as esophagogastroduodenoscopies and colonoscopies, allow for diagnosis and treatment of numerous gastrointestinal disorders. Advanced endoscopic procedures, such as endoscopic ultrasounds, endoscopic retrograde cholangiopancreatography, and balloon enteroscopies, offer therapeutic options that are minimally invasive and effective. As technology advances, the equipment and tools in an endoscopist's armamentarium continue to grow. This article highlights key endoscopic equipment and supplies, from simple to advanced.

> Quality improvement is a dynamic process that requires continuously monitoring quality indicators and benchmarking these with national and professional standards. Endoscopists have formed societal task forces to propose quality indicators and performance goals. Institutions are now incentivized by payers and value-based reimbursement agreements to have processes in place to measure, report, and act on these quality metrics. Nationwide registries, such as the Gastrointestinal Quality Improvement Consortium, are used to report quality data to these merit-based incentive payment systems. Quality improvement processes such as these are instrumental to improve patient safety, health, and satisfaction while decreasing costs and medical errors.

managed with an endolumenal approach. This article is an in-depth review of endoscopic management of surgical complications.

Endoscopic ultrasound provides high-resolution, real-time imaging of the gastrointestinal tract and surrounding extramural structures. In recent years, endoscopic ultrasound has played an increasing role as an adjunct or alternative method to conventional surgical therapies. The role of endoscopic ultrasound in diagnosis and management of gastrointestinal malignancy, pancreatic diseases, and biliary diseases continues to evolve. Therapeutic endoscopic ultrasound procedures for a variety of pancreatic and biliary indications shows a high technical and clinical success rate, with low rate of adverse events. Endoscopic ultrasound plays a key role in multidisciplinary management of complex surgical and oncology patients and those with pancreaticobiliary disorders.

The evolution of advanced pancreaticobiliary endoscopy in the past 50 years is remarkable. Endoscopic retrograde cholangiopancreatography (ERCP) has progressed from a diagnostic test to an almost entirely therapeutic procedure. The endoscopist must have a clear understanding of the indications for ERCP to avoid unnecessary complications, including post-ERCP pancreatitis. Endoscopic ultrasound initially was used as a diagnostic tool but now is equipped with accessary channels allowing endoscopic ultrasound–guided interventions in various pancreaticobiliary conditions. This review discusses the endoscopic management of common pancreatic and biliary diseases along with the techniques, indications, outcomes, and complications of pancreaticobiliary endoscopy.

Intramural surgery is a minimally invasive surgical technique based on flexible endoscopy. The first step involves the initial mucosal incision for entry point. Then a submucosal tunnel is dissected to the site of the target anatomy. The procedure performed may include myotomy or lesion removal. When complete, the initial mucosal incision is closed. This technique separates the mucosal flap from the surgical site, minimizing the risk of full-thickness perforation and gastrointestinal leakage. Peroral endoscopic myotomy is the most studied application of intramural surgery but other procedures have emerged. This article explores principles of intramural surgery and summarizes its applications.

Achalasia is a neurodegenerative disorder of the lower esophagus characterized by high lower esophageal pressures and aperistalsis of the

SURGICAL CLINICS
OF NORTH AMERICA

SERIES OF RELATED INTEREST

Advances in Surgery
https://www.advancessurgery.com/
Surgical Oncology Clinics
https://www.surgonc.theclinics.com/
Thoracic Surgery Clinics
http://www.thoracic.theclinics.com/

THE CLINICS ARE AVAILABLE ONLINE!
Access your subscription at:
www.theclinics.com

Foreword

Endoscopic Surgery

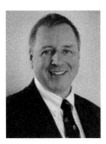

Ronald F. Martin, MD, FACS
Consulting Editor

While one might say that all issues of *Surgical Clinics* are special—and they are—this one is also special in a somewhat different way than others: this issue marks the completion of the 100th issue of the *Surgical Clinics* series. *Surgical Clinics* began as *Surgical Clinics of North America* in 1921. Over that time, there have been some changes, but the mission of the "*Clinics*" has remained the same: to have thoughtful experts explore the best informational content we have and put that information into clinical context that can be useful to anyone.

In the early years of *Surgical Clinics of North America*, the issues were developed in a given city by esteemed faculty. In fact, the first issue was produced out of Philadelphia, Pennsylvania and edited by Dr John Deaver. The foreword to that inaugural issue of *Surgical Clinics of North America* (February 1921) was written by a surgeon, Dr William Williams Keen, who was renowned for pioneering liver surgery in the United States. Dr Keen wrote, "It is a pleasure to survey the constantly growing medical literature by our American colleagues.... I have seen all of this luxuriant growth from Gross' 'System of Surgery' (1859) down to the present time."

Over the years, the way in which *Surgical Clinics* series were developed changed but the objectives remained the same. The issues became developed by multiple collaborators from various geographic locations, and the issues were based on thematic consistency rather than reports of developments in a specific center. Guest Editors were chosen by the publishers based on her/his ability to generate a collection of articles around an important topic.

The development of the Internet and its ability to disseminate information digitally changed the entire world but *really* changed the publishing world. The ability to instantly have an essentially infinite number of "copies" of printed work that could be delivered in fractions of a second to virtually anywhere toppled the concept of having "unique ownership" of an issue. The digital format also changed how people became acquainted with information as the art of browsing a book aside from your

Surg Clin N Am 100 (2020) xiii–xv
https://doi.org/10.1016/j.suc.2020.09.011
0039-6109/20/© 2020 Published by Elsevier Inc.

surgical.theclinics.com

main topic of interest (or search) rapidly vanished into the digital ether. *Surgical Clinics*, through its publishers, navigated these changes very well, and the series has continued to flourish in both print and digital format.

Like many of the contributors to this series, I received my introduction to it by using it as "required reading" during my residency in general surgery. Our professors would impress upon us that if we knew what was written in *Surgical Clinics*, we would have "no problems" taking care of our patients or taking our board examinations—that seemed like a strong endorsement. When I got my first chance to contribute an article to *Surgical Clinics*, I was a bit overwhelmed by the responsibility. Fortunately, my coauthor and professor, Ricardo L. Rossi, was significantly more accustomed to that kind of responsibility. After a series of unlikely events, I was offered the role as the first Consulting Editor for the series, for which I am eternally grateful.

One would be hard-pressed to find a more fitting issue for this centenary issue than this compilation from Drs Rodriquez, Ponsky, and their colleagues on Surgical Endoscopy. Drs Rodriquez and Ponsky represent the quintessential archetypes for *Surgical Clinics* contributors: they are absolute experts in their fields who have a deep understanding of the development of their discipline and are at the forefront of developing its frontiers. Their work at one of the most well-respected organizations in health care is world renowned. We are grateful for the excellent contributions of their team.

The topic of endoscopy is also very fitting for this issue, as it represents both the past and the future of our surgical discipline. Surgeons represent a huge part of the national capacity to provide endoscopic support for their patients, especially in rural communities. Even in centers with outstanding access to all subspecialty physicians, endoscopy is an essential part of the surgeon's toolkit to complement open, laparoscopic, robotic, or image-guided procedures.

As we close this 100th volume of *Surgical Clinics*, this issue is coincidentally my 100th issue as Consulting Editor. It has been an indescribable privilege and an honor to have had this role. The incredible people involved in *Surgical Clinics* have shown me the depth and breadth of collegiality and dedication to improving our discipline that is shared by surgeons and our publishing colleagues alike. It would not be possible to thank everyone individually who has contributed to this series. That said, I would like to acknowledge 2 specific individuals at Elsevier Publishing for their efforts in this series: Catherine Bewick, who was our publisher when I began as Consulting Editor, and John Vassallo, who succeeded Ms Bewick as publisher some years ago. They have been the glue that has kept everything going and going well. Our publishers and the teams that have supported them over the years have been absolutely professional and a joy to work with. Without their hard work, diligence, and patience, we would never be able to get these issues from concept stage to final distribution. Of course, my sincere gratitude goes to everyone who has contributed content to our series over the years. They have done so from their hearts as well as their heads. I cannot fathom how many patients and families they have helped by sharing their keen insights and teachings. Most importantly, though, I would like to express my deepest appreciation to our readership. Their thirst for knowledge is what makes this whole enterprise worthwhile.

In his inaugural foreword to *Surgical Clinics of North America* in 1921, Dr Keen concluded with a final wish, "May it always grow in value and be dedicated solely to the cause of Scientific Truth." As we enter the second century of this series, we shall remain mindful of this wish. We shall do our best to always provide a place where we can take the best content in the surgical literature and view it through the lens of expert analysis and reflection, always trying to better understand our past and present while helping to define the challenges that lie over the horizon.

Ronald F. Martin, MD, FACS
Colonel (retired)
United States Army Reserve
York, Maine

E-mail address:
rfmcescna@gmail.com

Preface

Operating with the Endoscope

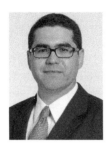 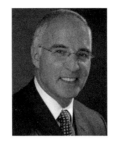

John H. Rodriguez, MD, FACS   Jeffrey L. Ponsky, MD, FACS
Editors

Since its introduction in the late 1950s, flexible endoscopy has revolutionized the evaluation and management of gastrointestinal disorders. Surgeons have always played a crucial role in the development and advancement of common endoscopic techniques. The never-ending quest to improve patient outcomes and minimize the physiologic impact of gastrointestinal interventions has created a perfect platform for the evolution of flexible endoscopy.

Many lessons have been learned throughout the years that have helped the evolution of flexible endoscopy. Diagnostic capabilities have discovered the potential for therapeutic interventions. From the early years of endoscopic management of bleeding and mucosal lesions, the discovery of biliary interventions, and most recently, "intramural surgery," endoscopy continues to prove its versatility and broadness. Innovation has been possible in this field thanks to the crossroads of physicians trying to address clinical challenges, and technology trying to satisfy those needs. As we move toward new applications and explore new boundaries, transparent data collection and reporting are critical.

Endoscopy has also proven to be a field for collaborative effort between specialties. The rapid advancement of this field has been possible due to the inquisitive nature, innovative personality, and ongoing effort to benefit our patients regardless of training background. The adoption and evolution of the techniques that will be covered in this issue of *Surgical Clinics of North America* have only been developed to its fullest potential in centers where this philosophy is practiced. We discourage the dishonest and retrograde practice of "territorial endoscopy." Not only does this pattern result in limited access and adoption of endoscopic interventions, but also, more importantly, this pattern is detrimental to patient care. Professional societies, medical industry, and academic institutions have made a significant effort to make training and skill acquisition easily accessible to physicians seeking those skills.

Surg Clin N Am 100 (2020) xvii–xviii
https://doi.org/10.1016/j.suc.2020.09.012
0039-6109/20/© 2020 Published by Elsevier Inc.

This issue covers several topics that range from basic equipment utilization all the way to advanced techniques. We hope that the reader can become more familiar with the available tools and all the potential applications. We also hope to inspire the future generations of surgeons in training to acquire the passion that the authors share toward this wonderful field.

John H. Rodriguez, MD, FACS
Department of General Surgery
Cleveland Clinic
Mail Code A100
1730 West 25th Street
Cleveland, OH 44113, USA

Jeffrey L. Ponsky, MD, FACS
Department of General Surgery
Cleveland Clinic
Mail Code A100
9500 Euclid Avenue
Cleveland, OH 44195, USA

E-mail addresses:
RODRIGJ3@ccf.org (J.H. Rodriguez)
ponskyj@ccf.org (J.L. Ponsky)

A History of Flexible Gastrointestinal Endoscopy

Jeffrey L. Ponsky, MD*, Andrew T. Strong, MD

KEYWORDS

- Gastrointestinal endoscopy • Flexible gastrointestinal endoscopy • Endoscopy
- Gastroscopy

KEY POINTS

- Early endoscopes were simple instruments with large lumens lacking any lens system.
- In the mid-twentieth century, the development of fiberoptic technology permitted the evolution of flexible endoscopes with transmission of light from an external source.
- Development of modern flexible endoscopes occurred in parallel with advances in computing, image capture and projection.

INTRODUCTION

Observation has been a foundational tenet of the practice of medicine since its earliest origins, a tenet challenged by the presence of intact skin and soft tissue obscuring pathologies beneath. The attempt to extend observation and physical examination to areas hidden from easy external view has resulted in every natural orifice being inspected and probed. The gastrointestinal tract, with 2 natural orifices, is logically a target for such inspection. The pursuit this internal examination has developed through a series of small innovations in technologies that have encompassed developments in illumination, lens making, optics, mechanics, fiberoptics, and image and video capture. The challenge of endoscopy is multifold. Various innovations have provided advantages in introducing a device into the natural openings, dilating the lumen, transmitting sufficient light to the interior, and transmitting an image. Once basic operability was established, further developments have come in the form of tissue resection and retrieval, tissue manipulation, dividing, and sealing.

EARLY ENDOSCOPY

Early endoscopes were simple instruments with large lumens lacking any lens system. Instruments unearthed in Greek and Roman archeological sites resembling speculums

Department of General Surgery, Cleveland Clinic, Desk A100, 9500 Euclid Avenue, Cleveland, OH 44195, USA
* Corresponding author.
E-mail address: ponskyj@ccf.org

Surg Clin N Am 100 (2020) 971–992
https://doi.org/10.1016/j.suc.2020.08.013
0039-6109/20/© 2020 Elsevier Inc. All rights reserved.

or funnel-shaped devices may have been in several natural orifices. Writings also indicate that copper funnel-shaped devices may be been passed into or through the abdominal wall, which may have been an ancient precursor to laparoscopy as well.

The earliest instrument resembling an illuminated endoscope is attributed to Philipp Bozzini in 1806.[1,2] The Bozzini endoscope was an internally lit device utilizing light from a candle flame reflected by an angled mirror to aim light down a polished tin tube (**Fig. 1**). Bozzini called this a *lichtleiter* (light conductor). Using this device, he was able to investigate the urethra, bladder, and vagina in his patients. Although this was an advance for the time, the design proved impractical for widespread use, and light was too dim to be used for deeper investigation. Moreover, Bozzini died of typhoid fever 3 years later, halting his own further development.

Several contemporaries of Bozzini added their own innovations to the field of endoscopy with similar devices using reflected light and tubular specula. Pierre Salomon Ségalas demonstrated the *speculum uretro-cystique* in Paris in 1826, and used the device to identify and destroy bladder stones.[1] In the United States, John D. Fisher produced a similar instrument. The added innovation was the addition of double convex lens to enlarge the image for the physician. In 1853, Antonin J. Desormeaux presented an improved endoscope to the Académie Impériale de Médecine in Paris. He

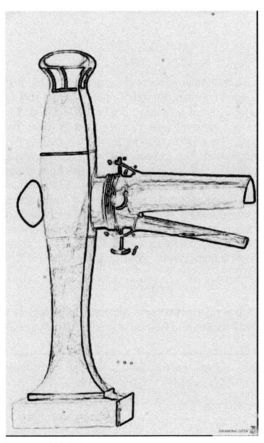

Fig. 1. Schematic of Bozzini lichtleiter.

employed a mixture of alcohol and turpentine, called *gazogene*, as a light source (**Fig. 2**). Desormeaux also is credited with coining the term, *endoscope*, which appeared in a monograph published in 1865 detailed the use of this instrument to diagnose and treat urologic disorders: *De L'endoscope Et De Ses Applications Au Diagnostic Et Au Traitement Des Affections De L'urèthre Et De La Vessie* (*The Endoscope and Its Application For Diagnosis and Treatment of Illnesses of the Urethra and Bladder*). This text and the new term were important in raising the profile of endoscopy in Europe and the United States. Contemporaries made other innovations, employing paraffin lamps, kerosene lamps, or burning magnesium to produce light. Many of these methods, while producing brighter lights, also produced greater amount of heat and problematic smoke.[1,2] Thomas Edison produced the first incandescent light bulb in 1879, which quickly was adapted for use for an early cystoscope within a decade. The stable and bright light source afforded by the incandescent bulbs allowed light penetration deeper into the body cavity and facilitated innovations that addressed other challenges in endoscopy over the next several decades.

EARLY ESOPHAGOSCOPY AND GASTROSCOPY: KUSSMAUL TO ELSNER

Between the 1870s and the 1910s there were numerous esophagoscope and gastroscope designs that were commercially produced, which generally fell into 3 categories. The earliest and the first was an open tube that employed illumination but no lenses or optics. Adolf Kussmaul was considered an early innovator of the open-tube gastroscope. Kussmaul employed a sword swallower to demonstrate gastroscopy at a meeting of the Society of Naturalists of Freiberg, Germany. This was a 47-cm rigid tube that was inserted down esophagus and introduced into the stomach with the patient's head fully extended (**Fig. 3**). Although this was a significant development, the parallel challenge of poor illumination made true gastroscopy difficult to accomplish with this device.

The city of Vienna hosted the next series of innovations endoscopy, both involving Josef Leiter, an instrument maker. Leiter initially collaborated with Maximilian Nitze to develop a function cystoscope. Their design had 2 key features. First a 30o bend in the

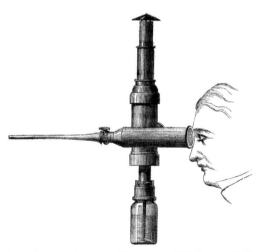

Fig. 2. Desormeaux's endoscope in use. (*Courtesy of* Wellcome Collection, London, UK. Available at: https://wellcomecollection.org/works/as2pqteq.)

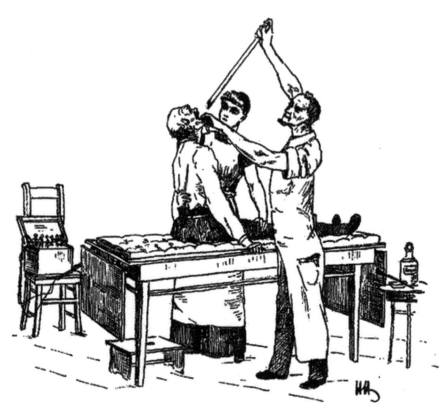

Fig. 3. Kussmaul's technique of introducing a rigid endoscope. (*From* Schindler R. Gastroscopy: The endoscopic study of gastric pathology (2nd ed.,1950), 3, Fig.1; and Victor R. von Hacker, Ueber die Technikder Oesophagoskopie, Wiener Klinische Wochenschrift 9 (1896):92,Fig.3.)

distal third of the instrument shaft facilitated visualization (**Fig. 4**). Second was the employment of a platinum wire loop lamp located in the distal tip and a water-cooling system.[1] This was lauded one of the first truly useable cystoscopes. They developed a gastroscope based on a similar design with a flexible shaft to be straightened after insertion; however, professional differences prevented further fine tuning and the instrument was later abandoned. Leiter soon found a new collaborator in Johann von Mikulicz. The 2 collaborated to develop an esophagus scope a gastroscope based on the Nitze design employing a platinum loop lamp and a distal angulated tip. Unfortunately, there was a growing thought that the principles of cystoscopy and gastroscopy were not interchangeable, and because the Mikulicz gastroscope had been based on a cystoscopic design, it was maligned in medical circles.[1] Mikulicz and Leiter also developed a esophagoscope based on Kussmaul's rigid open-tube design, initially employing the same platinum loop lamp. In 1886, however, the design was modified to employ the Edison incandescent lamp, which made for the first truly useful esophagoscope (**Fig. 5**). A similar design to the Mikulicz-Leiter esophagoscope was used by Chevalier Jackson, working as an otolaryngologist in the United States. Jackson became a well-known champion of bronchoscopy, esophagoscopy, and gastroscopy and their use in clinical practice. He almost exclusively used open-tube

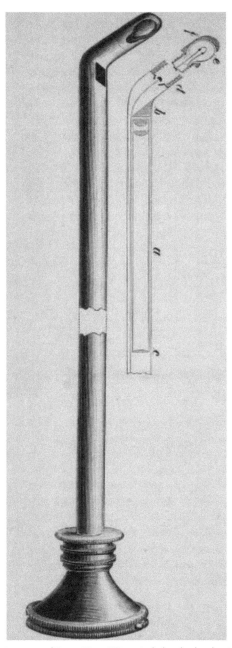

Fig. 4. Nitze-Leiter cystoscope. (*From* Max Nitze. Lehrbuch der kystoskopie : Ihre technik und klinische bedeutung. Wiesbaden: J F. Bergmann. 1889. Figure 14.)

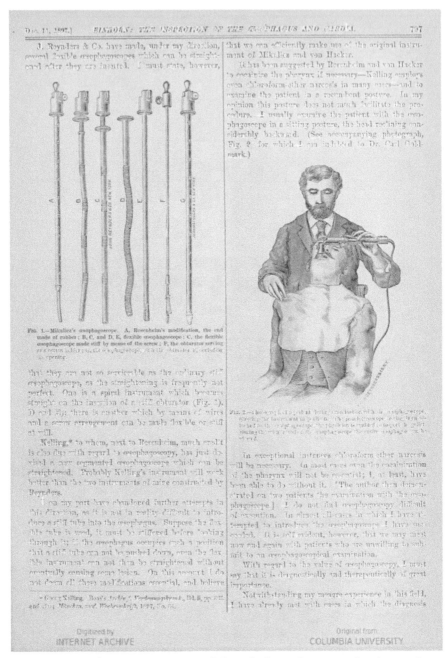

Fig. 5. Depiction of various components of the Mikulicz endoscope and endoscope in use. (*From* facsimile of Einhorn M. The inspection of the oesophagus and the cardia. New York Medical Journal 1897; 66: 797.)

endoscopes for both diagnostic and therapeutic purposes. He was described as a virtuoso of endoscopy, achieving a degree of technical acumen that none could reliably match. His zeal and proficiency with esophagoscopy, however, resulted in the shift of esophagoscopy into the domain of the otolaryngology departments in the United States for the next several decades.[1,2]

The term, *flexible*, was applied to endoscopic instruments in this era but did not conjure the same image as modern flexible endoscopes. Various designs employed tubes that had pliable sections, which were designed to facilitated the insertion of a rigid instrument, in many cases similar to an overtube used with modern fiberoptic endoscopes. Although these flexible tubes were easier to insert, they often necessitated the use of internal mirrors or prisms. These mirrors and prisms were quite fragile and further dimmed the already poor light, and as a result none saw wide use.

The introduction of optics to magnify objects and surfaces at the distal end of an endoscope was the next major development. The first device to employ this is credited to Theodor Rosenheim in 1895. This device contained 3 concentric tubes, one with the optical system, a second with the light source (in this case a platinum loop lamp with cooling system), and a third to mark the depth of insertion.[1] It was rumored that an accidental esophageal perforation caused Rosenheim to stop his work after completing more than 100 endoscopy procedures. In 1911, Henry Elsner produced a modification of the Rosenheim gastroscope, employing a flexible rubber tip affixed to the distal end to facilitate insertion. This innovation proved to be the most significant to improving safety of gastroscopy.

RUDOLF SCHINDLER AND SEMIFLEXIBLE ERA OF ENDOSCOPY

Rudolf Schindler worked in Germany following the close of World War I. He had cared for several soldiers during the war with complaints of various stomach maladies. On return from war he found women and children patients with similar complaints and became convinced that investigation of the stomach would be a valuable diagnostic procedure. Buoyed by the success and safety profile of the Elsner gastroscopic design, he set about performing gastroscopy. He quickly developed his own version of the Elsner scope, employing an additional air channel to clear secretions from the distal lens.[1] In addition to have a useable instrument, Schindler was meticulous in recording both his gastroscopy techniques and findings. He summarized his findings in the *Lehrbuch und Atlas der Gastroskopie*, published in 1923.[3]

Although Schindler demonstrated the utility of gastroscopy and trained many proselytes to promulgate gastroscopy techniques, he was well aware of the risk of perforation the rigid instruments introduced. He dedicated the next decade to improving on the design and ushered in an area of passively flexible/semiflexible endoscopes. He began a collaboration with Georg Wolf in 1928. Wolf was an instrument maker in Berlin and had previously worked to develop a flexible gastroscope with another physician that proved to be nonfunctional. Together Wolf and Schindler developed a semiflexible design for the tip of the gastroscope, utilizing a bronze wire coil with a protective rubber covering to allow for angulation.[4] They also employed a series of large lenses ground to have a very short focal distance and placed them close together, allowing up to 34° of flexion without distortion. A sixth version of the instrument was patented by Georg Wolf in 1932.

Schindler quickly employed this improved design into clinical practice and continued his meticulous documentation and study. Unfortunately, just as this academic work was beginning to spread throughout Europe, the political unrest that underpinned World War II gripped Germany. Schindler, who was of Jewish descent, was placed in "protective custody" by the Nazi party. His non-Jewish wife managed to secure release after 6 months. Schindler had erstwhile managed to communicate with American physicians Marie Ortmayer and Walter Palmer at the University of Chicago. With their help, and the aid of local philanthropists, Schindler was appointed as a visiting professor of medicine at the University of Chicago, and his family immigrated to Chicago.[1] This helped Chicago to become a center point in study and clinical application of gastroscopy. Several physicians in Massachusetts and Baltimore also had conducted early trials in 1933 to 1934 using the Wolf-Schindler gastroscope.

The period from 1932 to 1957 commonly is referred to as the Schindler era, which pays homage to the significant contributions Schindler made to the field of endoscopy. He continued to make improvements on design throughout his career. He was as well-known, however, for the detailed illustrations that allowed physicians to learn what pathologies could be diagnosed. He also was committed to training other physicians in techniques of gastroscopy, allowing them to carry them to academic centers in other parts of the country. There were several significant contributors to instrumentation and techniques in this era as well.

Geopolitics played a significant role in the adoption of gastroscopy in the United States. As discussed previously, protective custody under the Nazi party was the antecedent to Schindler's emigration. The onset of World War II also halted the flow of German-built Wolf-Schindler gastroscopes from Germany to the United States.[1] Although there were few companies that were equipped to manufacture such instruments at the time, 4 separate companies began to manufacture gastroscopes within the United States. Schindler worked directly with William J. Cameron of the of Cameron Surgical Specialty Company to produce the first gastroscope made in the United States in 1940 and became known as the Cameron-Schindler flexible gastroscope. An employee of Cameron Surgical Specialty, Louis Streifeneder left to found the Eder Instrument Co., which also began producing gastroscopes. Their designed, the Eder-Hufford gastroscope, was the first with a controllable distal flexible tip.[1] The American Cystoscope Makers Incorporated (ACMI) worked with Schindler to produce a useable esophagoscope. Schindler was convinced that 11 mm should be the maximal diameter of an esophagoscope, and their effort was largely to produce sufficient light and similar optical transmission, because a safer alternative to a competing rigid 15-mm device made by a competitor. These companies additional innovated in terms of tissue retrieval instruments, facilitating biopsy of gastric lumen as well.

The final noteworthy innovation in this era came as a result of collaboration between the Carl Zeiss company, the Eastman Kodak Company, and the Bausch & Lomb optical company. They jointly improved the capability to transmit light with less loss, which enhanced illumination for existing gastroscope models. They also created a mechanism that synchronized changes between a light supply, the gastroscope prism, and a camera shutter could be coordinated. The recently developed technology for color film then was applied, allowing for photographic capture of the gastrointestinal lumen.

FIBEROPTICS

In the mid-twentieth century, the development of fiberoptic technology permitted the evolution of flexible endoscopes with transmission of cold light from and external source. Fiberoptic technology is now familiar to endoscopists, but this was a nascent field in the 1950s. The principle of internal reflection for light condition has been established in 1930 and was even discussed with Schindler at that time point. Given lack of interest, however, this idea lay dormant for approximately 20 years. The primary problem was the proportion of light that escaped quartz fibers was too great to provide a useful image. Two Londoners published an article in 1954 using a glass fiber to transmit light.[5] This caught the attention of a Basil Hirschowitz, a fellow at the University of Michigan. After viewing the work in London in person, Hirschowitz worked with a graduate student named Larry Curtiss to produce glass fibers. Curtiss developed the technique that proved to the key innovation, wherein he coated glass fibers with a second layer of more optically dense glass, which optically insulated the inner fiber and allowed for total internal reflection to transmit light down the length of the fiber. The fibers could be arranged in a bundle, with each fiber transmitting a portion of the image. If the fibers as the proximal and distal end were arranged exactly the same in a "coherent bundle," then a near-complete image could be transmitted form the gastrointestinal lumen to the observer's eye. Demonstration of this instrument was made in Colorado Springs, Colorado, because the then-president of the American Gastroscopic Society yielded time originally allotted for his presidential address to Hirschowitz for demonstration his "fiberscope." The first publication followed in 1958.[6] Hirschowitz found a commercial partner in ACMI, and in 1960 the first commercial fiberoptic gastroscope was introduced (ACMI 4990). This was the first endoscope produced that would appear familiar to contemporary endoscopists. The major criticism of the ACMI 4990 was that it was too flexible. Although it was advertised a gastroduodenoscope, users found that that duodenum could not be visualized reliably. Control of the distal tip was the most requested design change. A side-viewing model with a 2-way deflectable tip was introduced later in the decade. Philip LoPresti produced a forward-viewing esophagoscope, which then was modified into a gastroscope, this additionally incorporated a channel for suction and air or water to clear the lens (**Fig. 6**). ACMI model 7089 then incorporated a 4-way deflectable tip by the early 1970s. Olympus, in Japan, began also producing competing endoscopes and the 2 companies continued to rapidly innovate throughout the 1970s.

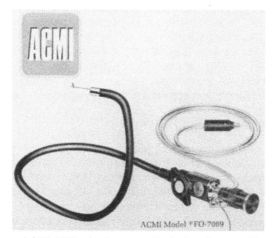

Fig. 6. ACMI early model FO-7089, also known as the LoPresti scope. (*From* Achord JL and VR Muthasamy. The History of Gastrointestinal Endoscopy. In: Chandrasekhara V, Elmunzer BJ, Khashab MA, Muthusamy VR, eds. Clinical Gastrointestinal Endoscopy. 3rd Ed. Philadelphia, PA: Elsevier. 2019: 2-11.e1. [redited in the Elsevier source as "(From advertisement in *Gastrointest Endosc* 16:79, 1970.)"]; with permission.)

COLONOSCOPY

The development of colonoscopy followed a pathway similar to development of the upper endoscopes, discussed previously. As discussed in the introduction, the interest in visual inspection of interior body cavity through natural orifices began in antiquity. Rudimentary devices that were likely used as anoscopes were discovered in the ruins of Pompeii, but there was little improvement until the late nineteenth century. A rigid sigmoidoscope was introduced in 1894 by Howard Kelly of Johns Hopkins.[1] This was a 30-cm tube illuminated by mirror reflected light from an ordinary lamp. Manufacturers in the United States and Germany continue to produce proctosigmoidoscopes with integrated electrical light and they still are used today. It was not until the 1960s, however with the advent fiberoptics and the ability to have a flexible, steerable tip that endoscopic visualization to the cecum became technically feasible. In 1963, Robert Turell reported on 2 innovations. The first was a rigid sigmoidoscope with fiberoptic illumination, and the second used a lightly modified Hirschowitz gastroscope, termed a *flexible fiberoptic coloscope*.[7] He was not enthusiastic about its diagnostic or therapeutic potential. Colonoscopy found a more enthusiastic and optimistic proponent in Bergein Overholt. He began not only to popularize colonoscopy as a diagnostic tool but also aided several companies in developing early instruments. He found that patients experience far less discomfort compared with rigid examinations and that he was able to view a greater extent of the sigmoid and descending colon. He reported the results of his first 40 patients in 1967.[8] Olympus soon released its CF-SB model and short the CF-LB model. The latter was the first flexible endoscope to incorporate a 4-way deflectable tip. Jerome Waye and Christopher Williams meticulously described the technique of colonoscopy. These early proponents who published on their early success included Paul Salmon, in England, and George Berci, Joel Panish and Leon Morgenstern, in the United States. The expertise afforded to them using fluoroscopy allowed to learn how to both reliably navigate the inherent curves of colon and identify the areas being observed.[2] As their skill increased, the need for fluoroscopy decreased, and efforts to train others in their choreographed movements were undertaken. Acquisition of the skills to achieve cecal intubation consistently continues to rely heavily on expert guidance and mentoring. It was only a few short years after the first flexible colonoscopy was performed that William Wolff and Hiromi Shinya described the use of a wire loop snare to resect colon polyps in 1971.[9,10] Additional advances in specimen retrieval added to the utility of this procedure, and colonoscopy quickly became the preferred approach to perform polypectomy. The use of India ink to mark the location of polypectomy was developed a few years later, which aided surgeons in identifying segments to remove.[11]

DIGITAL VIDEO CAPTURE AND TRANSMISSION

In 1984, the Welch Allyn company in New York, known more widely for its handheld illuminated ophthalmoscopes, implemented a light-sensitive computer chip called a charge-coupled device into a flexible endoscope. A lens with a short focal length and short depth of field projected the image on the chip and a video processor decoded the information and produced a video image on a television monitor.[2] With the exception of the eyepiece, the endoscope design and operation remained identical, with image quality that was equivalent. Initially there was resistance to the new technology, because it was much costlier. This was because the endoscopes themselves were more expensive and also necessitated the purchase of digital video processor, monitor, and the necessary attachments. The advantages, however, afforded soon were realized and were broad ranging. Videoendoscopy was adopted quickly for colonoscopy. This made for vastly improved ergonomics with the instrument held at waist level with the endoscopists standing upright. The useable length of the instrument also increased, because the scope did not need to reach to the eye level of the endoscopist. The introduction of television monitors also meant that anyone in the room could observe the examination, or, with the additional of available equipment, it could be broadcast, both of which proffered advances in teaching.[1,2] A less obvious advantage arguably was the most important, which was the introduction of computers into the endoscopy suite. This gave the ability to colocalize report generation, image production, storage and data management, and place them all at the fingertips of the endoscopist in the endoscopy suite. This later also enabled simultaneous storage of radiographic images obtained by roentgenography or fluoroscopy during endoscopic retrograde cholangiopancreatography (ERCP) as well. The standardization this afforded improved quality and reproducibility and eventually enabled automated data capture that has allowed studying rare events (complications) by accumulating thousands or tens of thousands of procedures and various data points to use for analysis.

THERAPEUTIC ADVANCES

Much of the history, discussed previously, details the development of a useable endoscope, that is, a tool or a platform with which procedures could performed. The initial development was focused squarely on observation and diagnosis by findings on the mucosal surface. As the platform became more familiar to the endoscopists employing it, however, they began to develop several additional adjuncts to facilitate performance of procedures.

Biopsy and Tissue Acquisition

The development of the esophagoscopy and gastroscopy was paralleled by the developed of x-ray technology (then roentgenography). Just as physicians began to rapidly make associations between findings observed on roentograms and the resultant pathology discovered on surgical exploration, so did endoscopists desire to establish such connections. Edward Benedict was a surgeon who transitioned away from surgical practice and into full-time endoscopy. He developed and introduced the Benedict operating gastroscope in 1948. This instrument placed a channel within the shaft of the gastroscope to allow tissue retrieval. It became clear that many illnesses needed as histologic examination, because superficial visual inspection was insufficient to make an accurate diagnosis. The Benedict operating scope, because of the introduction of this additional channel, had an outer diameter of 14 mm, and an ovoid cross-section, both of which made the instrument difficult to use.[2] Thus, it was not until biopsy instruments became easier to use with the later fiberscopes that biopsy became performed more routinely, in particular after 1971, with the advent of colonoscopic polypectomy.[9,10] Current endoscopic instrumentation includes various forceps, snares, and baskets to facilitate tissue retrieval.

Hemostasis

Evaluation and control of gastrointestinal hemorrhage now are among the most common indications for urgent or emergent endoscopy procedures. Esophageal varices were the first source that saw a new endoscopic solution. Sclerotherapy was developed by Greg Van Stiegmann.[12,13] At the time, standard therapy to reduce variceal bleeding was operation to create portosystemic shunts, and the new endoscopic approach rapidly reduced the need for these operations. Advances in numerous technologies to provide thermal coagulation followed, with significant contribution by John Papp and Walter Gaisford.[14,15] Currently employed technologies include monopolar and bipolar electrocautery, argon plasma coagulation, and a wide array of elastic bands and metallic clips.

Nonsurgical Enteral Access

In 1979, Michael Gauderer and Jeffrey Ponsky performed the first endoscopic percutaneous endoscopic gastrostomy (PEG).[16,17] In codeveloping and refining the procedure, the 2 identified 3 key goals to accomplish. The first was a to control the location within the stomach, where the tube was placed; the second, a mechanism to reliably approximate the stomach to anterior abdominal wall; and the third, to avoid injury to adjacent viscera. The technique reported in 1980 became known as the pull PEG technique.[16] Similar approaches were soon developed to introduce enteral access into the jejunum for patients unable to tolerate gastric feedings. Other endoscopists introduced additional techniques, including the push technique by Sacks and Vine[18] and the introducer technique by Russell and colleagues.[19] Enteral access is now one of the most common indications for therapeutic endoscopy in the world.

Endoscopic retrograde cholangiopancreatography

In the 1960s, some endeavoring (and, the authors argue, quite patient) physicians were using fluoroscopy to cannulate the duodenum and then blindly probe for the ampulla of Vater. The new advances fiberoptic endoscopy offered a remedy to this, to better facilitate cannulation. William McCune and Paul Schorb performed the first the first endoscopic cannulation of the ampulla of Vater using a modified duodenoscope in 1968 at George Washington Hospital.[20] A team of surgeons in Japan began to work closely with Olympus to developed endoscopes and instruments specifically for this purpose shortly thereafter. The procedure became called ERCP and found vocal champions in the United States in Peter Cotton, Steve Silvis, Jack Vennes, and Joseph Gennen. These individuals were instrumental in moving the tide of endoscopists to accept the procedure. The main critics cited high complication rates, including acute pancreatitis and sepsis. The utility and efficiency afforded by ERCP in diagnosing malignancies of the biliary tree and pancreas helped it to become more rapidly adopted. Then, 2 separate endoscopists, Keiichi Kawai in Japan and Meinhard Classen in Germany independently reported on similar techniques to complete biliary sphincterotomy in the 1970s.[21,22] Soon this led to several technologies to retrieve biliary stones including baskets, mechanical fragmenting devices, and lasers. Endoscopic stents were soon advanced and used to stent stricture and malignancies, pioneered by Nib Soehendra in Hamburg, Germany.[23] Further advances since that point have rendered the therapeutic value of ERCP far more advantageous than its diagnostic ability and included cholangioscopy, excision of periampullary masses, pancreatoscopy, and pancreatic duct stenting. Co-developed with these technologies have been large-scale studies that have worked to increase the safety of the procedure and mitigate potential complications, including periprocedural antibiotics, administration of nonsteroidal anti-inflammatory drugs, and temporary stenting.

Endoscopic Ultrasound

With fully functional endoscopes available that increasingly were user friendly, an additional tool was added to the endoscope, the ultrasound. John Julian Wild and John Reid,[24] who produced the first ultrasound devices for echocardiography, built a rotating echoprobe that they used to diagnose a recurrent rectal cancer in 1956. Several other articles similarly reported using rigid linear ultrasound probes to aid in detecting anal and distal rectal cancers, including determining depth of invasion. In 1976, 2 German physicians used a new 3-mm diameter ultrasound probe passed through the instrument channel of an operative endoscope to distinguish solid and cystic pancreatic lesions.[25] A group of physicians in the United States, including Philip Green (who later would develop the underpinnings for surgical robots) and Eugene DiMagno, affixed a linear ultrasound probe to a side viewing ACMI endoscope. This was the first instrument that combined ultrasound with the optical guidance and tip manipulation capabilities of the endoscope. A feasibility study was published in 1980, with a first in human study published 2 years later.[26,27] The early developers were quick to recognize the utility of endoluminal ultrasound. The concluding line of the abstract for the first reported human use of endoluminal ultrasound stated: "rapid differentiation among mucosal and intramural disease of the hollow gut and disease of extraluminal organs should be possible with this diagnostic technique."[27] Transesophageal echocardiography and endoluminal ultrasound primarily focused on pancreatic imaging codeveloped in the next decade. The utility of endoscopic ultrasound now includes staging for some gastrointestinal tract cancers and a visualization system for myriad diagnostic and therapeutic procedures.

Enteroscopy

In some ways, endoscopic examination and intervention beyond the ligament of Treitz is the final frontier of endoscopy, at least in terms of diagnosis. The sonde enteroscope was introduced in the late 1970s and went through several iterations as a technique to visualize mucosal surfaces beyond the duodenum.[28] The sonde small intestinal fiberoscope was long, flexible endoscope with a weighted balloon at the end, similar to the then popular Miller-Abbott tubes used for nasoenteric decompression, which used native intestinal peristalsis to push the balloon and endoscope forward. The endoscopist then slowly drew the instrument back, and could reliably inspect approximately half of the small bowel mucosa; however, there was no instrument channel for tissue sampling or therapeutic intervention.[29] In 2001, Yamamato revolutionized small bowel endoscopy with the advent of double-balloon enteroscopy.[30] This technique used the traction between 2 separate balloons on the endoscopy to provide a fixed fulcrum to advance the scope tip forward. Single-balloon versions were soon developed, which were simpler to maneuver but did not permit access as deep into the small bowel. Push enteroscopy was introduced as another option, with transoral introduction of a small caliber colonoscope.[31]

ENDSOCOPIC SURGERY

The development of endoscopy has been heavily influenced by surgeons, which explains why most new endoscopic developments in terms of visualization and diagnosis quickly were followed by therapeutic applications. The realization of the endoscope as a surgical tool, however, has started to come into its own only in the past 2 decades.

In 1997, a group of surgeons and gastroenterologists secured industry funding and infrastructure to found the Apollo Group with a goal to innovate in therapeutic endoscopy. After several high-profile presentations at major national meetings, representatives of the Society of American Gastrointestinal and Endoscopic Surgeons, the American Society for Gastrointestinal Endoscopy, and the Apollo Group organized under the broader consortium Natural Orifice Consortium for Assessment and Research (NOSCAR). They coined the term, *natural orifice translumenal surgery (NOTES)*, in a white paper.[32–34] This method involves gaining luminal access, then traversing the wall of the stomach, colon, vagina, or bladder with an endoscope to perform an intra-peritoneal procedures. Although the grand vision of this group ultimately failed to materialize in terms of common use, the concentrated effort into the development of new instrumentation gave endoscopists a new set of tools and vigorously fueled new imagination. The outgrowth of this has been the development of new endoscopic, and intramural surgical procedures.

Peroral Endoscopic Myotomy

Peroral endoscopic myotomy (POEM) emerged as an outgrowth of NOTES and is the most successful manifestation of NOSCAR. Christopher Gostout and colleagues were the first to suggest submucosal tunneling as a component of a natural orifice surgery. The technique was a midesophageal mucosal incision, with long tunnel, and was initially intended to facilitate peroral peritoneoscopy by exiting the submucosa from the gastric wall.[35] This technique offset the serosal and mucosal defects with the protection of a long submucosal tunnel that was meant to address the fear of enteric leak with full thickness division of the intestinal wall. The following year, the same technique was proposed as the tunneling technique as a way to divide the esophageal muscles as a therapy achalasia. Haruhiro Inoue became the first to perform the procedure in a human in 2008.[36,37] The POEM procedure is now well known and has become an accepted treatment of achalasia. The technique involves creating longitudinal mucosal incision in the midesophagus and engaging the submucosal plane. A plastic cap fitted on the end of a standard endoscope provides tissue traction and more importantly holds the tissue a few millimeters away from the endoscope lens. The tunnel is developed down to the esophagogastric junction. The circular muscle fibers then are divided from within the tunnel. Finally the mucosal entry point is closed with a series of endoscopic clips (**Fig. 7**).[38,39] The entry point for the tunnel in early experience was on the anterior surface of esophagus, although a posterior technique has also been described. Thousands of POEM procedures have been performed in the past decade. In many ways, the POEM not only has become the greatest legacy of but also the prototypical example of NOTES.[40]

The first natural offshoot of the POEM was a technique, called submucosal tunneled endoscopic resection, to treat esophageal leiomyomas. Leiomyomas of the esophagus are rare submucosal lesions found in the distal esophagus and can cause dysphagia even when small. Surgical resection offers the opportunity for cure but with a significant risk of complications, such that the benefit often was not outweighed. A submucosal tunnel offered access to the distal esophageal submucosal space with a much more favorable safety profile. This technique is increasingly employed to resect and retrieve these tumors.[41,42]

Peroral Pyloromyotomy

Another adaptation of submucosal tunneling has altered the treatment paradigm for gastroparesis, peroral pyloromyotomy (POP), alternately known as gastric POEM, although the former both more accurately describes the procedure and is less likely to be confused for the achalasia treatment. Part of the gastric emptying delay in gastroparesis may be related to pylorospasm and/or inappropriately timed pyloric relaxation. Prior therapies to correct this have been the temporary botulinum toxin injection and surgical pyloroplasty. POP offered an endoscopic corollary. POP involves the creation of a submucosal tunnel in the stomach antrum, identification and division of the pyloric muscular ring.[43] Retrospective series have demonstrated that this technique improves both gastric emptying and gastroparesis symptoms.[44–46] Comparative

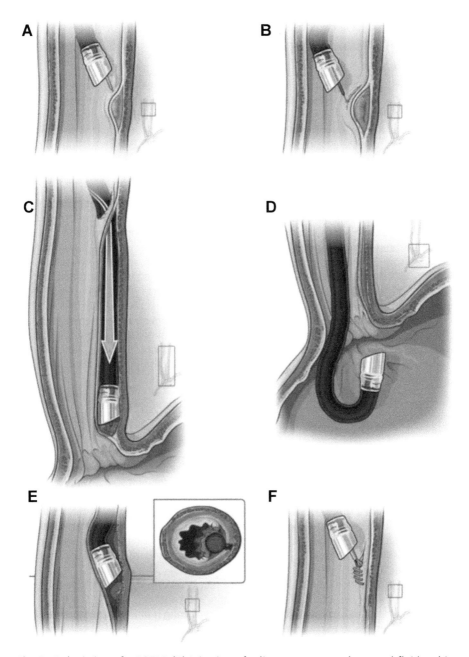

Fig. 7. A depiction of a POEM. (*A*) Injection of saline to create a submucosal fluid cushion; (*B*) longitudinal incision over the submucosal fluid cushion; (*C*) development of a submucosal tunnel as depicted by the *arrow*; (*D*) retroflexed view from within the stromch to view the distal extent of dye in the submucosal space; (*E*) division of the circular muscle fibers from within the submucosal tunnel; and (*F*) closure of the mucosal incision with endoscopic clips. (*From* Ponsky JL, Marks JM, Pauli EM. How I do it: per-oral endoscopic myotomy (POEM). J Gastrointest Surg. 2012; 16(6):1251-5; Printed with permission from © Novie Studio, 2020.)

retrospective data have demonstrated the therapeutic effect of POP to be similar to laparoscopic pyloroplasty.[47]

Flexible Endoscopic Zenker Diverticulotomy

Zenker diverticulum, or hypopharyngeal diverticulum, is another esophageal pathology that has seen application of therapeutic flexible endoscopy and submucosal tunneling. A Zenker diverticulum is a pseudodiverticulum that forms through a congenital point of the weakness in the cervical esophagus that results from hyperpressurization of the esophagus due to dysfunction of the cricopharyngeus muscle. The surgical treatment of a symptomatic Zenker diverticulum is either resection or suspension to prevent swallowed food from entering during deglutition, both of which traditionally were approached through a lateral neck incision and combined with a cricopharyngeal myotomy. Transoral routes were developed, using a variety of cutting and sealing devices, although most relied on being able to directly the diverticulum from the mouth. To accomplish this, a specially designed retractor was developed (Weerda scope) but involves extreme neck extension that not always was possible in the elderly patients that suffer from Zenker diverticula. Flexible endoscopic techniques were developed in the 1990s but failed to gain acceptance, at least partially due to limited instrumentation options.[48,49] A new approach to Zenker diverticulotomy has been to use endoscopic knives to divided both the septum between the esophageal lumen and the cricopharyngeus muscle contained therein.[50,51] The authors have developed a similar technique, where a submucosal tunnel is developed on either side of the cricopharyngeal bar with a goal to divide the muscle alone.[52] This is an endoscopic corollary to an acceptable treatment, where only the muscle is divided for small diverticula with minimal symptoms.

Endoscopic Mucosal Resection and Endoscopic Submucosal Dissection

Tissue acquisition for histology analysis came with the advent of the Benedict operating endoscope and later with the endoscopic polypectomy. The original snare polypectomy technique used today is well applied to pedunculated polyps throughout the gastrointestinal tract; however, lateral spreading and sessile polyps are more challenging to remove. Injection of fluid in the submucosa was introduced as a way to create a neopolyp or pseudopolyp. Once the lesion is raised with this submucosal fluid cushion, a snare has more tissue purchase in addition to a margin of safety from the fluid cushion, and the mucosal can be removed with a snare. Additional adjuncts, including suction, and rubber band application have been developed to assist with mucosal resection after saline lift and collectively are referred to as endoscopic mucosal resection (EMR).[53,54]

One of the challenges with EMR is the imprecise nature, in terms of both lateral margin and depth of resection. Furthermore, the thermal energy applied to the snare may obscure the edges on pathologic analysis, rendering it difficult to assess margin status. Endoscopic submucosal dissection (ESD) was developed as an outgrowth of EMR but relies on tunneling into a deeper layer of the submucosa similar to that achieved by submucosal tunneling in POEM. Because margin status, in particular, the deep margin, is able to be ascertained, ESD may be employed for curative intent of early gastrointestinal cancers.[55] To perform ESD, a lesion is identified that is suspicious for malignancy. Narrow-band imaging, chromoendoscopy, and high magnification endoscopy to examine surface architecture and pit patterns are employed to ascertain likely pathology without a biopsy to avoid the scarring from biopsy that may make ESD more difficult. The lesion then is marked circumferentially with an argon plasma coagulator or ESD specific monopolar knife. A circumferential mucosal incision then is made. A tunnel is developed in the submucosa beneath the entire lesion, until it is lifted free of the submucosa and then extracted. In Asia, gastric cancer occurs at a high rate and national screening programs exist that detect early gastric cancers. ESD has supplanted traditional surgical resection as the standard of care for early gastric cancers.[56,57] ESD has been slower promulgate outside Asia, where gastric cancer is less common. In the United States and Europe, where colon cancer is more endemic, ESD has hopeful application for resection of sessile and laterally spreading polyps. The greater difficulty in fine maneuvering and the thinner colonic wall, however, make ESD more challenging.[58]

ENDOLUMINAL THERAPY AND ENDOSCOPIC DELIVERY OF INTRALUMINAL DEVICES

The endoscope as a therapeutic tool is no longer limited to tissue sampling and resection. The endoscope increasingly is leveraged as a delivery platform for devices used to treat various maladies of the gastrointestinal tract. In addition, as endoscopic instrumentation continues to more closely resemble and replicate surgical instruments used in open or laparoscopic surgery, the endoscope has become a valuable surgical instrument. A brief overview of some examples of these innovations follows.

Endoscopic Treatment of Barrett esophagus

Until the past 3 decades, the progression from columnar metaplasia to esophageal adenocarcinoma was managed best by esophagectomy. A series of endoscopic therapeutic options, however, have moved the treatment of metaplasia, and even early-stage esophageal malignancy into the realm of endoscopy. The first ablative therapy applied to Barrett esophagus was argon plasma coagulation.[59] Now, numerous therapeutic devices exist, with an array of technologies that include electrocoagulation, laser ablation, photodynamic therapies, cryoablation, and radiofrequency ablation.[60] In addition to ablative technologies, endoscopic technologies have been developed to augment or reinforce the reflux barrier function of lower esophageal sphincter. These include endoscopic fundoplication, endoscopic suturing, mucosal resection and radiofrequency ablation.[61]

Endoscopic Management of Obesity

As obesity and its attendant co-morbidities afflict a growing proportion of the global population, there has been an increasing interest in non-surgical options for weight loss. Space-occupying, liquid-filled, endoscopically deployable, and retrievable intragastric balloons have been demonstrated to augment short-term weight loss.[62] Several commercial options exist, but their duration is limited to 3 months to 12 months in most cases. Other technologies have sought to divert chyme from the stomach and/or minimize its surface interactions with the mucosa of the proximal small intestine responsible for producing a number of metabolically active gut hormones. A watertight liner that shuttles food from the stomach to the jejunum has been studied in Europe, with a United States trial currently under way.[63] A device used to ablate the duodenal mucosa (termed, *duodenal mucosal resurfacing*) to restore insulin sensitivity has been used in feasibility studies, with randomized trial currently under way.[64]

Finally, endoscopists are actively experimenting with techniques that are familiar to surgeons: suturing and creation of anastomoses. Commercially available endoscopic suturing devices now have made sutured endoluminal gastric volume reduction possible. Endoscopic sleeve gastroplasty is a technique that uses a triangular suture pattern to plicate the greater curve of the stomach and reduce stomach volume.

Several devices that use self-assembling magnets also currently are in development to create nonsurgical anastomoses.[64]

TRANSLUMENAL ENDOSCOPIC SURGERY

Recent innovations in endoscopic technique have pushed the therapeutic endoscope as a tool that can be used to cross the wall of the gastrointestinal tract to perform procedures. Typically paired with endoscopic ultrasound guidance, new procedures have been introduced. The first technique in this category was transmural drainage of peripancreatic fluid collections. The first report was 19 patients, with pseudocysts resulting from pancreatitis. A diathermy needle was used to penetrate the wall of stomach or duodenum, where there was bulging from a cyst and make a 10-mm to 15-mm incision. A nasoenteric catheter was placed into the cyst with the endoscope for later irrigation.[65] This technique later was advanced with the use of endoscopic ultrasound guidance.[66] Soon, self-expanding metal stents, and later lumen-opposing metal stents were introduced to maintain patency between the cyst and the gastrointestinal tract to allow for internal drainage.[67] Endoscopic necrosectomy through these lumen-apposing metal stents is becoming an increasingly routine component of the management of necrotizing pancreatitis.[68,69]

Gallbladder decompression also has been accomplished with endoscopic guidance. In 2007, a report was published of a patient with advanced cholangiocarcinoma with acute cholecystitis caused by coverage of the cystic duct with a metal biliary stent. Using endoscopic ultrasound guidance, 2 double-pigtail stents were placed from the duodenum into the distended gallbladder.[70] Additional series have been published utilizing a similar technique to deploy self-expanding metal stents as well as lumen-apposing metal stents.[71] Both techniques provided a completely internal solution to biliary decompression in patients who are poor surgical candidates with acute cholecystitis.

FUTURE DEVELOPMENTS IN ENDOSCOPY

The future of endoscopy is likely to be one of exciting innovation. The endoscope, and the procedures performed with it, likely will appear more similar to operations currently performed with laparoscopic and open surgical instruments. The application of robotic technology to endoscopy will bring new capabilities, in particular with regard to tissue retraction, which has been a perpetual challenge to the performance of endoscopic surgical procedures. Increasingly, digital video displays will embed augmented reality and add tools to aid diagnosis and intraprocedural decision making. There may be new mechanisms to deliver therapeutic medications directly to their tissue targets and new advances to develop endoscopic analogs to formerly open or laparoscopic operations. The ever-increasing array of devices and procedures likely will demand new mechanisms to ascertain safety and efficacy as well as quality assurance and training.

SUMMARY

Surgeons have been involved in the development and evolution of endoscopy from is early origins using aluminum tubes and candle light to modern high definition flexible therapeutic endoscopes. They have been instrumental in developing new methods and have been actively involved in most of the therapeutic applications discussed previously. The continued evolution of endoscopic technique is inevitable and will involve the integration of new technology with innovative thinking.

CLINICS CARE POINTS

- Endoscopy began as a tool for observation and diagnosis.
- Advances in illumination, photography, video capture, and computing have paralleled the development of flexible endoscopes.
- Increasingly endoscopes are being used to perform operations.
- With the advent of endoscopic ultrasound and submucosal tunneling techniques, endoscopic surgery is no longer limited to intervening on mucosa based disease, full thickness, transmural, and intramural procedures are possible and increasingly common.

DISCLOSURE

The authors have nothing to disclose.

REFERENCES

1. Edmonson JM. History of the instruments for gastrointestinal endoscopy. Gastrointest Endosc 1991;37:S27–56.
2. Achord JL, Muthusamy VR. The history of gastrointestinal endoscopy. In: Chandrasekhara V, Elmunzer BJ, Khashab M, et al, editors. Clinical Gastrointestinal Endoscopy. Chapter 1. 3rd Edition. Philadelphia: Elsevier; 2019. p. 2–11.
3. Schindler R. Lehrbuch und Atlas der Gastroskopie. Muchen: Lehmann; 1923.
4. Schindler R. Gastroscopy with a flexible gastroscope. Am J Dig Dis Nutr 1935;2: 656, 63.
5. Hopkins HH, Kapany NS. A flexible fibrescope, using static scanning. Nature 1954;173:39–41.
6. Hirschowitz BI, Curtiss LE, Peters CW, et al. Demonstration of a new gastroscope, the fiberscope. Gastroenterology 1958;35:50 [discussion: 51–3].
7. Turell R. Fiber optic coloscope and sigmoidoscope. Am J Surg 1963;105:133–6.
8. Overholt BF. Clinical experience with the fibersigmoidoscope. Gastrointest Endosc 1968;15:27.
9. Wolff WI, Shinya H. Colonofiberoscopy. JAMA 1971;217:1509–12.
10. Wolff WI, Shinya H. Polypectomy via the fiberoptic colonoscope. Removal of neoplasms beyond reach of the sigmoidoscope. N Engl J Med 1973;288:329–32.
11. Ponsky JL, King JF. Endoscopic marking of colonic lesions. Gastrointest Endosc 1975;22:42–3.
12. Lilly JR, Van Stiegmann G, Stellin G. Esophageal endosclerosis in children with portal vein thrombosis. J Pediatr Surg 1982;17:571–5.
13. Van Stiegmann G, Goff JS. Endoscopic esophageal varix ligation: preliminary clinical experience. Gastrointest Endosc 1988;34:113–7.
14. Gaisford WD. Endoscopic electrohemostasis of active upper gastrointestinal bleeding. Am J Surg 1979;137:47–53.
15. Papp JP. Endoscopic electrocoagulation in the management of upper gastrointestinal tract bleeding. Surg Clin North Am 1982;62:797–806.
16. Gauderer MW, Ponsky JL, Izant RJ. Gastrostomy without laparotomy: a percutaneous endoscopic technique. J Pediatr Surg 1980;15:872–5.
17. Ponsky JL, Gauderer MW. Percutaneous endoscopic gastrostomy: a nonoperative technique for feeding gastrostomy. Gastrointest Endosc 1981;27:9–11.
18. Sacks BA, Vine HS, Palestrant AM, et al. A nonoperative technique for establishment of a gastrostomy in the dog. Invest Radiol 1983;18:485–7.

19. Russell TR, Brotman M, Norris F, et al. Percutaneous gastrostomy. A new simplified and cost-effective technique. Am J Surg 1984;148:132–7.
20. McCune WS, Shorb PE, Moscovitz H. Endoscopic cannulation of the ampulla of vater: a preliminary report. Ann Surg 1968;167:752–6.
21. Kawai K, Akasaka Y, Murakami K, et al. Endoscopic sphincterotomy of the ampulla of Vater. Gastrointest Endosc 1974;20:148–51.
22. Classen M, Demling L. [Endoscopic sphincterotomy of the papilla of vater and extraction of stones from the choledochal duct (author's transl)]. Dtsch Med Wochenschr 1974;99:496–7.
23. Soehendra N, Reynders-Frederix V. Palliative bile duct drainage - a new endoscopic method of introducing a transpapillary drain. Endoscopy 1980;12:8–11.
24. Wild JJ, Reid JM. Diagnostic use of ultrasound. Br J Phys Med Its Appl Ind 1956; 19:248–57, passim.
25. Lutz H, Rösch W. Transgastroscopic ultrasonography. Endoscopy 1976;8:203–5.
26. DiMagno EP, Buxton JL, Regan PT, et al. Ultrasonic endoscope. Lancet 1980;1: 629–31.
27. Dimagno EP, Regan PT, Clain JE, et al. Human endoscopic ultrasonography. Gastroenterology 1982;83:824–9.
28. Tada M, Akasaka Y, Misaki F, et al. Clinical evaluation of a sonde-type small intestinal fiberscope. Endoscopy 1977;9:33–8.
29. Tada M, Shimizu S, Kawai K. A new transnasal sonde type fiberscope (SSIF type VII) as a pan-enteroscope. Endoscopy 1986;18:121–4.
30. Yamamoto H, Sekine Y, Sato Y, et al. Total enteroscopy with a nonsurgical steerable double-balloon method. Gastrointest Endosc 2001;53:216–20.
31. Chong J, Tagle M, Barkin JS, et al. Small bowel push-type fiberoptic enteroscopy for patients with occult gastrointestinal bleeding or suspected small bowel pathology. Am J Gastroenterol 1994;89:2143–6.
32. Rattner D, Kalloo A, ASGE/SAGES Working Group. ASGE/SAGES Working Group on Natural Orifice Translumenal Endoscopic Surgery. October 2005. Surg Endosc 2006;20:329–33.
33. ASGE, SAGES. ASGE/SAGES Working Group on Natural Orifice Translumenal Endoscopic Surgery White Paper October 2005. Gastrointest Endosc 2006;63: 199–203.
34. Pearl JP, Ponsky JL. Natural orifice translumenal endoscopic surgery: a critical review. J Gastrointest Surg 2008;12:1293–300.
35. Sumiyama K, Tajiri H, Gostout CJ. Submucosal endoscopy with mucosal flap safety valve (SEMF) technique: a safe access method into the peritoneal cavity and mediastinum. Minim Invasive Ther Allied Technol 2008;17:365–9.
36. Pasricha PJ, Hawari R, Ahmed I, et al. Submucosal endoscopic esophageal myotomy: a novel experimental approach for the treatment of achalasia. Endoscopy 2007;39:761–4.
37. Inoue H, Minami H, Kobayashi Y, et al. Peroral endoscopic myotomy (POEM) for esophageal achalasia. Endoscopy 2010;42:265–71.
38. Ponsky JL, Marks JM, Pauli EM. How i do it: per-oral endoscopic myotomy (POEM). J Gastrointest Surg 2012;16:1251–5.
39. Grimes KL, Inoue H. Per oral endoscopic myotomy for achalasia: a detailed description of the technique and review of the literature. Thorac Surg Clin 2016;26:147–62.
40. Bechara R, Inoue H. POEM, the prototypical 'New NOTES' procedure and first successful NOTES procedure. Gastrointest Endosc Clin N Am 2016;26:237–55.

41. Liu B-R, Song J-T. Submucosal Tunneling Endoscopic Resection (STER) and other novel applications of submucosal tunneling in humans. Gastrointest Endosc Clin N Am 2016;26:271–82.
42. Xu M-D, Cai M-Y, Zhou P-H, et al. Submucosal tunneling endoscopic resection: a new technique for treating upper GI submucosal tumors originating from the muscularis propria layer (with videos). Gastrointest Endosc 2012;75:195–9.
43. Allemang MT, Strong AT, Haskins IN, et al. How I do it: Per-Oral Pyloromyotomy (POP). J Gastrointest Surg 2017;21:1963–8.
44. Rodriguez JH, Haskins IN, Strong AT, et al. Per oral endoscopic pyloromyotomy for refractory gastroparesis: initial results from a single institution. Surg Endosc 2017;31:5381–8.
45. Rodriguez J, Strong AT, Haskins IN, et al. Per-oral Pyloromyotomy (POP) for medically refractory gastroparesis: short term results from the first 100 patients at a high volume center. Ann Surg 2018;268:421–30.
46. Shlomovitz E, Pescarus R, Cassera MA, et al. Early human experience with per-oral endoscopic pyloromyotomy (POP). Surg Endosc 2015;29:543–51.
47. Landreneau JP, Strong AT, El-Hayek K, et al. Laparoscopic pyloroplasty versus endoscopic per-oral pyloromyotomy for the treatment of gastroparesis. Surg Endosc 2018. https://doi.org/10.1007/s00464-018-6342-6.
48. Mulder CJ, den Hartog G, Robijn RJ, et al. Flexible endoscopic treatment of Zenker's diverticulum: a new approach. Endoscopy 1995;27:438–42.
49. Ishioka S, Sakai P, Maluf Filho F, et al. Endoscopic incision of Zenker's diverticula. Endoscopy 1995;27:433–7.
50. Tang S-J. Flexible endoscopic Zenker's diverticulotomy: approach that involves thinking outside the box (with videos). Surg Endosc 2014;28:1355–9.
51. Tang S, Jazrawi SF, Chen E, et al. Flexible endoscopic clip-assisted Zenker's diverticulotomy: the first case series (with videos). Laryngoscope 2008;118: 1199–205.
52. Klingler MJ, Landreneau JP, Strong AT, et al. Endoscopic mucosal incision and muscle interruption (MIMI) for the treatment of Zenker's diverticulum. Surg Endosc 2020. https://doi.org/10.1007/s00464-020-07861-5.
53. Chandrasekhara V, Ginsberg GG. Endoscopic mucosal resection: not your father's polypectomy anymore. Gastroenterology 2011;141:42–9.
54. ASGE Technology Committee, Hwang JA, Konda V, et al. Endoscopic mucosal resection. Gastrointest Endosc 2015;82:215–26.
55. Lian J, Chen S, Zhang Y, et al. A meta-analysis of endoscopic submucosal dissection and EMR for early gastric cancer. Gastrointest Endosc 2012;76: 763–70.
56. ASGE Technology Committee, Maple JT, Abu Dayyeh BK, et al. Endoscopic submucosal dissection. Gastrointest Endosc 2015;81:1311–25.
57. Matsui N, Akahoshi K, Nakamura K, et al. Endoscopic submucosal dissection for removal of superficial gastrointestinal neoplasms: A technical review. World J Gastrointest Endosc 2012;4:123–36.
58. Draganov PV, Gotoda T, Chavalitdhamrong D, et al. Techniques of endoscopic submucosal dissection: application for the Western endoscopist? Gastrointest Endosc 2013;78:677–88.
59. Dumoulin FL, Terjung B, Neubrand M, et al. Treatment of Barrett's esophagus by endoscopic argon plasma coagulation. Endoscopy 1997;29:751–3.
60. Sharma P, Shaheen NJ, Katzka D, et al. AGA clinical practice update on endoscopic treatment of Barrett's Esophagus with dysplasia and/or early cancer: expert review. Gastroenterology 2020;158:760–9.

61. Mayor MA, Fernando HC. Endoluminal approaches to gastroesophageal reflux disease. Thorac Surg Clin 2018;28:527–32.
62. Bazerbachi F, Vargas EJ, Abu Dayyeh BK. Endoscopic bariatric therapy: a guide to the intragastric balloon. Am J Gastroenterol 2019;114:1421–31.
63. Glaysher MA, Mohanaruban A, Prechtl CG, et al. A randomised controlled trial of a duodenal-jejunal bypass sleeve device (EndoBarrier) compared with standard medical therapy for the management of obese subjects with type 2 diabetes mellitus. BMJ Open 2017;7:e018598.
64. McCarty TR, Thompson CC. The current state of bariatric endoscopy. Dig Endosc 2020. https://doi.org/10.1111/den.13698.
65. Sahel J, Bastid C, Pellat B, et al. Endoscopic cystoduodenostomy of cysts of chronic calcifying pancreatitis: a report of 20 cases. Pancreas 1987;2:447–53.
66. Giovannini M, Bernardini D, Seitz JF. Cystogastrotomy entirely performed under endosonography guidance for pancreatic pseudocyst: results in six patients. Gastrointest Endosc 1998;48:200–3.
67. Shah RJ, Shah JN, Waxman I, et al. Safety and efficacy of endoscopic ultrasound-guided drainage of pancreatic fluid collections with lumen-apposing covered self-expanding metal stents. Clin Gastroenterol Hepatol 2015;13:747–52.
68. Seewald S, Groth S, Omar S, et al. Aggressive endoscopic therapy for pancreatic necrosis and pancreatic abscess: a new safe and effective treatment algorithm (videos). Gastrointest Endosc 2005;62:92–100.
69. Seifert H, Wehrmann T, Schmitt T, et al. Retroperitoneal endoscopic debridement for infected peripancreatic necrosis. Lancet 2000;356:653–5.
70. Baron TH, Topazian MD. Endoscopic transduodenal drainage of the gallbladder: implications for endoluminal treatment of gallbladder disease. Gastrointest Endosc 2007;65:735–7.
71. Law R, Baron TH. Endoscopic ultrasound-guided gallbladder drainage. Gastrointest Endosc Clin N Am 2018;28:187–95.

Endoscopic Equipment— From Simple to Advanced

Sarah Choi, MD[a], Kevin El-Hayek, MD[b,c,d],*

KEYWORDS

- Endoscopic equipment • Endoscopic instruments • Endoscopic surgery

KEY POINTS

- Endoscopy plays a paramount role in the diagnosis and treatment of gastrointestinal diseases.
- Knowledge of simple and advanced endoscopic equipment and tools is crucial prior to performing endoscopic procedures.
- Advanced endoscopic surgery is minimally invasive and effective in treatment of gastrointestinal disorders that previously required surgery.

INTRODUCTION

From the introduction of the first semiflexible gastroscope in the 1930s to the development of the fiberoptic endoscope in the 1950s to the evolution of the current video endoscope, flexible endoscopy has played a critical role in the management of gastrointestinal (GI) diseases. Flexible endoscopy not only allows for diagnosis of GI disorders but also offers therapeutic options that are minimally invasive and effective. As technology advances, the equipment and tools in an endoscopist's armamentarium continue to grow. This article highlights key endoscopic equipment and supplies, from simple to advanced.

THE FLEXIBLE ENDOSCOPE

The basic design of today's flexible endoscope consists of 3 main components: the control section, the insertion tube, and the umbilical cord (**Fig. 1**). The control section (**Fig. 2**) is held in the endoscopist's left hand and controls the movement and function

[a] Department of General Surgery, Cleveland Clinic, 9500 Euclid Avenue, Cleveland, OH 44195, USA; [b] Section of Endoscopic Surgery, Division of General Surgery, MetroHealth System, 2500 MetroHealth Drive, H924, Cleveland, OH 44109, USA; [c] Section of Hepato-Pancreato-Biliary Surgery, Division of Surgical Oncology, MetroHealth System, 2500 MetroHealth Drive, H924, Cleveland, OH 44109, USA; [d] Case Western Reserve University School of Medicine, 9501 Euclid Ave, Cleveland, OH 44106, USA
* Corresponding author. Division of General Surgery, MetroHealth System, 2500 MetroHealth Drive, H924, Cleveland, OH 44109.
E-mail address: kelhayek@metrohealth.org

Surg Clin N Am 100 (2020) 993–1019
https://doi.org/10.1016/j.suc.2020.08.002
0039-6109/20/© 2020 Elsevier Inc. All rights reserved.
surgical.theclinics.com

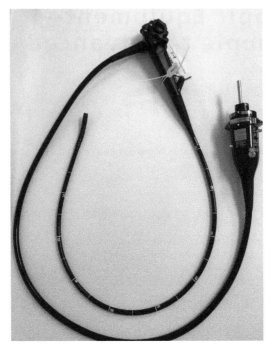

Fig. 1. Standard gastroscope.

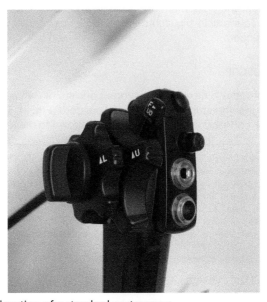

Fig. 2. The control section of a standard gastroscope.

of the insertion tube. Two dials located on the side of the control section allow for manipulation of the scope tip and can be locked into place for prolonged tip deflections. The larger inner wheel allows for upward and downward tip deflection whereas the smaller outer wheel allows for left and right tip deflection. In addition to manipulation of the control dials, torqueing the insertion tube and rotating the control section can help acquire the desired image.[1] Two buttons on the front of the control section allow for tip cleaning, suction, and air or carbon dioxide (CO_2) insufflation, while additional buttons allow for image freeze and capture. An entry channel located distally on the control section allows for passage of various instruments toward the tip of the scope. Additionally, for colonoscopes, a variable stiffness control feature located at the base of the control section allows the endoscopist to adjust the insertion tube coil elasticity to easily reduce loops and freely maneuver through the angulations of the colon (**Fig. 3**).

The insertion tube is a flexible shaft attached to the control section that usually is grasped with the endoscopist's right hand and inserted into the patient. It can vary in length, diameter, direction of view, degree of tip angulation, and number of working channels, with newer endoscopes including an auxiliary water channel that allows for a foot-controlled water pump for extra flushing capabilities.[2] The working channel allows for passage of accessory instruments while acting simultaneously as a suction channel. The shaft also contains angulation wires to enable deflection of the

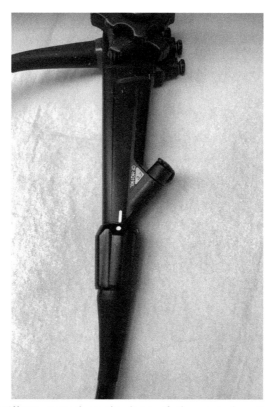

Fig. 3. Variable stiffness control at the base of the control section on a standard colonoscope.

instrument tip while the tip itself contains the objective lens, light guide illumination system, working channel opening, auxiliary water nozzle, and air/water channel nozzle.[2] Most importantly, for videoscopes, the tip contains a mounted image sensor called a charge-coupled device, which allows an image to be transmitted via an electronic signal to an external image processor for display onto a video monitor.[2] Charge-coupled device technology allows for high-resolution images and requires high-definition processors and monitors for accurate and comprehensive information.

The umbilical cord connects the endoscope to the light source, electrical source, and video processor and includes ports for insufflation (air/CO_2), irrigation (water), and suction.

ENDOSCOPY TOWER BASICS

The endoscopy tower is a fundamental element of an endoscopic unit and houses all the components necessary for a successful endoscopic procedure. The basic tower includes the image processor, light source, monitor, and insufflator (**Fig. 4**). Additional components include a CO_2 insufflator, water pump, and energy source. Room air insufflation is provided by an air pump, located in the video processor or light source, that is connected to a bottle filled with sterile water and to the umbilical cord. It is free and does not require medical gas lines or gas cylinders. In contrast, CO_2 insufflation is established by a CO_2 insufflator machine that is connected directly to the umbilical cord and a gas cylinder containing compressed CO_2.[3] Illumination is provided by an external light source, which the umbilical cord plugs into, and the brightness and intensity of the light can be controlled by the endoscopist.

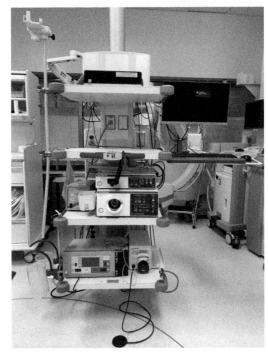

Fig. 4. Basic endoscopy tower.

An electrosurgical unit (**Fig. 5**) is necessary for most therapeutic endoscopic interventions and works by converting electrical energy to a high-frequency electrical current, which then is transformed to a desired voltage. The final effect leads to either coagulation or cutting of tissue with different modes (pure and blend), adjusted by the endoscopist to produce the desired effect.[4]

SIMPLE ENDOSCOPIC TOOLS

A forward-viewing gastroscope is used to survey the oropharynx, esophagus, stomach, and proximal duodenum whereas a forward-viewing colonoscope or sigmoidoscope is used to survey the colon and rectum. Esophagogastroduodenoscopies and colonoscopies often are indicated for diagnostic purposes in patients with a persistent or unknown cause of abdominal symptoms refractory to medical therapy, concerning findings on radiography indicative of strictures or neoplasms, and surveillance of known premalignant conditions, such as Barrett esophagus (BE) and familial adenomatous polyposis syndromes.

Endoscopic Diagnostic Tissue Sampling

If abnormalities, such as ulcers, lesions, masses, polyps, inflammation, and so forth, are observed, endoscopic tissue sampling is done to further evaluate these pathologies. Endoscopic instruments used for tissue sampling include biopsy forceps, snares, and brush cytology.

Biopsy forceps (**Fig. 6**) are used for tissue sampling and come in different sizes and shapes. The standard cold biopsy forceps with or without a needle spike can go through a standard working channel whereas the jumbo forceps, which open up

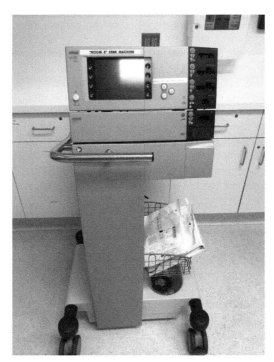

Fig. 5. Electrosurgical unit.

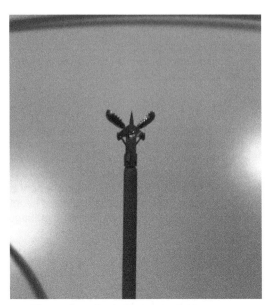

Fig. 6. Biopsy forceps with needle spike in an open position.

2-times to 3-times the span of the standard forceps, allow for a larger tissue sample, and require a slightly larger working channel (**Fig. 7**).[5] Hot biopsy forceps use monopolar electrocautery to simultaneously coagulate tissue while taking a biopsy, but these can be associated with complications, such as delayed bleeding, perforation, and submucosal scarring, especially in patients taking anticoagulant and antiplatelet agents.[6]

Endoscopic snares (**Fig. 8**) are wires configured in different shapes (oval, hexagonal, and round) and diameters that serve to resect polyps and can take larger samples of tissue using the lift and cut, suction and cut, or endoscopic mucosal resection (EMR) techniques.[5] These single or multiuse instruments come in monofilament or braided wires and can be used with or without electrocautery. They are loaded in a plastic catheter, passed through the working channel, and deployed once outside the tip of the endoscope. The open portion of the snare encompasses the target tissue and is closed gradually using the handle, which often is controlled by an assistant (**Fig. 9**). Retrieval of larger specimens can be completed by using a Roth Net® (**Fig. 10**) or a trap (**Fig. 11**) that is connected between the scope and the suction canister for easier retrieval.

Endoscopic cytology brushes (**Fig. 12**) also are used for tissue sampling, can vary in diameters and lengths, and are used with or without a guide wire. The brush tip is placed in a plastic catheter, advanced to the tip of the scope, and brushed against the target tissue multiple times before being swabbed onto glass slides or washed in a cytology solution on retrieval.

Endoscopic Therapeutic Interventions

In addition to diagnostic surveillance of the GI mucosa and tissue sampling, upper and lower endoscopies can be done for therapeutic interventions in the setting of bleeding, foreign body retrieval, strictures, palliation for obstructive neoplasms, and need for enteral access.

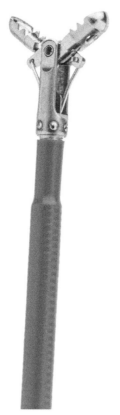

Fig. 7. Jumbo forceps. (*Courtesy of* Olympus, Center Valley, PA.)

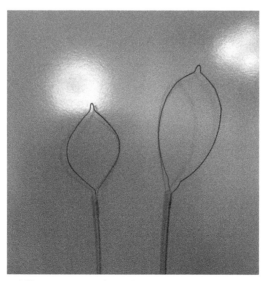

Fig. 8. Two snares in different sizes. *Left,* oval snare (15 mm); *Right,* oval snare (25 mm).

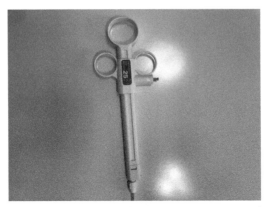

Fig. 9. Handle portion of snare that the endoscopist's assistant controls to open and close the instrument. Electrosurgical energy can be connected.

Thermal tools for gastrointestinal hemostasis

Ablative therapies allow for tissue coagulation, coaptation of blood vessels, and activation of the coagulation cascade for thrombosis. The ablative process is achieved by application of intense energy delivered by means of the electrosurgical unit and instruments that fit into the working channel and transfer energy by contact or noncontact methods.[5] Contact methods include both thermocoagulation using a heater probe (**Fig. 13**) to deliver direct heat transfer (cautery) and electrocoagulation, which uses

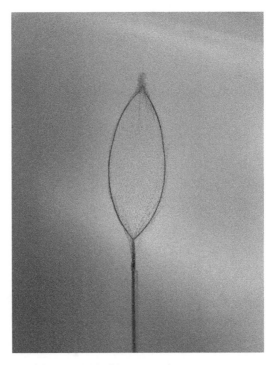

Fig. 10. Roth net.

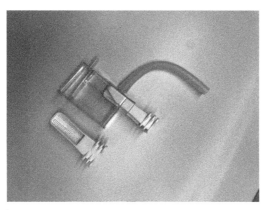

Fig. 11. Endoscopy trap.

monopolar and bipolar electrical energy. Both function by applying pressure to the tissue for tamponade effect in addition to energy transfer to the tissue causing coagulation. Noncontact methods include argon plasma coagulation—a monopolar electrocoagulation technique that works by applying high-frequency current to the tissues through ionized argon gas.[4] Argon plasma coagulation has a decreased risk of perforation compared with standard electrocautery due to shallower depth of penetration and typically is used for more superficial lesions or vascular abnormalities, such as angiodysplasias or radiation proctitis.

Nonthermal tools for gastrointestinal hemostasis
Chemical hemostasis is achieved by injection therapy, using an injector needle (**Fig. 14**) threaded through the working channel for infiltration of agents in the submucosa near the bleeding regions. The handle controlling the in-and-out motion of the needle (**Fig. 15**) from its protective sheath is held by the endoscopist's assistant and communication between the 2 is crucial in safely injecting agents, such as epinephrine and/or sclerosing agents, for both nonvariceal and variceal bleeding.

Mechanical hemostasis is achieved by use of endoscopic clips, rubber band ligation, and tissue adhesives. Hemostatic clips (**Fig. 16**) come in different sizes and can be deployed with or without rotational capabilities to grasp the mucosa and

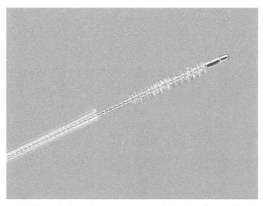

Fig. 12. Cytology brush. (Permission for use granted by Cook Medical, Bloomington, IN.)

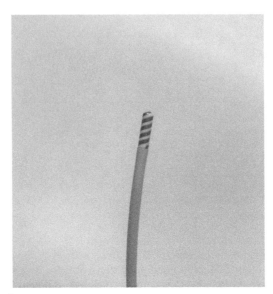

Fig. 13. Heater probe.

submucosa, approximating healthy tissue on either side of the bleeding vessel and subsequently creating an occlusive pressure. Endoclips are best used for bleeding secondary to Mallory-Weiss tears, postpolypectomy bleeds, Dieulafoy lesions, and bleeding ulcers and are left in place with natural sloughing of the clips from the mucosa in 10 days to 14 days. Rubber band ligation, used for variceal or hemorrhoidal bleeding, mechanically occludes vessels. Rubber bands are loaded onto a clear cap (**Fig. 17**) at the tip of the endoscope and deployed around the bleeding vessel.

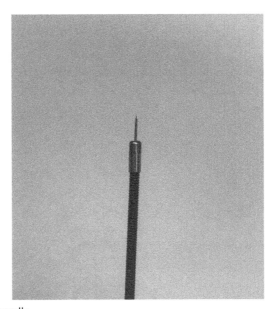

Fig. 14. Injector needle.

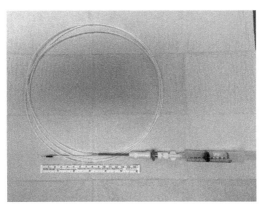

Fig. 15. Injector needle with the handle.

Less common hemostasis techniques include fibrin and cyanoacrylate injections, which polymerize rapidly once injected into tissue and cause thrombosis and obliteration vessels. Additionally, agents like Hemospray (Cook Medical, Bloomington, Indiana) (**Fig. 18**) can be applied directly onto tissues, providing a barrier over the bleeding and encouraging thrombus formation by increasing local concentration of clotting factors.[7]

Foreign body retrieval
Among foreign body ingestions, 80% do not require endoscopic intervention and pass distally without consequence; however, 20% require intervention secondary to concern for injury to the GI tract.[5] An endoscopic overtube is available for protection

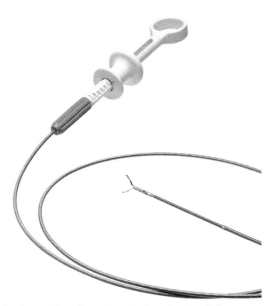

Fig. 16. Hemostatic clip and handle prior to being deployed. (Images provided courtesy of Boston Scientific.)

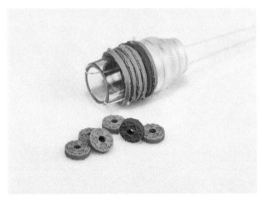

Fig. 17. Rubber bands loaded onto a clear cap. (*Courtesy of* Intelligent Endoscopy, Clemmons, NC.)

of the airway and oropharynx during removal of sharp objects. Various tools are available for retrieval of foreign bodies for both the upper and lower GI tract and range from forceps (ie, rat tooth, alligator, and raptor) (**Fig. 19**), graspers (**Fig. 20**), baskets (**Fig. 21**), Roth nets, and snares to through-the-scope (TTS) balloons that are placed distal to foreign object and propelled proximally.

Enteral strictures

Enteral strictures often are secondary to ischemia, inflammation, neoplasm, radiation, and postsurgical scar tissue. Strictures that can be accessed endoscopically in the esophagus or pylorus can undergo endoscopic dilation, with the risk of perforation reported between 0.1% and 0.4%.[8] Colorectal anastomotic strictures also can be treated using endoscopic dilation, with success rates upwards of 86%.[9] Various types of dilation techniques exist, including those performed with a rigid versus balloon dilator, with or without a guide wire, and with or without fluoroscopy.[9] Endoscopic dilations using TTS balloon dilators (**Fig. 22**) are as effective as dilations using rigid dilators and provide the advantage of not requiring fluoroscopy or repeated esophageal intubations.[10] TTS balloon dilators come in multiple diameters, can be

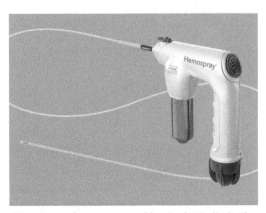

Fig. 18. Hemospray. (Permission for use granted by Cook Medical, Bloomington, IN.)

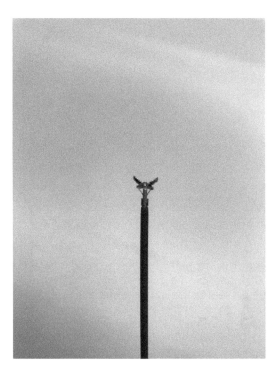

Fig. 19. Forceps.

hydrostatic or pneumatic, and work by exerting controlled radial forces during expansion at the level of the stricture, with incremental dilation as needed.

Enteral stents

Endoscopic stenting increasingly is used for fistula closure, anastomotic leaks, obstructing neoplasms, and strictures. Stents are deployed either endoscopically TTS or via a guide wire with or without fluoroscopy. TTS stents are self-expanding whereas wire-guided stents can be deployed in a proximal or distal approach under

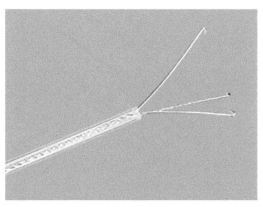

Fig. 20. Grasper. (Permission for use granted by Cook Medical, Bloomington, IN.)

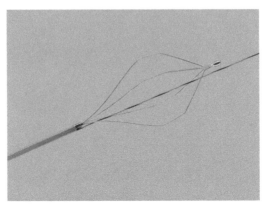

Fig. 21. Basket. (Permission for use granted by Cook Medical, Bloomington, IN.)

fluoroscopic guidance. The stents themselves come in different diameters, lengths, and (plastic and metal) and can be covered fully, covered partially, or uncovered (**Fig. 23**). They can be used for benign or malignant esophageal, gastroduodenal, pancreatic, biliary, and colorectal diseases. Covered stents have the advantage of preventing tissue ingrowth and allow for easier removal once the treated leaks or fistulas resolve whereas uncovered stents usually are not intended for removal and are used for palliative purposes in the setting of malignant strictures and obstructive neoplasms.[1] One disadvantage to fully covered stents is an increased risk of distal migration, with reported rates between 20% and 40% in fully covered stents used for the treatment of benign and malignant esophageal disease.[11]

Enteral access

Percutaneous endoscopic gastrostomy (PEG) tubes have become the standard of care for nutritional support in patients with the inability to swallow or tolerate oral intake and patients with the need for long-term gastric decompression. Additional percutaneous enteral access includes direct percutaneous endoscopic jejunostomy

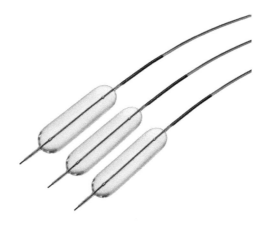

Fig. 22. TTS balloons in 3 different sizes. (Images provided courtesy of Boston Scientific.)

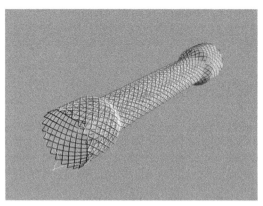

Fig. 23. Esophageal stent. (Permission for use granted by Cook Medical, Bloomington, IN.)

(PEJ) tubes and PEG with jejunal extension. All endoscopic percutaneous techniques allow for safe and feasible enteral access without the need for general anesthesia and laparoscopic or open surgery.[5] Three types of PEG techniques are described: pull-type, push-type, and introducer-type. All 3 techniques start with a diagnostic endoscopy, gastric insufflation for apposition to the anterior abdominal wall, transillumination, finger indentation, and the safe-tract technique.[5] The safe-tract technique is used when the bedside assistant slowly advances a needle into the abdominal wall and verbalizes "air" once it is aspirated into a syringe filled with local anesthetic while the endoscopist clearly verbalizes "needle" once it is visualized in the stomach. In the pull-type technique (**Fig. 24**), a polypectomy snare is passed through the working channel and encircles a looped wire that is passed through the needle. The endoscope, snare, and looped wire are withdrawn from the patient's mouth and the gastrostomy tube is fastened to the looped wire. The assistant then pulls the PEG and endoscope into the GI tract until the bumper of the PEG tube is snug against the stomach wall.[5] The position of the PEG should be confirmed by visualization before the assistant secures the catheter externally. In the push-type technique, a guide wire, rather than a looped wire, is passed through the needle and pulled out through the mouth. The gastrostomy tube, which has a tapered tip for dilation, is pushed over the wire until it exits the anterior abdominal wall. Lastly, in the introducer-type technique, a stiff guide wire is passed through the needle, and the Seldinger technique is used to

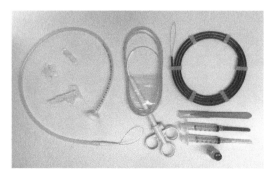

Fig. 24. PEG tube and supplies (20 Fr PEG tube, one piece bolster, external star bolster, dual port feeding adapter, grasping snare, insertion wire, scalpel, 5 cc syringe with blunt fill needle, 5 cc syringe with 25 gauge needle, 5 cc ampule Lidocaine HCL 1%) required for the pull-type technique.

pass the dilator and then the peel-away sheath, through which the gastrostomy tube is advanced into the stomach with subsequent inflation of its balloon. T-fasteners can be placed prior to placement of the introducer PEG to help secure the stomach to the abdominal wall.[1]

ADVANCED ENDOSCOPIC EQUIPMENT AND TOOLS
Endoscopic Ultrasound

Endoscopic ultrasound (EUS) is used in various diagnostic and therapeutic interventions involving esophageal, gastric, ampullary, pancreaticobiliary, and colorectal diseases. Echoendoscopes are forward-viewing or oblique-viewing endoscopes fitted with an ultrasound (US) transducer at the tip, which can be radial or linear.[2] Radial echoendoscopes (**Fig. 25**) provide a circumferential image of structures perpendicular to the axis of the insertion tube and have higher frequency capability allowing for finer mucosal detail. These do not have a working channel and primarily are used for diagnostic purposes, such as assessing submucosal lesions, staging malignancy in the pancreaticobiliary and anorectal regions, and identification of vascular structures with Doppler imaging. In contrast, the curvilinear echoendoscope (**Fig. 26**) produces 100° to 180° images that are parallel to the axis of the insertion tube.[2] It has a working channel allowing for passage of instruments, termed the EUS workhorse, due to its ability to sample tissues via fine-needle aspiration (FNA) and guide therapeutic interventions, such as pseudocyst drainage, pancreaticobiliary access, celiac plexus interventions, oncologic interventions, and vascular interventions.[9] EUS-guided transmural drainage of pancreatic pseudocysts has been shown to be noninferior to open surgical drainage with a shorter length of stay and lower cost.[12] Lumen-apposing metal stents (LAMSs) (**Fig. 27**), double-pigtail plastic stents, and self-expanding metal stents (SEMSs) are used to facilitate drainage and debridement of pancreatic walled-off necrosis.[13] The walled-off necrosis is identified sonographically using a linear echoendoscope and punctured with a needle, through which a guide wire is threaded and used for deployment of the stent.

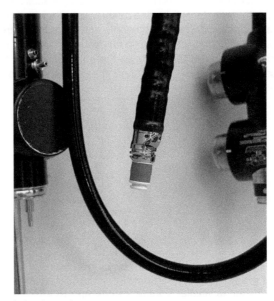

Fig. 25. Tip of a radial echoendoscope.

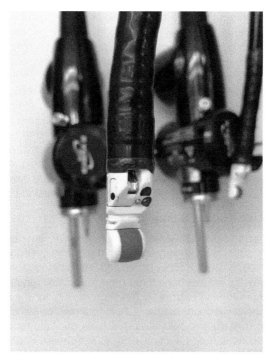

Fig. 26. Tip of a curvilinear echoendoscope.

Similarly, EUS-guided pancreaticobiliary access includes procedures, such as rendezvous, choledochoduodenostomy, hepaticogastrostomy, and gastrogastric anastomoses, and uses the linear echoendoscope and various tools, including puncture needles, guide wires, tapered or balloon dilators, and stents (LAMSs or SEMSs).[3]

EUS-guided celiac plexus interventions include celiac plexus blocks and celiac plexus neurolysis for pain relief in patients with chronic pancreatitis and pancreatic cancer. The origin of the celiac trunk off the aorta is identified and a 19-gauge or 22-gauge FNA needle is advanced cephalad to this region and aspirated for

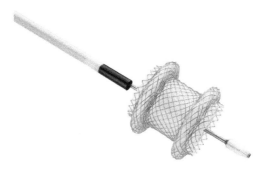

Fig. 27. LAMS (Axios), once fully deployed. (Images provided courtesy of Boston Scientific.)

confirmation that the needle is not within a blood vessel.[9] Once confirmed, the anesthetic agent (with or without steroids) or neurolytic agent (most commonly alcohol) is injected into the celiac plexus to complete the celiac plexus block or celiac plexus neurolysis, respectively. An advantage of EUS-guided over percutaneous celiac interventions is the ability to directly visualize and inject substances into the celiac ganglion. One study showed that pain relief was 73% when absolute ethanol was injected directly into the celiac ganglion versus 45% when injected diffusely near the celiac plexus.[14] EUS-guided oncologic interventions include needle injection of chemotherapeutic agents, placement of fiducials for radiotherapy using an FNA needle and stylet, and implantation of radioactive seeds for brachytherapy. EUS-guided vascular interventions include injection of cyanoacrylate and thrombin to treat GI bleeding and pseudoaneurysms; however, these interventions have been described only in smaller studies and case reports and are not standard of care at this time.

Endoscopic Retrograde Cholangiopancreatography

Endoscopic retrograde cholangiopancreatography (ERCP) is used to evaluate and treat diseases in the gallbladder, biliary tree, pancreas, and liver and is accomplished using the duodenoscope, choledochoscope, and pancreatoscope. Duodenoscopes (**Fig. 28**) are side-viewing endoscopes that come in variable lengths, diameters, and channel sizes. A large working channel is needed not only for the passage of instruments but also for the choledochoscope.[2] Choledochoscopes and pancreatoscopes are forward-viewing miniature endoscopes that have controls for tip deflection, buttons for air/water insufflation and suction, and an instrument channel for tools, such as biopsy forceps.[2] They require a separate light source and image processor and are used for direct visualization of biliary and pancreatic duct lumens.

ERCP generally is performed for diagnosis and treatment of biliary and pancreatic pathologies, such as obstructive stones, benign or malignant strictures, inflammatory processes, neoplasms, and postsurgical complications, such as biliary leaks or

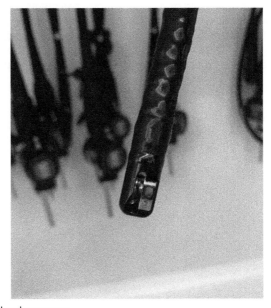

Fig. 28. Tip of a duodenoscope.

injuries. Tissue sampling can be done for diagnostic purposes using a cytology brush, biopsy forceps, or FNA. For therapeutic interventions in ERCP, a sphincterotomy may be needed facilitate access to biliary or pancreatic ducts for instrumentation. The most commonly used sphincterotome is made of a solid or braided wire that is attached to an electrosurgical unit and bowed across the tissue to be divided by the electrical energy current (**Fig. 29**). The needle knife sphincterotome is used less frequently due to increased risk of perforation but can be useful when ductal cannulation cannot be achieved.[3] Sphincteroplasty can be done in place of or in addition to sphincterotomies and is done using TTS balloon dilation, which also can be used to treat benign and malignant strictures. Endoscopic stenting is used to establish patency of the biliary and pancreatic ducts in the setting of strictures, obstructions, malignancies, and duct injuries. Stents comes in various sizes, lengths, diameters, and configurations. Biliary stents commonly are straight or curved stents with anchor flaps whereas pancreatic stents are narrower, have multiple side holes for accommodation of pancreatic juices from side branches of duct, and have a pigtail curve on duodenal side to prevent migration into the pancreatic duct (**Fig. 30**).[3] Clearance of the ducts and retrieval of stones are done using balloons and wire baskets and are successful 80% of the time[15]; however, lithotripsy may be required for larger stones. Mechanical lithotripsy uses a wire basket, metal sheath, and a handle to capture the large stone and mechanically fracture the stone for easier retrieval.[3] Electrohydraulic lithotripsy bathes the stone in fluid and sparks it using a bipolar probe, creating a oscillating shock wave that breaks up the stone.[5] This procedure is done under direct visualization using a choledochoscope. Laser lithotripsy uses a laser, which creates a plasma bubble on the surface of the stone and oscillates, leading to fragmentation of the stone.[3]

Balloon Enteroscopy

Enteroscopes are forward-viewing endoscopes, similar in design to gastroscopes, but with a longer insertion tube that serves to examine the duodenum, jejunum, and ileum.[2] They have various insertion tube lengths, diameters, and working channel diameters and also are available in forms of single-balloon, double-balloon, and spiral enteroscopes. Double-balloon enteroscopes have 2 balloons, 1 located at the tip of the enteroscope and another located at end of an overtube backloaded onto the enteroscope. Double-balloon enteroscopy uses alternating inflation and deflation of the balloons to serve as anchors, allowing the bowel to pleat over the endoscope

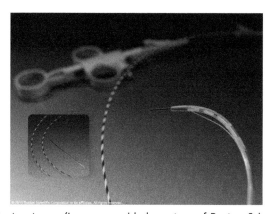

Fig. 29. Wire sphincterotome. (Images provided courtesy of Boston Scientific.)

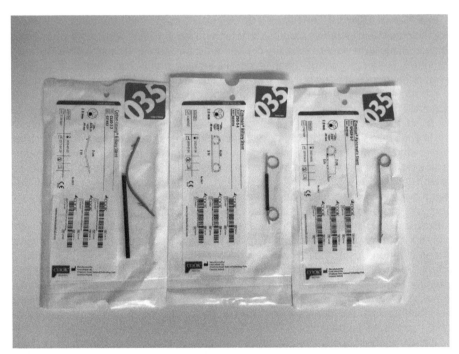

Fig. 30. Three different pancreaticobiliary stents. Cotton-Leung® biliary stent, Zimmon® biliary stent, Zimmon® pancreatic stent.

and reduce loop formation while progressively advancing the overtube and endo-scope to a greater insertion depth.[16] Single-balloon enteroscopes have only 1 balloon located at the end of the backloaded overtube and use tip deflection, instead of the second balloon, to serve as an anchor while the overtube is advanced.

In contrast, spiral enteroscopes have no balloons and use a mechanism of coupling and uncoupling of the overtube and enteroscope in addition to the rotational move-ments of the helical overtube that cause the small bowel to pleat over the overtube and allow it to be advanced (clockwise) or withdrawn (counterclockwise).[16] Entero-scopy commonly is indicated for evaluation and treatment of small bowel pathologies. Enteroscopes have working channels for various instruments used to diagnose Crohn disease and small bowel malignancies using tissue sampling, dilate small bowel stric-tures using TTS balloons, investigate occult GI bleeding and treat it using injection therapy, retrieve foreign bodies using graspers and nets, and remove polyps using snares.

ADVANCED ENDOSCOPIC SURGERY
Tissue Resection Methods

Advanced endoscopic approaches, such as EMR and endoscopic submucosal dissection (ESD), have allowed for more noninvasive tissue removal of mucosal le-sions, both benign and malignant, of the esophagus, stomach, colon, and rectum. Endoscopic resectability of lesions, determined by factors, such as size, depth of invasion, and risk of nodal metastasis, is crucial to determining the appropriate procedure. EMR is indicated for lesions limited to the mucosa or submucosa and less than 2 cm in size, with attempts to accomplish a complete en bloc resection of specimen for accurate histopathologic analysis and curative intent, although a piecemeal technique may be unavoidable at times.[9] Equipment and tools required include a flexible endoscope, electrosurgical unit, CO_2 insufflator, injection needle, injection solution, snares, and nets. Three techniques of EMR have been described: injection-assisted, suction-assisted, and band-assisted. Injection-assisted EMR requires injection of a solution (hypertonic saline, sodium hyaluronate, dextrose, and so forth, with or without blue staining using indigo carmine) into the submucosa, which raises the lesion off the submucosa. The lesion then isgrasped using forceps, encircled at its base using a snare, resected by the electrical current, and retrieved using a net. Suction-assisted EMR requires injection of a solution to lift the lesion and aspiration of the mucosa into the scope using a plastic clear cap that is attached to the tip of the endoscope (**Fig. 31**). The snare again is tightened around the base of the suctioned lesion and excised using the electrical current. Lastly, the band-assisted technique uses a variceal band ligator, attached at the tip of the endoscope, that suctions the mucosal lesion into the clear cap and bands it, creating a pseudopolyp that can be excised using a snare and electrical current either above or below the band.[5] ESD is indicated for larger en bloc specimens and has been shown more effective in achieving R0 resection and lowering risk of local recurrence in gastric cancers but is associated with longer procedure times and increased risk of perforation.[17] ESD uses similar equipment and tools to EMR; however, it includes hemostatic forceps, a clear cap, and, most importantly, an electrosurgical knife. Multiple electrosurgical knives exist, including needle knives, insulated tip knives, hook knives, flex knives, and triangle tip (TT) knives (**Figs. 32** and **33**). Needle knives have a fine tip and are sharp whereas insulated tip knives are covered by a ceramic ball and are blunt at the tip. Hook knives have the tip bent at a right angle whereas flex knives have a rounded tip made of twisted wire like a snare. Lastly, TT knives have a conductive tip in triangular shape that facilitates cutting mucosa.[5] Regardless of which knife is used, the steps of performing ESD include marking the lateral margins of the tumor using cautery, injecting a lifting solution, making an incision to separate the mucosa from submucosa, and continuing the submucosal dissection using the electrosurgical knife. The cap assists in elevating the specimen to provide retraction and visualization during dissection.[3] Hemostasis during and after the ESD is controlled by cautery using the knife and forceps or placement of hemostatic clips.

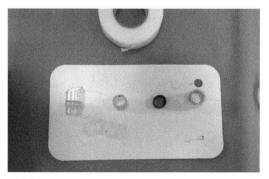

Fig. 31. Various plastic clear caps.

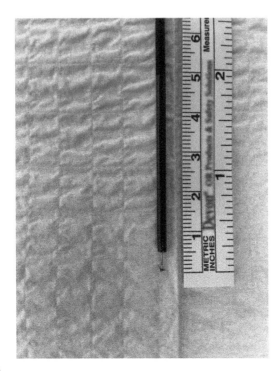

Fig. 32. TT knife.

Tissue Ablation

Mucosal ablation is used to treat mucosal-based diseases, such as BE, to prevent the progression of low-grade dysplasia to high-grade dysplasia and, ultimately, to esophageal adenocarcinoma. The diseased mucosa is removed down to the muscularis propria layer and replaced with nondiseased mucosa.[5] Photodynamic therapy (PDT) and bipolar radiofrequency ablation employ thermal modalities for ablation whereas cryotherapy employs a cryogenic modality. PDT uses a photosensitizing agent,

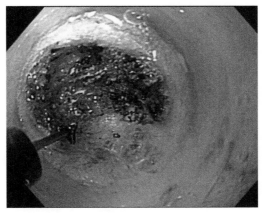

Fig. 33. TT knife being used for a POP procedure.

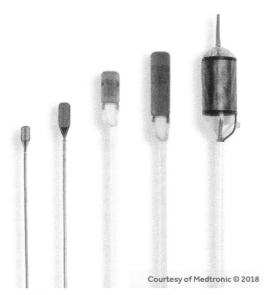

Courtesy of Medtronic © 2018

Fig. 34. HALO ablation balloon catheters. (Provided courtesy of Medtronic, Minneapolis, MN.)

such as sodium porfimer, that is given intravenously 48 hours to 72 hours prior to planned endoscopy and is preferentially taken up by the abnormal BE, which has a higher metabolic activity.[9] Laser light is targeted at the area of abnormality and delivers photoradiation, resulting in tissue destruction. Due to its association with side effects, such as strictures refractory to dilation and photosensitivity reactions, PDT has been replaced with use of radiofrequency ablation.[18] Radiofrequency ablation uses balloon-based bipolar electrode arrays to produce thermal energy and ablate the diseased mucosa down to the muscularis mucosa.[3] The HALO System (BarrX Medical, Sunnyvale, California) includes a circumferential HALO[360] ablation catheter as well as focal ablation catheters, HALO[60] and HALO[90], to circumferentially or focally treat segments of BE (**Fig. 34**). An initial endoscopic evaluation of the BE to size the HALO balloon catheter, which is advanced over a guide wire and inflated under direct visualization. Energy is delivered at 300 W and 10 J/cm^2 or 12 J/cm^2 (10 J/cm^2 for non-dysplastic BE; 12 J/cm^2 for low-grade dysplasia, high-grade dysplasia, or intramucosal esophageal adenocarcinoma) at a uniform, superficial depth between 500 μm

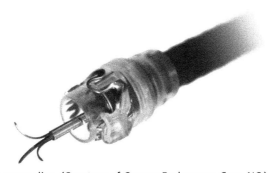

Fig. 35. Over-the-scope clips. (Courtesy of Ovesco Endoscopy, Cary, NC.)

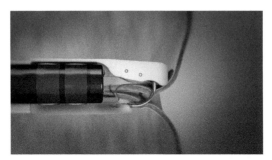

Fig. 36. OverStitch Sx™. (Courtesy of Apollo Endosurgery, Austin, TX.)

and 1000 μm, deflated, and advanced distally for repeated ablations.[5] Cryotherapy uses extreme cold via low-pressure liquid nitrogen or high-pressure nitrous oxide to ablate the mucosa.[5] The cryogenic agent is sprayed onto the targeted mucosa and induces ischemia and stimulation of the immune system, leading to cellular apoptosis and tissue necrosis.[9]

Endoscopic Closure of Full-thickness Defects

The development of endoscopic closure tools has changed drastically the management of full-thickness GI defects, such as spontaneous or iatrogenic perforations, anastomotic leaks, and inflammatory or neoplastic fistulas. These defects, which historically required surgery, now are treated using definitive closure tools, including over-the-scope clips, endoscopic suturing system, and cardiac septal defect occluders. Over-the-scope clips (**Fig. 35**) are made of biocompatible nitinol, are larger in size than endoscopic clips, and can close defects up to 2 cm in diameter with a single application.[20] They attach to the end of the endoscope via a large cap in an open position and are deployed by sliding off the cap and onto the target tissue after it is drawn up into the cap via suction or graspers.[3] The endoscopic suture system, OverStitch Sx™ (Apollo Endosurgery, Austin, Texas) (**Fig. 36**), is a disposable, single-use suturing device that is composed of an end cap that mounts at the tip of the gastroscope, a needle driver handle, and an anchor exchange catheter. Advantages of the endoscopic suture system is its versatility in allowing the endoscopist to choose the suture material (permanent or absorbable), suture pattern (running or interrupted), and depth of bites (full-thickness) in a free-handed technique.[3] The Amplatzer Septal Occluder (**Fig. 37**) (Abbott Laboratories, St. Paul,

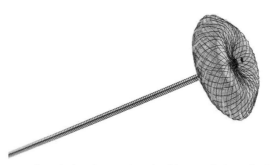

Fig. 37. Amplatzer Septal Occluder. (Reproduced with permission of Abbott, © 2020. All rights reserved.)

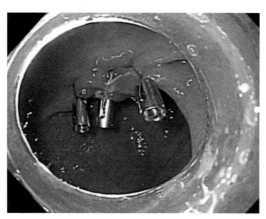

Fig. 38. Closure of mucosotomy in a POP procedure using endoscopic clips.

Minnesota), originally meant for occlusion of cardiac septal defects, has been used off-label for closure of fistulas in the GI tract.[19] The Amplatzer Septal Occluder is composed of 2 self-expandable, umbrella-shaped disks made of nitinol mesh with polyester fabric and shaped like a dumbbell. It is deployed over a guide wire and apposes the wall on each side of the defect, occluding it and creating a platform for tissue ingrowth and epithelization.[19]

Peroral Myotomy

Peroral esophageal myotomy (POEM) is an endoscopic procedure that divides the circular muscle fibers across the gastroesophageal junction and into the stomach to treat esophageal dysmotility disorders, such as achalasia, distal esophageal spasm, hypercontractile (jackhammer) esophagus, and hypertensive lower esophageal sphincter.[9] It requires a standard gastroscope, CO_2 insufflation, injection solution, a clear cap, TT knife, and an electrosurgical unit. A submucosal injection of a saline-based dye solution is performed, followed by a mucosotomy, creation of submucosal tunnel, and myotomy using the TT knife, and finally closure of the mucosotomy using endoclips.[3] Studies have shown a reduction in both the Eckardt score and lower esophageal sphincter pressure, with symptom relief maintained at 1 month, 6 months, and 12 months after treatment.[21] Not long after the introduction of POEM, the peroral pyloromyotomy (POP) procedure was described for treatment of medically refractory gastroparesis.[3] It uses a technique similar to the POEM procedure, including creation of a submucosal bleb at the pylorus, mucosotomy, submucosal tunneling, myotomy of the pyloric muscle fibers, and closure of the mucosotomy (**Fig. 38**). POP has been shown to improve Gastroparesis Cardinal Symptom Index scores and gastric emptying and is an effective procedure, even after previous gastric electric simulation.[22,23]

SUMMARY

Advanced endoscopic surgeries have transformed management of GI disease by providing minimally invasive but effective methods of treating pathologies that previously required surgery. As the number of advanced diagnostic and therapeutic endoscopic procedures continues to grow, endoscopists must be familiar not only with existing equipment and tools but also with novel endoscopic instruments.

CLINICS CARE POINTS

- It is important to be familiar with both current and cutting-edge endoscopic equipment as the use of endoscopy to diagnose, treat, and manage GI diseases and complications is increasing.
- Proficiency of performing advanced endoscopic surgery and learning novel therapeutic techniques requires time and practice.
- Knowledge of available equipment and appropriate techniques combined with sound surgical judgment will aid clinicians in offering minimally invasive, endoscopic options to diagnose and treat patients.

DISCLOSURE

The authors have nothing to disclose.

REFERENCES

1. Zinner MJ. Maingot's abdominal operations. New York: McGraw-Hill Education; 2019.
2. Varadarajulu S, Banerjee S, Barth BA, et al. GI Endoscopes. Gastrointest Endosc 2011;74(1):1–6.
3. Nau P, Pauli EM, Sandler BJ, et al. The Sages manual of flexible endoscopy. Cham (Switzerland): Springer; 2020.
4. Supancek S, Grega T, Zavoral M. The role of equipment in endoscopic complications. Best Pract Res Clin Gastroenterol 2016;30(5):667–78.
5. Marks JM, Dunkin BJ. Principles of flexible endoscopy for surgeons. New York: Springer Verlag; 2016. https://doi.org/10.1007/978-1-4614-6330-6.
6. Wadas DD, Sanowski RA. Complications of the hot biopsy forceps technique. Gastrointest Endosc 1988;34(1):32–7.
7. Babiuc RD, Purcarea M, Sadagurschi R, et al. Use of Hemospray in the treatment of patients with acute UGIB – short review. J Med Life 2013;6(2):117–9.
8. Parrillo JE, Dellinger RP. Critical care medicine: principles of diagnosis and management in the adult. Philadelphia: Elsevier/Saunders; 2014.
9. Kroh M, Reavis KM. The Sages manual: operating through the endoscope. Cham (Switzerland): Springer; 2016. https://doi.org/10.1007/978-3-319-24145-6.
10. Scolapio JS, Pasha TM, Gostout CJ, et al. A randomized prospective study comparing rigid to balloon dilators for benign esophageal strictures and rings. Gastrointest Endosc 1999;50(1):13–7.
11. Thomas S, Siddiqui AA, Taylor LJ, et al. Fully-covered esophageal stent migration rates in benign and malignant disease: a multicenter retrospective study. Endosc Int Open 2019;7(6):E751–6.
12. Varadarajulu S, Bang JY, Sutton BS, et al. Equal efficacy of endoscopic and surgical cystogastrostomy for pancreatic pseudocyst drainage in a randomized trial. Gastroenterology 2013;145(3):583–90.e1.
13. Siddiqui AA, Kowalski TE, Loren DE, et al. Fully covered self-expanding metal stents versus lumen-apposing fully covered self-expanding metal stent versus plastic stents for endoscopic drainage of pancreatic walled-off necrosis: clinical outcomes and success. Gastrointest Endosc 2017;85(4):758–65.
14. Doi S, Yasuda I, Kawakami H, et al. Endoscopic ultrasound-guided celiac ganglia neurolysis vs. celiac plexus neurolysis: a randomized multicenter trial. Endoscopy 2013;45(5):362–9.

15. McHenry L, Lehman G. Difficult bile duct stones. Curr Treat Options Gastroenterol 2006;9(2):123–32.
16. Chauhan SS, Manfredi MA, Abu Dayyeh BK, et al. Enteroscopy. Gastrointest Endosc 2015;82(6):975–90.
17. Lian J, Chen S, Zhang Y, et al. A meta-analysis of endoscopic submucosal dissection and EMR for early gastric cancer. Gastrointest Endosc 2012;76(4): 763–70.
18. Overholt BF, Lightdale CJ, Wang KK, et al. Photodynamic therapy with porfimer sodium for ablation of high-grade dysplasia in Barrett's esophagus: international, partially blinded, randomized phase III trial. Gastrointest Endosc 2005;62(4): 488–98.
19. Kumta NA, Boumitri C, Kahaleh M. New devices and techniques for handling adverse events: claw, suture, or cover? Gastrointest Endosc Clin N Am 2015; 25(1):159–68.
20. Al Ghossaini N, Lucidarme D, Bulois P. Endoscopic treatment of iatrogenic gastrointestinal perforations: an overview. Dig Liver Dis 2014;46(3):195–203.
21. Cho YK, Kim SH. Current status of peroral endoscopic myotomy. Clin Endosc 2018;15(1):13–8.
22. Rodriguez J, Strong AT, Haskins IN, et al. Per-oral Pyloromyotomy (POP) for Medically Refractory Gastroparesis: Short Term Results From the First 100 Patients at a High Volume Center. Ann Surg 2018;268(3):421–30.
23. Strong AT, Rodriguez J, Kroh M, et al. Safety and Feasibility of Per-Oral Pyloromyotomy as Augmentative Therapy after Prior Gastric Electrical Stimulation for Gastroparesis. J Am Coll Surg 2019;229(6):589–95.

Quality in Endoscopy

Chaitanya Vadlamudi, MD, MBA[a], Stacy Brethauer, MD[b],*

KEYWORDS

- Quality • Indicators • Metrics • Endoscopy • Benchmark • Task force • Registry

KEY POINTS

- Quality improvement is a dynamic process that requires continuous monitoring of several quality indicators and benchmarking to national and professional standards.
- Institutions and practices are now incentivized by payers and professional guidelines to have processes in place to measure, report, and act on quality metrics.
- The ACG/ASGE Task Force has laid out proposed quality indicators and performance goals common to all endoscopic procedures, along with those specific to EGD, colonoscopy, ERCP, EUS, and to the endoscopy unit as a whole.
- Multiple nationwide benchmarking and reporting methods, such as the GIQuIC, are approved as CMS registries to report quality data to merit-based incentive payment systems.
- Use of quality metrics and benchmarks leads to improved patient outcomes, reduced adverse events, improved patient satisfaction, and reduced cost.

INTRODUCTION

The Institute of Medicine report on medical errors, "To Err Is Human; Building a Safer Health System," found that 44,000 to 98,000 Americans die each year from medical errors. This has since generated a keen interest in quality measures in health care.[1] That report identified three major quality domains: (1) safety, (2) practice consistency based on present medical knowledge, and (3) customization.[1]

Since the report was published in 2000, there has been a push to embed quality measure within reimbursement schemes and performance evaluations of health care systems, hospitals, and practitioners. Value-based care that ties payment to the quality of care and bundled payments and rewards providers for efficient care have become the driver of multiple new payment models. Financial incentives and penalties now exist within Medicare for providers to report quality

[a] Department of Surgery, MedStar Georgetown University Hospital, 3800 Reservoir Road NW, Gorman 2051, Washington DC 20007, USA; [b] Department of Surgery, The Ohio State University, 410 West 10th Avenue, N721 Doan Hall, Columbus, OH 43210, USA
* Corresponding author.
E-mail address: stacy.brethauer@osumc.edu
Twitter: @StacyBrethauer (S.B.)

Surg Clin N Am 100 (2020) 1021–1047
https://doi.org/10.1016/j.suc.2020.08.008
0039-6109/20/© 2020 Elsevier Inc. All rights reserved.

surgical.theclinics.com

measures.[2,3] Stakeholders influenced by this shift in focus include patients, providers, professional societies, payors, regulatory bodies and accrediting organizations, the National Quality Forum, and the Centers for Medicare and Medicaid Services (CMS).[3]

In response to this new focus on quality, endoscopists have formed societal task forces to identify and develop quality indicators and suggest methods to collect, report, and empirically analyze endoscopy data. The goal of these task forces was to provide valid and reliable comparative information for consumers and payers. It was the hope that these data would provide a practical, objective method to grade performance and prepare the industry for future reporting requirements from public and private insurers and to optimize patient care.

DEFINITIONS
Quality Indicators and Measures

The ultimate goal of all quality indicators is improved patient health and satisfaction by continuously monitoring, evaluating, and improving the value of care provided to individual patients and populations using evidence-based metrics.[4] Broadly speaking, quality measures work toward this end by evaluating the following: receipt of appropriate indicated procedure or treatment, establishment of the correct diagnosis, use of established strategies to minimize risk/morbidity, treatment in an appropriate facility, treatment with appropriate equipment, treatment by trained and credentialed staff, and implementation of known measures to improve outcomes and avoid unintended adverse consequences.[3,5]

Quality indicators are separated into three categories: (1) structural, (2) process, and (3) outcome-based measures.[6-10] Structural measures assess characteristics of the entire health care environment (eg, rates at which physicians participate in a clinical database registry that include quality measures, the overall culture of safety). Process measures assess performance during the delivery of care (eg, rate of cannulation of the desired duct, adherence to safety checklists). Outcome measures assess the results of the care that was delivered (eg, rates of adverse events, such as bowel perforation, polypectomy detection rate). All three are reported as ratios or proportions, often as ratios of the incidence of correct performances to the opportunities for correct performances or the proportion of interventions that achieve a predefined goal. All quality indicators should be concrete, measurable, rapidly actionable items, which are regularly, if not continuously, evaluated and acted on.

Competency

The increased focus on quality has highlighted the need to ensure competency among all endoscopists. This is especially true when considering that endoscopists often arise from multiple specialties with varied training and backgrounds. Competency is defined as the minimum level of skill, knowledge, and/or experience required to safely and proficiently perform a task or procedure.[5] This is often established by the respective presiding societal bodies, such as the American College of Gastroenterology (ACG), the American Society for Gastrointestinal Endoscopy (ASGE), the American Board of Surgery, the Society of American Gastrointestinal and Endoscopic Surgeons, or the European Society of Gastrointestinal Endoscopy (ESGE). Therefore, the criteria for competency may vary depending on specialty, indication, procedure, and geographic location. Most institutions now base their local credentialing standards on these competency definitions.

Benchmarking

Benchmarking, with regards to quality, is the process of measuring, reporting, and comparing quality measures against set standards. Internal benchmarking involves regularly evaluating an endoscopist's own quality measures over time and comparing quality measures between endoscopists within the same institution. External benchmarking involves comparing an individual's or organization's own quality metrics with national or practice wide standards.

SOCIETY GUIDELINES

Multiple professional societies have taken a lead on establishing and implementing quality measures. A joint task force of the ASG and ASGE has proposed several quality metrics to establish competence and help define areas of continuous quality improvement for endoscopic procedures. These metrics have been conveniently separated into quality indicators pertinent to preprocedural, intraprocedural, and postprocedural periods for all endoscopic procedures universally, and for those specific to esophagogastroduodenoscopy (EGD), colonoscopy, endoscopic retrograde cholangiopancreatography (ERCP), and endoscopic ultrasound (EUS).[5–10] Additionally, the ASGE and the United Kingdom's National Health Service's Global Rating Scale (GRS) have separately published guidelines of quality metrics for endoscopy units.[5,11] Finally, the ESGE has published guidelines for facilitating quality improvement for reporting systems in gastrointestinal (GI) endoscopy and for quality control of image documentation in upper and lower endoscopy.[12,13]

AMERICAN COLLEGE OF GASTROENTEROLOGY/AMERICAN SOCIETY FOR GASTROINTESTINAL ENDOSCOPY TASK FORCE ON QUALITY IN ENDOSCOPY

In 2006, the ASGE/ACG Task Force on Quality in Endoscopy published a list of quality indicators common to all endoscopic procedures that covered assessment of the preprocedural, intraprocedural, and post-procedural periods. These were subsequently updated in 2015 and now include metrics specific to EGD, colonoscopy, ERCP, and EUS.[5–11]

Preprocedural

The preprocedure period starts when a patient's endoscopy is planned and ends at the time of the administration of sedation or insertion of the endoscope.[5] A list of preprocedural metrics universal to all endoscopic procedures is detailed in **Table 1**, all of which are process measures.[5,8–10] A list of indications for EGD and colonoscopy are listed in **Table 2** and **Box 1**.

Intraprocedural

The intraprocedural period starts with the administration of sedation or insertion of the endoscope to its removal. This period includes all technical aspects of the procedure, such as complete diagnostic examination and therapeutic maneuvers.[5] **Table 3** provides a list of intraprocedural metrics universal to all procedures, all of which are process measures.[5,8–10]

Post-procedural

The post-procedural period extends from the time the endoscope is removed to subsequent follow-up. **Table 4** lists the post-procedural quality metrics common to all procedures, most of which are process measures.[5,8–10]

Table 1
Preprocedural quality indicators common to all endoscopic procedures

Quality Indicator	Measure Type	Performance Target (%)
Preprocedure		
1. Frequency with which endoscopy is performed for an indication that is included in a published standard list of appropriate indications, and the indication is documented (priority indicator)	Process	>80
2. Frequency with which informed consent is obtained and fully documented	Process	>98
3. Frequency with which preprocedure history and directed physical examination are performed and documented	Process	>98
4. Frequency with which risk for adverse events is assessed and documented before sedation is started	Process	>98
5. Frequency with which prophylactic antibiotics are administered for appropriate indication (priority indicator)	Process	>98
6. Frequency with which a sedation plan is documented	Process	>98
7. Frequency with which management of antithrombotic therapy is formulated and documented before the procedure (priority indicator)	Process	N/A
8. Frequency with which a team pause is conducted and documented	Process	>98
9. Frequency with which endoscopy is performed by an individual who is fully trained and credentialed to perform that particular procedure	Process	>98

Abbreviation: N/A, Not available.
From Rizk MK, Sawhney MS, Cohen J, et al. Quality indicators common to all GI endoscopic procedures. Gastrointest Endosc. 2015;81(1):3-16; with permission.

Esophagogastroduodenoscopy-Specific Quality Indicators

In 2009, an estimated 6.9 million EGD procedures were performed in the United States at an estimated cost of $12.3 billion dollars. From 2000 to 2010, a 50% increase in EGD use was observed among Medicare recipients.[8] This increased use of EGD for diagnostic and therapeutic purposes and their associated cost has resulted in several EGD-specific quality measures. **Table 5** provides a list of the ACG/ASGE Task Force quality measures specific to EGD.[5,8] Some proposed quality indicators not specifically outlined by the task force include the biopsy of small bowel ulcers in setting of unexplained diarrhea, rates of rebleeding after gastrointestinal bleeds, and rates of postpolypectomy bleeding.[5]

Barrett Esophagus Relevant Quality Indicators

Patients with intestinalized metaplasia of the esophagus are at 40-fold increased risk of progression to high-grade dysplasia or cancer.[8] This has prompted the

Table 2
Indications and contraindications for EGD

1. EGD is generally indicated for evaluating:	A. Upper abdominal symptoms, which persist despite an appropriate trial of therapy
	B. Upper abdominal symptoms associated with other symptoms or signs suggesting serious organic disease (eg, anorexia and weight loss) or in patients aged >45 y
	C. Dysphagia or odynophagia
	D. Esophageal reflux symptoms, which are persistent or recurrent despite appropriate therapy
	E. Persistent vomiting of unknown cause
	F. Other diseases where the presence of upper GI pathology might modify other planned management (eg, patients who have a history of ulcer or GI bleeding who are scheduled for organ transplantation, long-term anticoagulation, or chronic nonsteroidal anti-inflammatory drug therapy for arthritis and those with cancer of the head and neck)
	G. Familial adenomatous polyposis syndromes
	H. For confirmation and specific histologic diagnosis of radiologically demonstrated lesions:
	  1. Suspected neoplastic lesion
	  2. Gastric or esophageal ulcer
	  3. Upper tract stricture or obstruction
	I. GI bleeding:
	  1. In patients with active or recent bleeding
	  2. For presumed chronic blood loss and for iron deficiency anemia when the clinical situation suggests an upper GI source or when colonoscopy result is negative
	J. When sampling of tissue or fluid is indicated
	K. In patients with suspected portal hypertension to document or treat esophageal varices
	L. To assess acute injury after caustic ingestion
	M. Treatment of bleeding lesions, such as ulcers, tumors, vascular abnormalities (eg, electrocoagulation, heater probe, laser photocoagulation, or injection therapy)
	N. Banding or sclerotherapy of varices

(continued on next page)

Table 2 *(continued)*	
	O. Removal of foreign bodies
	P. Removal of selected polypoid lesions
	Q. Placement of feeding or drainage tubes (peroral, PEG, or percutaneous endoscopic jejunostomy)
	R. Dilation of stenotic lesions (eg, with transendoscopic balloon dilators or dilation systems by using guidewires)
	S. Management of achalasia (eg, botulinum toxin, balloon dilation)
	T. Palliative treatment of stenosing neoplasms (eg, laser, multipolar electrocoagulation, stent placement)
	U. Endoscopic therapy for intestinal metaplasia
	V. Intraoperative evaluation of anatomic reconstructions typical of modern foregut surgery (eg, evaluation of anastomotic leak and patency, fundoplication formation, pouch configuration during bariatric surgery)
	W. Management of operative adverse events (eg, dilation of anastomotic strictures, stenting of anastomotic disruption, fistula, or leak in selected circumstances)
2. EGD is generally not indicated for evaluating:	A. Symptoms that are considered functional in origin (there are exceptions in which an endoscopic examination may be done once to rule out organic disease, especially if symptoms are unresponsive to therapy) B. Metastatic adenocarcinoma of unknown primary site when the results will not alter management Radiographic findings of: 1. Asymptomatic or uncomplicated sliding hiatal hernia 2. Uncomplicated duodenal ulcer that has responded to therapy 3. Deformed duodenal bulb when symptoms are absent or respond adequately to ulcer therapy
3. Sequential or periodic EGD may be indicated:	A. Surveillance for malignancy in patients with premalignant conditions (ie, Barrett esophagus)
	(continued on next page)

Table 2 (continued)	
4. Sequential or periodic EGD is generally not indicated for:	A. Surveillance for malignancy in patients with gastric atrophy, pernicious anemia, or prior gastric operations for benign disease B. Surveillance of healed benign disease, such as esophagitis or gastric or duodenal ulcer C. Surveillance during repeated dilations of benign strictures unless there is a change in status

Abbreviation: PEG, percutaneous endoscopic gastrostomy; N/A, Not available.
From Park WG, Shaheen NJ, Cohen J, et al. Quality indicators for EGD. Am J Gastroenterol. 2015;110(1):60–71; with permission.

development of additional quality measures specific to Barrett esophagus (BE). Appropriate biopsy of BE with four-quadrant biopsies every 1 to 2 cm throughout the length of BE tissue is of key importance because acquisition of fewer biopsy specimens is associated with a reduced likelihood of detecting dysplasia, after controlling for segment length. This has been included in the ACG/ASGE quality measures for endoscopy with a target of greater than or equal to 90%.[5,8] No other BE-relevant quality indicators were mentioned by the ACG/ASGE Task Force because of a lack of consensus. Most of this stems from a lack of prospective evidence showing improvement in survival or earlier detection with any other specific quality measure.[14] Still it has been proposed that three additional quality measures be included.[14]

Barrett inspection time
Some studies have shown a direct link between time spent during endoscopic inspection and diagnosis of neoplasm for esophageal and gastric cancerous lesions.[14] No benchmark time has been proposed.

Neoplasm detection rate
This measure is defined as the proportion of patients with one or more biopsies positive for neoplasia during their index endoscopy identifying BE, similar to adenoma detection rate (ADR) for colonoscopies. This stems from several studies, including a meta-analysis, which have shown that patients with BE are highly likely to have neoplasia detected at the time of the BE diagnosis (index endoscopy).[14] In fact, neoplasia rates at index endoscopy have increased over the last 25 years.[14] It has been estimated that the neoplasm detection rate is approximately 4% in these patients at index endoscopy, but no benchmark has been officially proposed as of yet.[14]

Appropriate surveillance guidelines
This measure stems from the overuse of surveillance endoscopy for follow-up of BE. Current guidelines recommend follow-up for nondysplastic BE at 3 to 5 years, yet approximately 30% of nondysplastic BE underwent an upper endoscopy within 6 months to 2 years instead.[14]

Colonoscopy-Specific Quality Measures
Colonoscopy provides an excellent arena for quality improvement because of its high volume, significant associated risk and expense, and evidence that variability in its performance affects outcomes.[3] Colonoscopy is the most common endoscopic

---

Box 1
Indications for colonoscopy

Evaluation of an abnormality on barium enema or other imaging study that is likely to be clinically significant, such as a filling defect or stricture

Evaluation of unexplained GI bleeding
  Hematochezia
  Melena after an upper GI source has been excluded
  Presence of fecal occult blood

Unexplained iron deficiency anemia

Screening and surveillance for colon neoplasia
  Screening of asymptomatic, average-risk patients for colon neoplasia
  Examination to evaluate the entire colon for synchronous cancer or neoplastic polyps in a patient with treatable cancer or neoplastic polyp
  Colonoscopy to remove synchronous neoplastic lesions at or around the time of curative resection of cancer followed by colonoscopy at 1 year, if examination normal then 3 years, and if normal then 5 years thereafter to detect metachronous cancer
  Surveillance of patients with neoplastic polyps
  Surveillance of patients with a significant family history of colorectal neoplasia

For dysplasia and cancer surveillance in select patients with long-standing ulcerative or Crohn colitis

For evaluation of patients with chronic inflammatory bowel disease of the colon, if more precise diagnosis or determination of the extent of activity of disease will influence management

Clinically significant diarrhea of unexplained origin

Intraoperative identification of a lesion not apparent at surgery (eg, polypectomy site, location of a bleeding site)

Treatment of bleeding from such lesions as vascular malformation, ulceration, neoplasia, and polypectomy site

Intraoperative evaluation of anastomotic reconstructions (eg, evaluation for anastomotic leak and patency, bleeding, pouch formation)

As an adjunct to minimally invasive surgery for the treatment of diseases of the colon and rectum

Management or evaluation of operative adverse events (eg, dilation of anastomotic strictures)

Foreign body removal

Excision or ablation of lesions

Decompression of acute megacolon or sigmoid volvulus

Balloon dilation of stenotic lesions (eg, anastomotic strictures)

Palliative treatment of stenosing or bleeding neoplasms (eg, laser, electrocoagulation, stenting)

Marking a neoplasm for localization

From Rex DK, Schoenfeld PS, Cohen J, et al. Quality indicators for colonoscopy. Am J Gastroenterol. 2015;110(1):72–90; with permission.

---

procedure performed in the United States and colonoscopy-related quality measures are the best studied and validated within the realm of endoscopy.[3,5] Colorectal cancer (CRC) incidence and mortality are the most relevant and important outcomes with regard to colonoscopy but these remain difficult to measure because of the low

Table 3
Intraprocedural quality indicators common to all endoscopic procedures

Quality Indicator	Measure Type	Performance Target (%)
Intraprocedure		
10. Frequency with which photodocumentation is performed	Process	N/A
11. Frequency with which patient monitoring during sedation is performed and documented	Process	>98
12. Frequency with which the doses and routes of administration of all medications used during the procedure are documented	Process	>98
13. Frequency with which use of reversal agents is documented	Process	>98
14. Frequency with which procedure interruption and premature termination because of sedation-related issues is documented	Process	>98

From Rizk MK, Sawhney MS, Cohen J, et al. Quality indicators common to all GI endoscopic procedures. Gastrointest Endosc. 2015;81(1):3-16; with permission.

Table 4
Intraprocedural quality indicators common to all endoscopic procedures

Quality Indicator	Measure Type	Performance Target (%)
Post-procedure		
15. Frequency with which discharge from the endoscopy unit according to predetermined discharge criteria is documented	Process	>98
16. Frequency with which patient instructions are provided	Process	>98
17. Frequency with which the plan for pathology follow-up is specified and documented	Process	>98
18. Frequency with which a complete procedure report is created	Process	>98
19. Frequency with which adverse events are documented	Process	>98
20. Frequency with which adverse events occur	Outcome	N/A
21. Frequency with which post-procedure and late adverse events occur and are documented	Outcome	N/A
22. Frequency with which patient satisfaction data are obtained	Process	N/A
23. Frequency with which communication with referring providers is documented	Process	N/A

Abbreviation: N/A, Not available.
From Rizk MK, Sawhney MS, Cohen J, et al. Quality indicators common to all GI endoscopic procedures. Gastrointest Endosc. 2015;81(1):3-16; with permission.

Table 5
Quality indicators specific to EGD (ACG-ASGE)

Summary of Proposed Quality Indicators for EGD		
Quality Indicator	**Type of Measure**	**Performance Target (%)**
Preprocedure		
1. Frequency with which EGD is performed for an indication that is included in a published standard list of appropriate indications, and the indication is documented	Process	>80
2. Frequency with which informed consent is obtained, including specific discussions of risks associated with EGD, and fully documented	Process	>98
3. Frequency with which appropriate prophylactic antibiotics are given in patients with cirrhosis with acute upper GI bleeding before EGD (priority indicator)	Process	>98
4. Frequency with which appropriate prophylactic antibiotics are given before placement of a PEG tube	Process	>98
5. Frequency with which a PPI is used for suspected peptic ulcer bleeding (priority indicator)	Process	>98
6. Frequency with which vasoactive drugs are initiated before EGD for suspected variceal bleeding	Process	>98
Intraprocedure		
7. Frequency with which a complete examination of the esophagus, stomach, and duodenum, including retroflexion in the stomach, is conducted and documented	Process	>98
8. Among those with nonbleeding gastric ulcers, frequency with which gastric biopsies are done to exclude malignancy	Process	>80
9. Frequency with which Barrett esophagus is appropriately measured when present	Process	>98
10. Frequency with which biopsies are obtained in cases of suspected Barrett esophagus	Process	>90
11. Frequency with which type of upper GI bleeding lesion is described, and the location is documented	Process	>80
12. Frequency with which, during EGD examination revealing peptic ulcers, at least one of the following stigmata is noted: active bleeding, nonbleeding visible vessels (pigmented protuberance), adherent dot flat spot, and clean-based	Process	>98
13. Frequency with which, unless contraindicated, endoscopic treatment is given to ulcers with active bleeding or with nonbleeding visible vessels (priority indicator)	Process	>98
14. Frequency with which achievement of primary hemostasis in cases of attempted hemostasis of upper GI bleeding lesions is documented	Process	>98

(*continued on next page*)

Table 5
(continued)

Summary of Proposed Quality Indicators for EGD

Quality Indicator	Type of Measure	Performance Target (%)
15. Frequency with which a second treatment modality is used (eg, coagulation or clipping) when epinephrine injection is used to treat actively bleeding or nonbleeding visible vessels in patients with bleeding peptic ulcers	Process	>98

Abbreviations: PEG, percutaneous endoscopic gastrostomy; PPI, proton pump inhibitor.
From Park WG, Shaheen NJ, Cohen J, et al. Quality indicators for EGD. Am J Gastroenterol. 2015;110(1):60–71; with permission.

incidence.[3] Furthermore, years of data collection are not often feasible with regards to quality improvement because data collection, results, and adjustments are made much more rapidly than in classical clinical research. Therefore, multiple surrogate markers, such as cecal intubation rates (CIR), ADR, and withdrawal time, have been identified for quality improvement. Most of the measures proposed by the ACG/ASGE task force are process measures rather than outcome measures and occur at the level of the endoscopist, rather than the endoscopy unit or hospital. The over-arching goals of all screening and surveillance colonoscopies are to consistently reach the cecum, identify all mucosal lesions, and safely removal of all polyps.[5] This has been reflected among the 15 quality metrics proposed by the joint ASGE/ACG Task Force on Quality Indicators for Colonoscopy (**Table 6**).[3,9] A few of the key metrics and their rationale are explored next.

Cecal intubation rate
Cecal intubation is defined as passage of the colonoscope tip proximal to the ileocecal valve, so that the entire cecal caput, including the medial wall of the cecum between the ileocecal valve and appendiceal orifice, is visible.[9] The ACG/ASGE Task Force published performance targets for photodocumentation of cecal intubation in greater than or equal to 90% in all colonoscopies and greater than or equal to 95% of all screening colonoscopies.[3,5,9] Photodocumentation should include the ileocecal valve and appendiceal orifice on every colonoscopy.[5,9] Photographs of the terminal ileum are used if they convincingly show villi, circular valvulae connivents, and lymphoid hyperplasia.[9]

These recommendations stem from data showing that incomplete colonoscopies are one of the most important factors associated with missed lesions and interval cancers.[3,5] Higher CIRs led to higher ADR and lower right-sided cancers. Conversely, low CIRs have been associated with higher rates of interval proximal colon cancer.[3,9]

Adenoma detection rate
Because of the aforementioned difficulties with using CRC incidence and mortality as a quality measure for colonoscopy, a more feasible and readily accessible metric, the ADR, has been used as a surrogate.[3] ADR is defined as the proportion of patients undergoing a complete screening colonoscopy who have one or more adenomas detected.[3] There is no defined time period or number of cases over which ADR is calculated, although it has been suggested that 500 cases are required for a reliable ADR.[3]

Table 6
Quality indicators specific to ERCP

Summary of Proposed Quality Indicators for ERCP		
Quality Indicator	Type	Performance Target (%)
Preprocedure		
1. Frequency with which colonoscopy is performed for an indication that is included in a published standard list of appropriate indications, and the indication is documented	Process	>80
2. Frequency with which informed consent is obtained, including specific discussions of risks associated with colonoscopy, and fully documented	Process	>98
3. Frequency with which colonoscopies follow recommended postpolypectomy and postcancer resection surveillance intervals and 10-y intervals between screening colonoscopies in average-risk patients and have negative examination results and adequate bowel cleaning (priority indicator)	Process	≥90
4. Frequency with which ulcerative colitis and Crohn colitis surveillance is recommended within proper intervals	Process	≥90
Intraprocedure		
5. Frequency with which the procedure note documents the quality of preparation	Process	>98
6. Frequency with which bowel preparation is adequate to allow the use of recommended surveillance or screening intervals	Process	≥85 of outpatient examinations
7. Frequency with which visualization of the cecum by notation of landmarks and photodocumentation of landmarks is documented in every procedure (priority indicated)	Process	
Cecal intubation rate with photography (all examinations)		≥90
Cecal intubation rate with photography (screening)		≥95
8. Frequency with which adenomas are detected in asymptomatic average risk individuals (screening) (priority indicator)	Outcome	
Adenoma detection rate for male/female population		≥25
Adenoma detection rate for male patients		≥30
Adenoma detection rate for female patients		≥20
9a. Frequency with which withdrawal time is measured	Process	>98
9b. Average withdrawal time in negative result screening colonoscopies	Process	≥6 min

(continued on next page)

Table 6 (continued)		
Summary of Proposed Quality Indicators for ERCP		
Quality Indicator	**Type**	**Performance Target (%)**
10. Frequency with which biopsy specimens are obtained when colonoscopy is performed for an indication of chronic diarrhea	Process	>98
11. Frequency of recommended tissue sampling when colonoscopy is performed for surveillance in ulcerative colitis and Crohn colitis	Process	>98
12. Frequency with which endoscopic removal of pedunculated polyps and sessile polyps <2 cm is attempted before surgical referral	Outcome	>98
Post-procedure		
13. Incidence of perforation by procedure type (all indications vs colorectal cancer screening/polyp surveillance) and postpolypectomy bleeding	Outcome	
Incidence of perforation, all examinations		<1:500
Incidence of perforation, screening		<1:1000
Incidence of postpolypectomy bleeding		<1
14. Frequency with which postpolypectomy bleeding is managed without surgery	Outcome	≥90
15. Frequency with which appropriate recommendation for timing of repeat colonoscopy is documented and provided to the patient after histologic findings are reviewed	Process	≥90

From Rex DK, Schoenfeld PS, Cohen J, et al. Quality indicators for colonoscopy. Am J Gastroenterol. 2015;110(1):72–90; with permission.

Again, the main goal of a screening colonoscopy is detection and removal of all neoplastic polyps.[3,5] Missed adenomas may be one of many factors responsible for the increased incidence of CRC seen in recent years.[3,5] The rate of interval cancers has been shown to be inversely related to ADR.[3–5,15] Endoscopists with less than 20% ADR have significantly higher rates of interval cancers.[5] Every 1% increase in ADR was associated with a 3% decrease in CRC risk and a 5% decrease in CRC mortality.[4,9,15] These findings have led the ACG/ASGE Task Force to set performance targets for ADR in screening colonoscopies (age ≥50) at greater than or equal to 20% in women and greater than or equal to 30% in men.[3,5,9] The ADR is the most important and best validated quality metric in colonoscopy.[3,5] It has been found to correlate directly with CRC and predicts the effective prevention of CRC.[9]

As a quality metric the ADR remains time consuming and cumbersome because health systems must follow-up the pathology of all resected polyps and associate them with each individual endoscopy. Furthermore, some question of whether ADR is an accurate predictor of adenoma miss rate continues to be debated, with one recent study using tandem colonoscopies finding that a high ADR was not predictive of a low adenoma miss rate.[4] Additionally, as far as quality metrics are concerned, the ADR is difficult to improve. Few if any studies have shown improvement in ADR by focusing on endoscopist-related factors, such as withdrawal time, financial incentives, re-education, or identification of poor performers.[9] Others have expressed concerns that the ADR incentivizes endoscopists to be less vigilant after finding one adenoma.

This may be ultimately addressed by switching to an adenomas per colonoscopy. This measure (adenomas per colonoscopy) is currently being evaluated in clinical trials.[9]

Polyp detection rate

Polyp detection rate (PDR) has been proposed as a less labor-intensive and time-consuming alternative to the ADR. The PDR is defined as the number of patients with greater than or equal to one polyp removed during screening colonoscopy in patients aged greater than or equal to 50 years.[9] These data are already logged and recorded at the completion of each colonoscopy, do not require manual entry of pathology data, and correlate well with ADR in several studies.[3,5,9] Furthermore, unlike ADR, the PDR can be measured by anyone with access to claims data.[9] This enables payers or even those outside the institution to perform fast, effective, reliable, and complete reviews for any endoscopists at any point in time.[9]

Currently the PDR is not an official quality metric proposed by the ACGE/ACG Task Force. Proposed performance measures include a PDR greater than or equal to 40% in men and a PDR greater than 30% in women.[3,5] Concerns exists that this measure can also be manipulated (eg, by the removal of diminutive hyperplastic or nonneoplastic polyps in the rectosigmoid).[3,5,9] If PDR is used, the periodic audits are used to deter this practice.[3] In fact, PDR of the proximal colon, rather than the entire colon, has better correlation with ADR and may ultimately be the suggested quality metric.[5] Other have suggested the use of polyps greater than or equal to 9 mm only in the PDR. The use of polyps greater than or equal to 9 mm as a surrogate for advanced neoplasia is 84% specific.[3]

Withdrawal time

Withdrawal time is defined as the time elapsed between reaching the cecum and complete withdraw of the scope from the patient.[5] It is presumed that careful inspection of colonic mucosa occurs during this time. The US Multi-Society Task Force on Colorectal Cancer and ACG/ASGE Task Force recommends at least 6 minutes for withdrawal and mucosal evaluation.[3,5,9] This should not include time spent for biopsy or polypectomy and should be averaged over multiple cases.[3] This benchmark results from studies that revealed withdrawal times of greater than or equal to 6 minutes led to higher polypectomy rates, ADR rates, and increased detection of significant neoplastic lesions.[3,9,16]

Despite this, a mandatory withdrawal time has not been shown to improve ADR.[5,16] It is likely that withdrawal time is simply a surrogate marker for ADR and has limited value if endoscopists are already performing careful inspections (ie, appropriate ADR).[3,9] However, for those with low ADR, short withdrawal time might be a modifiable factor for improvement.[3,9]

Other Quality Indicators

The ACG/ASGE Task Force has proposed quality indicators specific to ERCP (**Table 7**) and EUS (**Table 8**). For a list of appropriate indications for ERCP and EUS see **Boxes 2** and **3**, respectively.

Quality Metrics in Endoscopy Training

Currently most quality indicators for training purposes work on the presumption that competence is attained across the board for all learners after a threshold number of procedures have been performed. Suggested thresholds from the ACG and the ASGE are as follows[5]:

- 130 EGDs

Table 7
Quality indicators specific to EUS

Summary of Proposed Quality Indicators for ERCP

Quality Indicator	Measure Type	Performance Target (%)
Preprocedure		
1. Frequency with which ERCP is performed for an indication that is included in a published standard fist of appropriate indications and the indication is documented (priority indicator)	Process	>90
2. Frequency with which informed consent is obtained, including specific discussions of risks associated with ERCP, and fully documented	Process	>98
3. Frequency with which appropriate antibiotics for ERCP are administered for setting in which they are indicated	Process	>98
4. Frequency with which ERCP is performed by an endoscopist who is fully trained and credentialed to perform ERCP	Process	>98
5. Frequency with which the volume of ERCPs performed per year is recorded per endoscopist	Process	>98
Intraprocedure		
6a. Frequency with which deep cannulation of the ducts of interest is documented	Process	>98
6b. Frequency with which deep cannulation of the ducts of interest in patients with native papillae without surgically altered anatomy is achieved and documented (priority indicator)	Process	>90
7. Frequency with which fluoroscopy time and radiation dose are measured and documented	Process	>98
8. Frequency with which common bile duct stones <1 cm in patients with normal bile duct anatomy are extracted successfully and documented (priority indicator)	Outcome	$\geq$90
9. Frequency with which stent placement for biliary obstruction in patients with normal anatomy whose obstruction is below the bifurcation successfully achieved and documented (priority indicator)	Outcome	$\geq$90
Post-procedure		
10. Frequency with which a complete ERCP report that details the specific techniques performed, particular accessories used, and all intended outcomes is prepared	Process	>98
11. Frequency with which acute adverse events and hospital transfers are documented	Process	>98
12. Rate of post-ERCP pancreatitis (priority indicator)	Outcome	N/A
13. Rate and type of perforation	Outcome	$\leq$0.2
14. Rate of clinically significant hemorrhage after sphincterotomy or sphincteroplasty in patients undergoing ERCP	Outcome	$\leq$1

(*continued on next page*)

Table 7 (continued)		
Summary of Proposed Quality Indicators for ERCP		
Quality Indicator	**Measure Type**	**Performance Target (%)**
15. Frequency with which patents are contacted at or >14 d to detect and record the occurrence of delayed adverse events after ERCP	Process	>90

Adapted from Adler DG, Lieb II JG, Cohen J, et al. Quality indicators for ERCP. Gastrointest Endosc. 2015; 81(1):54-66; with permission.

- 200 colonoscopies
- 25 to 30 flexible sigmoidoscopies
- 180 to 200 ERCPs
- 100 EUS

Similarly, the American College of Surgeons requires 50 colonoscopies and 35 EGDs for graduation from general surgery residency. It has been widely acknowledged that the number required to attain competence varies wildly between trainee, specialty, and procedure. Over time these quality indicators may shift toward true competency assessments, such as evaluations by experts regarding the ability to cannulate the biliary duct in a native papilla without verbal instruction in greater than or equal to 80% of cases.

Quality Indicators for Gastrointestinal Endoscopy Unit

The UK National Health Services developed the GRS in 2004.[11] It was created with the goal of enhancing quality while also developing uniformity in endoscopy unit processes and operations.[11] This was truly the first attempt to assess quality and service at the level of the endoscopy unit.[11] Multiple evaluations after implementation have found that it has successfully aided in reducing wait times, identifying service gaps, increasing patient satisfaction, and reducing adverse events within endoscopy units in the United Kingdom.[11] This demonstrated and confirmed that measuring an endoscopy unit parameter repeatedly and incorporating it into a quality improvement program leads to improvement.[11]

The ASGE task force for quality indicators in GI endoscopy units was inspired by the GRS and is the first comprehensive list of quality indicators for US endoscopy units.[11] They identified 29 quality indicators with five domains, only one of which is procedure related. The domains evaluate patient experience (informed consent and communication about results), employee experience (feedback, evaluations, education), efficiency and operations (defined leadership structure, designated quality officer, self-governance), a procedure-related domain, and a safety and infection control domain (disinfection and equipment maintenance, credentialing of staff). The ASGE also identified the five most compelling endoscopy unit quality indicators to measure and track for a high-quality endoscopy unit:

- Endoscopy unit has a defined leadership structure.
- Endoscopy unit has regular education, training programs, and continuous quality improvement for all staff on new equipment/devices and endoscopic techniques.
- Endoscopy unit records, tracks, and monitors procedure quality indicators for the endoscopy unit and individual endoscopists.

| Table 8 |
| Indications for ERCP |

| Summary of Proposed Quality Indicators for EUS | | |
Quality Indicator	Type of Measure	Performance Target (%)
Preprocedure		
1. Frequency with which EUS is performed for an indication that is included in a published standard list of appropriate indications and the indication is documented	Process	>80
2. Frequency with which consent is obtained, including specific discussions of risks associated with EUS, and fully documented	Process	>98
3. Frequency with which appropriate antibiotics are administered in the setting of FNA of cystic lesions	Process	N/A
4. Frequency with which EUS examinations are performed by trained endosonographers	Process	>98
Intraprocedure		
5. Frequency with which the appearance of relevant structures, specific to the indication for the EUS, is documented	Process	>98
6a. Frequency with which all gastrointestinal cancers are staged with the American Joint Committee on Cancer/Union for International Cancer Control TNM staging system (priority indicator)	Process	>98
6b. Frequency with which pancreatic mass measurements are documented along with evaluation for vascular involvement, lymphadenopathy, and distant metastases	Process	>98
6c. Frequency with which EUS wall layers involved by subepithelial masses are documented	Process	>98
		(continued on next page)

Table 8		
(continued)		

Summary of Proposed Quality Indicators for EUS		
Quality Indicator	**Type of Measure**	**Performance Target (%)**
7a. Percentage of patients with distant metastasis, ascites, and lymphadenopathy undergoing EUS-guided FNA who have tissue sampling of the primary tumor diagnosis and lesions outside of the primary field when this would alter patient management	Process	>98
7b. Diagnostic rate of adequate sample in all solid lesions undergoing EUS-FNA (adequate sample is defined by the presence of cells/tissue from the representative lesion in question)	Outcome	≥85
7c. Diagnostic rates and sensitivity for malignancy in patients undergoing EUS-FNA of pancreatic masses (priority indicator)	Outcome	Diagnostic rate: ≥70 Sensitivity: ≥85
Post-procedure		
8. Frequency with which the incidence of adverse events after EUS-FNA (acute pancreatitis, bleeding, perforation, and infection) is documented	Process	>98
9. Incidence of adverse events after EUS-FNA (acute pancreatitis, bleeding, perforation, and infection) (priority indicator)	Outcome	Acute pancreatitis: <2% Perforation: <0.5% Clinically significant bleeding: <1%

Abbreviation: FNA, fine-needle aspiration; N/A, Not available.

Adapted from Wani S, Wallace MB, Cohen J, et al. Quality indicators for EUS. Gastrointest Endosc. 2015; 81(1):67-80; with permission.

- Procedure reports are communicated to referring providers, and a process is in place for patients to receive a copy of their endoscopy report.
- Process is in place to track each specific endoscope from storage, use, reprocessing, and back to storage.

Quality Indicators for Reporting Systems

Quality indicators rely on accurate and timely reporting to be effective agents of quality improvement. Additionally, with the large variety of reporting systems available, some need for uniformity and transferability is required. To address these needs the ESGE has published guidelines facilitating quality improvement for reporting systems in GI endoscopy (**Box 4**).[12] Additionally, they have also published guidelines for quality

---

Box 2
Indications for EUS

Appropriate indications for ERCP

The jaundiced patient suspected of having biliary obstruction (appropriate therapeutic maneuvers should be performed during the procedure)

The patient without jaundice whose clinical and biochemical or imaging data suggest pancreatic duct or biliary tract disease

Evaluation of signs or symptoms suggesting pancreatic malignancy when results of direct imaging (eg, EUS, ultrasound, computed tomography, MRI) are equivocal or normal

Evaluation of pancreatitis of unknown cause

Preoperative evaluation of the patient with chronic pancreatitis and/or pseudocyst evaluation of the sphincter of Oddi by manometry

Empirical biliary sphincterotomy without sphincter of Oddi manometry is not recommended in patients with suspected type III sphincter of Oddi dysfunction
  Endoscopic sphincterotomy:
  Choledocholithiasis
  Papillary stenosis or sphincter of Oddi dysfunction
  To facilitate placement of biliary stents or dilation of biliary strictures
  Sump syndrome
  Choledochocele involving the major papilla
  Ampullary carcinoma in patients who are not candidates for surgery
  Facilitate access to the pancreatic duct

Stent placement across benign or malignant strictures, fistulae, postoperative bile leak, or in high-risk patients with large unremovable common duct stones

Dilation of ductal strictures

Balloon dilation of the papilla

Nasobiliary drain placement

Pancreatic pseudocyst drainage in appropriate cases

Tissue sampling from pancreatic or bile ducts

Ampullectomy of adenomatous neoplasms of the major papilla

Therapy for disorders of the biliary and pancreatic ducts

Facilitation of cholangioscopy and/or pancreatoscopy

From Adler DG, Lieb II JG, Cohen J, et al. Quality indicators for ERCP. Gastrointest Endosc. 2015; 81(1):54-66; with permission.

---

control in image documentation.[13] For upper endoscopy (EGD) they recommend eight images total (**Fig. 1**) including 20 cm from incisors, 2 cm above squamocolumnar junction or "Z-line" line, retroflexion view of cardia, upper portion of lesser curve, incisura angularis, antrum, duodenal bulb, and the second portion of the duodenum. They also recommend at least eight images for colonoscopies including the rectum 2 cm above dentate line, middle portion of sigmoid, descending colon distal to splenic flexure, transverse colon just proximal to splenic flexure, transverse colon proximal to hepatic flexure, ascending colon distal to hepatic flexure, ileocecal valve, and cecum with visualization of appendiceal orifice (**Fig. 2**).

Benchmarking Methods

Benchmarking is an essential element of quality improvement. Practices should implement internal and external benchmarking through data collection and implementation

---

Box 3
Proposed requirements for endoscopic reporting systems (ESGE)

Appropriate indications for EUS

Staging of tumors of the GI tract, pancreas, bile ducts, and mediastinum including lung cancer

Evaluating abnormalities of the GI tract wall or adjacent structures

Tissue sampling of lesions within, or adjacent to, the wall of the GI tract

Evaluation of abnormalities of the pancreas, including masses, pseudocysts, and chronic pancreatitis

Evaluation of abnormalities of the biliary tree

Placement of radiologic (fiducial) markers into tumors within or adjacent to the wall of the GI tract

Treatment of symptomatic pseudocysts by creating an enteral-cyst communication

Providing access into the bile ducts or pancreatic duct, either independently or as an adjunct to ERCP

Evaluation for perianal and perirectal disorders (anal sphincter injuries, fistulae, abscesses)

Evaluation of patients at increased risk of pancreatic cancer

Celiac plexus block or neurolysis

From Wani S, Wallace MB, Cohen J, et al. Quality indicators for EUS. Gastrointest Endosc. 2015; 81(1):67-80; with permission.

---

of quality assurance programs. This practice has become widely accepted and implemented because of the Patient Protection and Affordable Care Act of 2010. Within the act was the Physician Quality Reporting Initiative, which incentivized physicians and organizations financially for reporting health care quality data to CMS. This pay for performance program used specific approved Physician Quality Reporting Systems (PQRS), some of which are detailed next. These include certified electronic health record (EHR) products, qualified PQRS registries, qualified clinical data registries (QCDR), and Medicare part B claims submitted to CMS. There are currently five endoscopy-related measures endorsed by CMS for use in merit-based incentive payment systems.[4] These include age-appropriate screening colonoscopy, appropriate follow-up interval for a normal colonoscopy in an average-risk patient, appropriate colonoscopy interval for patients with a history of adenomatous polyps, ADR rates, and photodocumentation of cecal intubation.

Broadly speaking, there are three common mechanisms for measuring, reporting, and benchmarking endoscopic quality: (1) claims-based administrative data, (2) clinical data registries, and (3) measurement within a health system EHR.[3,4]

Clinical Data Registries

Clinical data registries were specifically designed for research and quality reporting and therefore avoid some of the biases seen in other administrative databases.[3] However, they are not passive processes and require significant investment from individual participants for data collection and control.[3] The GI Quality Improvement Consortium (GIQuIC) by the ASGE/ACG is a clinical data registry that tracks upper and lower endoscopic quality measures and allows organizations and individuals to benchmark internally and against registry averages.[4,5,10,11] See **Fig. 3** for a sample ADR report. The GIQuIC Registry has been approved as a QCDR by CMS for purposes of reporting

---

Box 4
Proposed requirements for endoscopic reporting systems (ESGE)

The following requirements for endoscopic reporting systems are crucial to help in developing high-quality patient care in endoscopy and in ensuring continuous measurement and reporting of endoscopy quality for individuals, centers, and countries.

These requirements should serve as guidance for manufacturers of electronic endoscopy software systems, caregivers, and policymakers alike.

1. Endoscopy reporting systems must be electronic.
2. Endoscopy reporting systems should be integrated into hospitals' patient record systems.
3. Endoscopy reporting systems should include patient identifiers to facilitate data linkage to other data sources.
4. Endoscopy reporting systems shall restrict the use of free-text entry to a minimum, and mainly be based on structured data entry.
5. Separate entry of data for quality or research purposes is discouraged. Automatic data transfer for quality and research purposes must be facilitated.
6. Double entry of data by the endoscopist or associate personnel is discouraged. Available data from outside sources (administrative or medical) must be made available automatically.
7. Endoscopy reporting systems shall facilitate the inclusion of information on:
   • Histopathology of detected lesions
   • Patient satisfaction
   • Adverse events
   • Surveillance recommendations
8. Endoscopy reporting systems must facilitate easy data retrieval at any time in a universally compatible format.
9. Endoscopy reporting systems must include data fields for key performance indicators as defined by the ESCE Quality Improvement Committee.
10. Endoscopy reporting systems must facilitate changes in indicators and data entry fields as required by professional organizations.

From Bretthauer M, Aabakken L, Dekker E, et al. Requirements and standards facilitating quality improvement for reporting systems in gastrointestinal endoscopy: European Society of Gastrointestinal Endoscopy (ESGE) Position Statement. Endoscopy. 2016;48(03):291-294; with permission.

---

quality data to the Merit-based Incentive Payment Systems (MIPS). Over the coming years GIQuIC is expected to expand its registry to include ERCP quality measures.[5]

The GRS is a clinical data registry that focuses on the endoscopy unit rather than the endoscopist or procedure.[5] The GRS has four domains: (1) clinical quality, (2) patient-centered care, (3) workforce, and (4) training. The GRS has been shown to reduce wait times, identify service gaps, increase patient satisfaction, and reduce adverse events.[11] Similar to the GIQuIC the GRS remains time consuming and costly, often requiring data collection from multiple sources.[5] Other clinical data registries include the New Hampshire Colonoscopy Registry, the Clinical Outcomes Research Initiative Registry, and the American Gastroenterology Association Digestive Health Outcomes Registry. The latter is also certified by CMS as an official PQRS registry.

Claims-Based Administrative Data

Claims-based administrative data come from insurance companies, billing records, and national databases. It is less labor intensive, cumbersome, and costly because the data have already been collected. These databases have extremely large sample sizes, powering them to detect lower rate events. Finally, they also often have the granularity to detect geographic differences, changes over time, compare different providers, and compare different settings (hospital vs surgery center).[4]

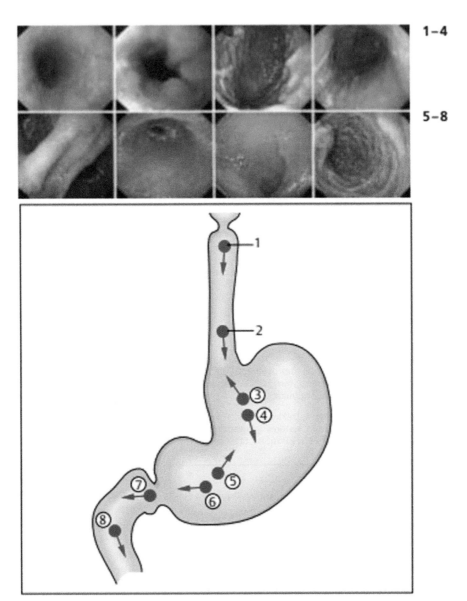

Fig. 1. Recommended imaging for upper endoscopy (ESGE). (*From* Rey J-F, Lambert R. ESGE Recommendations for Quality Control in Gastrointestinal Endoscopy: Guidelines for Image Documentation in Upper and Lower GI Endoscopy. Endoscopy. 2001;33(10):901-903; with permission.)

Unfortunately they rarely include clinical outcomes, final pathology, or complications. The coding used for billing often lacks clinical nuances. It is also well acknowledged that the coding accuracy is often suboptimal because billing and coding definitions were not designed for quality measurements. Questions often arise when using these data for clinical decision making, because they are subject to attribution errors and inaccurate risk adjustment.[4] Ultimately these data may be better suited

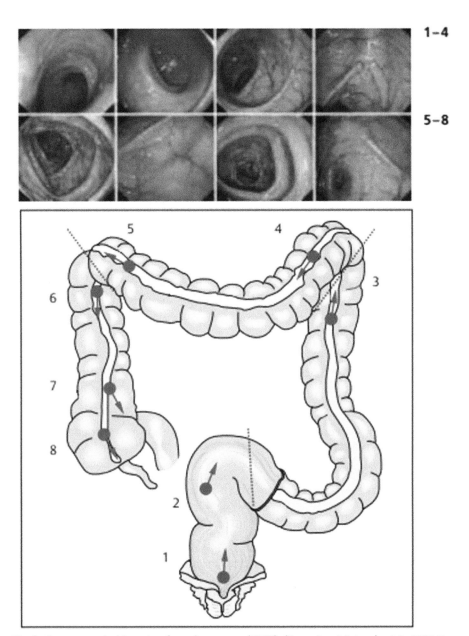

Fig. 2. Recommended imaging for colonoscopy (ESGE). (*From* Rey J-F, Lambert R. ESGE Recommendations for Quality Control in Gastrointestinal Endoscopy: Guidelines for Image Documentation in Upper and Lower GI Endoscopy. Endoscopy. 2001;33(10):901-903; with permission.)

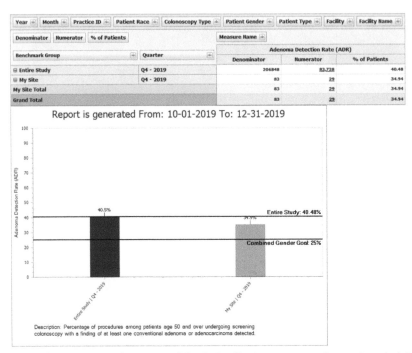

Fig. 3. Sample ADR report. (*Courtesy of* the GI Quality Improvement Consortium, Ltd, 2013; with permission.)

for process rather than outcome measures. Still, many CMS pay for performance or merit-based pay programs often rely on claims-based data.[4]

Electronic Health Systems

EHR-based measurement has the greatest promise for clinically accurate data that can be reported passively, or at the least in a less cumbersome manner than current clinical data registries. Using EHRs would enable real-time data capture while incorporating a wide range of outcomes, including those that are patient reported. All needed data are already entered into the EHR during clinical encounters and includes the full scope of care without the limitations encountered from coding-based insurance or administrative databases.[3,4] The biggest roadblock, however, is that the data have yet to be standardized in any way. Multiple EHRs exists, none of which are interoperable. Even within a single EHR, there remains large variability in terminology, missing or inconsistent documentation, and a lack of a standardized data structure.[3,4] One hope is that as technology progresses, natural language processing to extract data from electronic records will increasingly be used. The Veterans Affairs health administration is developing EHR-dependent quality measurements, including a recently validated e-measure assessing overuse of screening colonoscopy.[4]

SUMMARY

Measuring endoscopic quality is of little use if it does not lead to enhanced patient outcomes. Quality improvement requires continuous monitoring of several quality indicators reflecting all aspects of endoscopic care and benchmarking these against national and professional standards. Additionally, quality indicators themselves should be re-evaluated on an iterative basis. Measurement of quality indicators must also be combined with continuous training, feedback loops, and documented improvement or protective actions. Measurement and reporting of quality, and achieving performance benchmarks will become increasingly relevant as more financial incentives and penalties emerge. Endoscopy unit level quality measures also will likely become increasingly important. Future research should focus on bolstering evidence to support how particular metrics correlate with clinically relevant outcomes, and on identifying the types of interventions that improve these metrics.

CLINICS CARE POINTS

- Quality improvement is a dynamic process that requires continuously monitoring quality indicators and benchmarking these with national and professional standards.
- A joint task force of the ASG and ASGE has proposed several quality metrics to establish competence and help define areas of continuous quality improvement for endoscopic procedures.[5–10]
- Appropriate biopsy of BE with four quadrant biopsies every 1 to 2 cm throughout the length of BE tissue is associated with increased likelihood of detecting dysplasia.
- Appropriate biopsy of BE should be achieved in more than 90% of surveillance endoscopies with BE.[5,8]
- CIR of greater than or equal to 90% in all colonoscopies and greater than or equal to 95% of all screening colonoscopies should be achieved.[3,5,9] Photodocumentation should include the ileocecal valve and appendiceal orifice on every colonoscopy.[5,9]
- Higher CIRs led to higher adenoma detection rates and lower right-sided cancers. Conversely, low CIRs have been associated with higher rates of interval proximal colon cancer.[3,9]
- The rate of interval cancers has been shown to be inversely related to ADR.[3–5,15]
- Endoscopists with less than 20% ADR have significantly higher rates of interval cancers.[5]
- Every 1% increase in ADR was associated with a 3% decrease in CRC risk and a 5% decrease in CRC mortality.[4,9,15]
- Performance targets for ADR in screening colonoscopies (age ≥50) are set at greater than or equal to 20% in women and greater than or equal to 30% in men.[3,5,9]
- The US Multi-Society Task Force on Colorectal Cancer and ACG/ASGE Task Force recommends at least 6 minutes for withdrawal and mucosal evaluation.[3,5,9]
- Withdrawal times of greater than 6 minutes led to higher polypectomy rates, ADR rates, and increased detection of significant neoplastic lesions.[3,9,16]
- The UK GRS evaluated quality of endoscopy unit processes and operations. Implementation of the GRS was seen to successfully aid in reducing wait times, identifying service gaps, increasing patient satisfaction, and reducing adverse events within endoscopy units in the United Kingdom.[11]
- The GRS demonstrated and confirmed that measuring an endoscopy unit parameter repeatedly and incorporating it into a quality improvement program leads to improvement.[11]

- The ASGE task force for quality indicators in GI endoscopy units was inspired by the GRS and is the first comprehensive list of quality indicators for US endoscopy units.[11]
- The ESGE published guidelines for quality control in image documentation. For upper endoscopy (EGD) they recommend eight images total (see **Fig. 1**) and they recommend at least eight images for colonoscopies (see **Fig. 2**).
- The Physician Quality Reporting Initiative incentivized physicians and organizations financially for reporting health care quality data to CMS.
- There are currently five endoscopy-related measures endorsed by CMS for use in merit-based incentive payment systems.[4]
  - Age-appropriate screening colonoscopy.
  - Appropriate follow-up interval for a normal colonoscopy in an average-risk patient.
  - Appropriate colonoscopy interval for patients with a history of adenomatous polyps.
  - ADR rates.
  - Photodocumentation of cecal intubation.
- The GIQuIC is a national clinical data registry that tracks upper and lower endoscopic quality measures and allows organizations and individuals to benchmark internally and against national averages.[4,5,10,11]
- The GIQuIC Registry has been approved as a QCDR by CMS registry for purposes of reporting quality data to merit-based incentive payment systems.

DISCLOSURE

Dr S. Brethauer consults with GI Windows and receives speaking honoraria from Medtronic.

REFERENCES

1. Institute of Medicine (US) Committee on Quality of Health Care in America. To Err is Human: Building a Safer Health System. Kohn LT, Corrigan JM, Donaldson MS, editors. Washington (DC): National Academies Press (US); 2000. PMID: 25077248.
2. Sharma P, Parasa S, Shaheen N. Developing quality metrics for upper endoscopy. Gastroenterology 2020;158(1):9–13.
3. Calderwood AH, Jacobson BC. Colonoscopy quality: metrics and implementation. Gastroenterol Clin North Am 2013;42(3):599–618.
4. Adams M, Saini S, Allen J. Quality measures in gastrointestinal endoscopy: the current state. Curr Opin Gastroenterol 2017;33(5):352–7.
5. Gurudu SR, Ramirez FC. Quality metrics in endoscopy. Gastroenterol Hepatol (N Y) 2013;9(4):228–33.
6. Adler DG, Lieb JG, Cohen J, et al. Quality indicators for ERCP. Gastrointest Endosc 2015;81(1):54–66.
7. Wani S, Wallace MB, Cohen J, et al. Quality indicators for EUS. Gastrointest Endosc 2015;81(1):67–80.
8. Park WG, Shaheen NJ, Cohen J, et al. Quality indicators for EGD. Am J Gastroenterol 2015;110(1):60–71.
9. Rex DK, Schoenfeld PS, Cohen J, et al. Quality indicators for colonoscopy. Am J Gastroenterol 2015;110(1):72–90.
10. Cohen J, Pike IM. Defining and measuring quality in endoscopy. Gastrointest Endosc 2015;81(1):1–2.

11. Day LW, Cohen J, Greenwald D, et al. Quality indicators for gastrointestinal endoscopy units. VideoGIE 2017;2(6):119–40.
12. Bretthauer M, Aabakken L, Dekker E, et al. Requirements and standards facilitating quality improvement for reporting systems in gastrointestinal endoscopy: European Society of Gastrointestinal Endoscopy (ESGE) Position Statement. Endoscopy 2016;48(03):291–4.
13. Rey J-F, Lambert R. ESGE recommendations for quality control in gastrointestinal endoscopy: guidelines for image documentation in upper and lower GI endoscopy. Endoscopy 2001;33(10):901–3.
14. Desai M, Sharma P. What quality metrics should we apply in Barrett's esophagus? Am J Gastroenterol 2019;114(8):1197–8.
15. Corley DA, Jensen CD, Marks AR, et al. Adenoma detection rate and risk of colorectal cancer and death. N Engl J Med 2014;370(14):1298–306.
16. Barclay RL, Vicari JJ, Doughty AS, et al. Colonoscopic withdrawal times and adenoma detection during screening colonoscopy. N Engl J Med 2006. https://doi.org/10.1056/NEJMoa055498.

Polypectomy Techniques

Kelly T. Wagner, MD[a],*, Eleanor Fung, MD[b]

KEYWORDS

- Polypectomy • Cold snare • Hot snare • Cold forceps

KEY POINTS

- Gastrointestinal cancers are a leading cause of morbidity and mortality worldwide and their impact can be mitigated with endoscopic polypectomy.
- Dedicated cold snare polypectomy is the superior resection technique for polyps ≤10mm.
- Hot snare polypectomy or endoscopic mucosal resection is recommended for polyps >10mm.
- Polyps greater than 20mm require advanced endoscopic resection techniques or surgery.
- Perioperative complications are best managed by appropriate procedure and technique selection in addition to specific endoscopic techniques to both prevent and treat incomplete resection, bleeding, and/or perforation.

INTRODUCTION/HISTORY/DEFINITIONS/BACKGROUND

Cancers of the gastrointestinal system, which begin as either mucosal or submucosal lesions, have the benefit of being visible and accessible with modern endoscopic technologies. Endoscopic polypectomy procedures serve to detect and treat premalignant and malignant lesions early in the disease course, preventing morbidity and mortality or more invasive treatments.[1]

Polypectomy techniques are described based on whether they are done with or without cautery, with or without submucosal injections, and whether in an en bloc or piecemeal manner. The leading techniques include cold snare polypectomy (CSP) and hot snare polypectomy (HSP), both of which can be done with or without submucosal injections and either en bloc or piecemeal. Beyond these techniques are more advanced techniques used for larger lesions, including endoscopic mucosal resection (EMR), endoscopic submucosal dissection (ESD), endoscopic full-thickness resection (EFTR), and combined laparoendoscopic approaches, which are described

Disclosures: E. Fung is a consultant for Boston Scientific and an advisor for Arch Therapeutics.
[a] Department of Surgery, University at Buffalo, 100 High Street D350, Buffalo, NY 14203, USA;
[b] Department of Surgery, University at Buffalo, 462 Grider Street, DK Miller Building, 3rd Floor, Buffalo, NY 14215, USA
* Corresponding author.
E-mail address: Kelly.t.wagner@gmail.com
Twitter: @kellytwagner (K.T.W.)

in more detail in MacKenzie D. Landin and A. Daniel Guerrón's article, "Endoscopic Mucosal Resection and Endoscopic Submucosal Dissection"; and Christine Tat and colleagues' article, "Principles of Intramural Surgery," elsewhere in this issue.

NATURE OF THE PROBLEM/DIAGNOSIS

In the upper gastrointestinal tract, the stomach is a common location to incidentally identify premalignant and malignant lesions. A gastric polyp is identified in approximately 0.34% to 3.3% of esophagogastroduodenoscopies.[2] Of all polypectomies performed, the incidence of adenocarcinoma was 1%, carcinoid 0.5%, adenomatous polyp 2.6%, fundic gland polyp (FGP) 1.6%, focal alveolar hyperplasia 4.7%, and hyperplastic polyps 88%.[3] In populations taking proton pumps inhibitors, the incidence of FGPs is increased, whereas, in patient populations with high incidence of *Helicobacter pylori* infection, hyperplastic polyps are more common. Gastric hyperplastic polyps harboring dysplasia or cancer have a wide range of reported incidence, from as low as 0.6% to as high as 19%.[2,4] Although this risk is yet to be clearly defined, what is clear is that hyperplastic polyps carry some risk of malignancy, and, with their being among the most common gastric polyps, the consequences of missed lesions or failure to diagnose can be fatal. As such, early recognition and removal of all lesions of the upper gastrointestinal tract is essential.[4] Although the burden of gastric cancer in the United States is low compared with other cancers, gastric cancer remains the third most common cause of cancer-related death, responsible for more than 8% of deaths worldwide in 2018.[5]

The lower gastrointestinal tract has been studied to a much greater extent because colorectal cancer is the third leading cause of cancer death worldwide.[6] Colorectal polypectomy has been shown to reduce the rates of colorectal cancer. In a long-term follow-up study, polypectomy was shown to reduce the risk of developing colorectal cancer by 53%, whereas untreated colon polyps greater than or equal to 10 mm had a nearly 25% chance of harboring invasive adenocarcinoma at 20 years.[1,7] Such statistics are the reason why screening colonoscopy and endoscopic polypectomy of the lower gastrointestinal tract are of the utmost importance in health maintenance and preventive medicine.

ANATOMY

The upper gastrointestinal tract poses a unique anatomic challenge for endoscopy. The shape of the stomach alone requires retroflexion for complete visualization in patients with standard anatomy. There are additional complexities in patients with large esophageal or gastroesophageal junction lesions or paraesophageal hernias, which can complicate the ability to enter the stomach and visualize the mucosal surface. Beyond these natural challenges, a large portion of the population requires upper endoscopy on a background of surgical manipulation, whether in the form of a sleeve gastrectomy, Billroth, or Roux-en-Y reconstruction. More than 90% of gastric polyps resected were discovered incidentally on esophagogastroduodenoscopy (EGD) for other reasons, with most of these polyps being found in the antrum (35.9%) or the corpus (46.2%).[2,3]

The lower gastrointestinal tract generally has fewer natural and surgical anatomic challenges; however, it is faced with its own set of difficulties. For example, the cecum and ascending colon are known for their thin walls, making these areas especially prone to bleeding and perforation. The colon is also riddled with a greater number of hyperplastic polyps, which, in contrast with gastric polyps, have a very low risk of harboring dysplasia or malignancy. The most common types of polyp found in the colon and rectum are adenomatous and hyperplastic polyps. Adenomatous polyps can be either sessile (flat, laterally spreading) or pedunculated (hanging from a stalk). Adenomatous polyps carry a risk of harboring underlying dysplasia or malignancy, particularly the sessile serrated adenomatous histologic subtype.

PREOPERATIVE/PREPROCEDURE PLANNING

In preparing for endoscopy, there are various preprocedure considerations. From a patient perspective, anticoagulation, bowel preparation, and preprocedure diet must be addressed. From a procedural perspective, room setup, staffing, and equipment needs must be addressed.

Anticoagulation

Postpolypectomy bleeding is generally accepted to occur at a rate of 1% in all comers and can be as high as 10% in patients on anticoagulation.[8] As such, it is important to be aware of patients on anticoagulation and have a management plan (**Table 1**). In general, it is recommended to discontinue anticoagulation for an appropriate interval before endoscopy in patients with a low risk of thromboembolic events if chances of polypectomy are high. If the patient is on short-term anticoagulation or antiplatelet therapy, the recommendation is to delay any elective endoscopic procedure until the anticoagulation/antiplatelet therapy is completed.[9] In 1 prospective randomized controlled trial (RCT), 70 patients were continued on warfarin and polyps less than 10 mm were resected. This trial showed improved safety with CSP versus HSP regarding risk of delayed bleeding (0% vs 14%, $P = .027$). For lesions greater than 10 mm, the authors recommend bringing the patient back for resection after holding anticoagulation or antiplatelet agents.[8] The value of prophylactic clipping is unclear

Table 1
Recommendations for anticoagulation and antiplatelet medications for endoscopic polypectomy

	Low-Risk Procedure		High-Risk Procedure	
	Low-Risk Patient	High-Risk Patient	Low-Risk Patient	High-Risk Patient
Antiplatelet	Continue	Continue	Continue ASA, NSAIDs, hold thienopyridines	Continue ASA, NSAIDs, hold thienopyridines
Anticoagulation	Continue	Continue	Discontinue	Hold anticoagulation with bridging therapy
Identify lesion ≥10 mm while on anticoagulation	Return for resection	Return for resection with bridging therapy	Return for resection after holding	Return for resection with bridging therapy

Low-risk procedure = screening examination, polypectomy of lesions less than or equal to 10 mm.
   High-risk procedure = planned polypectomy or EMR.
   Low-risk patient = anticoagulation for atrial fibrillation, antiplatelets for peripheral vascular disease.
   High-risk patient = anticoagulation for mechanical valve or pulmonary embolism, antiplatelets for coronary stents, history of ischemic stroke.
   Abbreviations: ASA, acetylsalicylic acid; NSAIDs, nonsteroidal antiinflammatory drugs.

in the literature, and, at this time, the decision to clip is at the discretion of the endo-scopist. If patients are at high risk of thromboembolic events, we recommend the use of bridging therapy.[9]

Bowel Preparation

Rates of polyp detection have been found to improve with adequate bowel prepara-tion. There are a variety of bowel preparation agents on the market, including isos-motic, hyperosmotic, and hypo-osmotic preparations. There is significant evidence to support the efficacy of split bowel preparations, in which half to two-thirds of the solution is consumed the night prior and the remaining solution is consumed 4 to 6 hours before the procedure. There has also been evidence to support a low-fiber or fully liquid diet until the evening before the procedure and a clear liquid diet starting the night before the procedure.[10] The most commonly used solution is the isosmotic high-volume (4 L) polyethylene glycol split-dose regimen, which has been found to have good efficacy but is sometimes poorly tolerated. Alternate solutions include the hypo-osmotic low-volume polyethylene glycol plus electrolyte sports drink, or hyperosmotic magnesium citrate. Although these are generally better tolerated by pa-tients, the evidence for their efficacy is mixed. In addition, hyperosmotic agents can result in clinically significant fluid and electrolyte shifts, making them less desirable in the elderly or patients with congestive heart failure, liver failure, and especially renal failure. Overall, the choice of bowel preparation should be individualized based on pa-tient and provider preference, and care should be taken to communicate instructions verbally and in written format in the patient's native language.[10]

Staff/procedure room setup

The setup of the room for endoscopic polypectomy does not significantly differ from the standard setup for a screening endoscopy (**Fig. 1**). The room should be adequately equipped in preparation for airway protection as well as with tools for endoscopic polypectomy and hemostasis, as outlined later in this article.

PREPARATION AND PATIENT POSITIONING
Sedation Techniques

Although there are some reports of successful endoscopy in fully awake patients, most endoscopic procedures require either moderate or deep sedation and some advanced procedures may even require general anesthesia.[11] The main sources of morbidity from procedural sedation are hypoxemia and aspiration, and all efforts should be made to mitigate these risks. For moderate sedation, the most commonly used agents are benzodiazepines (midazolam) and opiates (fentanyl). The use of moderate sedation does not require a dedicated anesthesia specialist or a person dedicated to patient monitoring. Another commonly used agent, propofol, easily achieves deep sedation; however, this does require a per-son trained in emergency airway management dedicated to patient monitoring. For moderate sedation, the minimal monitoring required includes pulse oximetry and noninvasive blood pressure every 5 minutes. Capnography is a helpful adjunct in all cases; however, it is only required for deep sedation. Electrocardio-gram monitoring is recommended for deep sedation and any level of sedation in patient with a cardiac history. In addition, antagonists for sedatives should be readily available in the procedure room, including flumazenil and naloxone. Regardless of level of sedation, in patients with American Society of

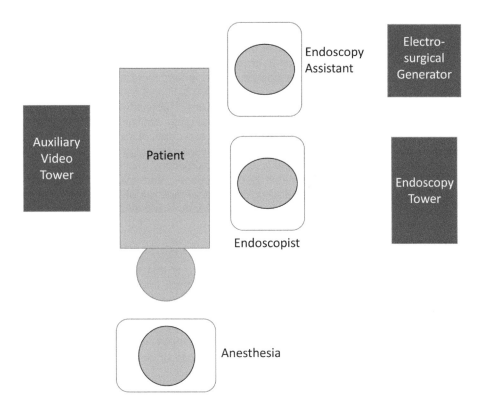

Fig. 1. Room setup for colonoscopy.

Anesthesiologists score greater than 3, the presence of a dedicated anesthesia provider is recommended.[12]

Patient Positioning

For upper endoscopy, the patient is generally positioned in the left lateral decubitus position. A prone or semiprone position is often used for more advanced duodenal and biliary procedures. For lower endoscopy, the patient is generally placed in the left lateral decubitus position. The patient may be transitioned to the supine position if needed to aid in advancing to the proximal colon. Sigmoid pressure performed by the bedside assistant may also need to be considered to improve scope maneuverability.

EQUIPMENT AND MATERIALS

For standard polypectomy, the required equipment includes a fiber-optic endoscope with a working channel, dedicated cold snares, traditional snares, endoscopic hemostatic clips, injection needles, and injectable agents. A more detailed discussion of this topic can be found in Sarah Choi and Kevin El-Hayek's article, "Endoscopic Equipment – From Simple to Advanced," elsewhere in this issue.

Endoscopes and Advanced Imaging

The camera of the endoscope is either front viewing, which is common for standard endoscopy, or side viewing, which is used when there is need for access into the ampulla of Vater. In addition to the location of the camera, there is also consideration of the light used to illuminate the mucosal surface. Traditional endoscopes use white light and rely on reflected light in the visible spectrum.[13] More advanced technologies include narrow-band imaging, which uses blue and green optical fibers that enhance vasculature for ease of delineating polyp margins and depth of invasion and can help determine the resectability of a lesion.[14] More advanced imaging modalities that are not as widely used include confocal laser endomicroscopy, multimodal endoscopy, photoacoustic endoscopy, volumetric laser endoscopy, and scanning fiber endoscopy.[15] Because these emerging technologies either fade out of vogue or earn their place in a standard endoscopy suite, recommendations will evolve to reflect those changes.

Resection Tools

Dedicated cold snares differ from traditional snares in that they are stiff, monofilament, and thin wired compared with the braided thick traditional snares (**Fig. 2**). Dedicated cold snares do not have the capacity to be connected to cautery. A prospective RCT comparing dedicated with traditional CSP showed significantly higher complete resection rates (CRRs) for lesions less than or equal to 10 mm with use of a dedicated snare versus a traditional snare (91% vs 79%, $P = .015$) with no significant difference in immediate or delayed bleeding rates.[8]

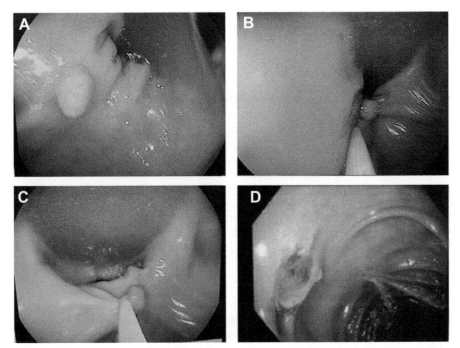

Fig. 2. Treatment of an adenomatous polyp by CSP technique. (*A*) Adenomatous polyp in the sigmoid colon, (*B, C*) cold snare resection of the polyp, (*D*) postpolypectomy resection bed.

In addition, some dedicated cold snares are thin enough that the resected specimen can be retrieved through the working channel without removal of the snare.[14] Although cold biopsy forceps were shown to be used in 62.3% of all gastric polypectomies, including 41.3% of gastric polyps greater than 10 mm, their use was associated with incomplete resection and failure to reveal dysplastic histology, suggesting their inferiority to CSP.[2] In colonoscopy, there is also strong evidence against the use of cold forceps polypectomy (CFP) for any polyp larger than 4 mm. Although these data show noninferiority of CFP versus CSP for complete resection of polyps less than or equal to 4 mm (96.9% vs 100%, P = 1.00), this requires accurate visual size assessment and the use of 2 different tools.[16] As such, the use of a dedicated cold snare for the resection of all diminutive polyps is recommended. Although hot biopsy forceps are an option for polypectomy, it has been associated with increased adverse event rates and decreased CRRs and, as such, it is generally not recommended.[14,17]

Submucosal Injection

Submucosal injection works by infiltrating the submucosal layer with a solution that lifts and separates the lesion from the underlying muscularis propria. This method serves the dual purpose of reducing the risk of injury to the muscular layer while improving chances of a complete resection and determining the level of invasion of the polyp. Submucosal injection is a required step for EMR, ESD, and intramural surgery, which are discussed in MacKenzie D. Landin and A. Daniel Guerrón's article, "Endoscopic Mucosal Resection and Endoscopic Submucosal Dissection"; and Ipek Sapci and Emre Gorgun's article, "Advanced Colonic Polypectomy"; and Christine Tat and colleagues' article, "Principles of Intramural Surgery," elsewhere in this issue. Solutions may also contain a dye that helps delineate lesion margins as well as residual polypoid tissue. Staining dyes have also been shown to aid in identifying perforations at the time of procedure when repair is easiest to perform.[18] In endoscopic polypectomy, submucosal injection is generally recommended for HSP and CSP of lesions greater than or equal to 10 mm undergoing en bloc or piecemeal resection or for pedunculated polyps with a head greater than or equal to 20 mm or a stalk greater than or equal to 10 mm.[19,20] There are currently numerous injectable agents available on the market, which vary in their availability, duration of cushion, cost, and damage to specimen. Some of the available solutions have unusual risks associated, such as an ability to stimulate residual tumor cell growth with hyaluronic acid, potential for antibody-antigen reaction with hydroxylpropyl methylcellulose, and potential to transmit infectious agents with fibrinogen, making them generally less desirable.[18] Normal saline is the most commonly used injectate because it is inexpensive and readily available. However, it has rapid absorption, making it less useful for piecemeal resection or long procedures. If a longer-lasting submucosal cushion is required, injectates such as glycerol, succinylated gelatin, or hydroxylethyl starch are good alternatives. Additives to these solutions include epinephrine (diluted to between 1:50,000 and 1:200,000) and staining dyes (80 mg of indigo carmine or 20 mg of methylene blue in 500 mL of normal saline). Although epinephrine has not been shown to decrease delayed bleeding, it has been shown to decrease immediate bleeding, which may improve visualization and therefore improve outcomes. There are more expensive synthetic injectates that incorporate the epinephrine and stain into premeasured aliquots, such as Eleview and O-RISE. However, these are limited by availability and cost. Future considerations that require further research include the use of needleless injections (ERBE-Lift) and dissecting gels.[18]

INDICATIONS AND CONTRAINDICATIONS
Esophagogastroduodenoscopy

All gastric polyps have malignant potential and should all be resected for histologic evaluation. For lesions less than or equal to 4 mm, complete resection with either CFP or CSP is recommended. For lesions greater than or equal to 5 mm and less than 20 mm, CSP is recommended. For lesions greater than or equal to 20 mm in the stomach or duodenum, the authors recommend advanced polypectomy techniques.[3,21] The American Society for Gastrointestinal Endoscopy (ASGE) has also released the following recommendations for gastric polyps:

- Complete polypectomy for:
  - FGP greater than 10 mm
  - HP (hyperplastic polyps) greater than 5 mm
  - All APs (adenomatous polyps)
  - All lesions greater than 10 mm
- Multiple polyps require complete resection of the largest lesion with sampling biopsies of smaller polyps[4]

Colonoscopy

In the colon and rectum, the indications for polypectomy are straightforward in that, if a polyp is visualized, it should be resected.[22] Although diminutive polyps are prone to neglect for their high chances of being benign, they still may harbor premalignant or malignant tissue and are associated with a very low adverse event rate and merit resection.[23] Large lesions (>20 mm) often require advanced techniques and possibly advanced work-up and are discussed in greater detail in MacKenzie D. Landin and A. Daniel Guerrón's article, "Endoscopic Mucosal Resection and Endoscopic Submucosal Dissection"; and Christine Tat and colleagues' article, "Principles of Intramural Surgery," elsewhere in this issue.

The techniques recommended based on the size and morphology of a lesion are discussed next. For a summary of recommendations, please refer to **Table 2**.

Diminutive Polyps 1 to 3 mm: Cold Snare Polypectomy

When directly comparing CSP with CFP for lesions less than or equal to 4 mm, there was no significant difference in CRR (96.9% vs 100%, $P = 1.00$) or adverse events.[16] However, because this is not true for slightly larger lesions, it would be inefficient and more expensive to use 2 different tools when 1 would suffice.[23] As such, CSP is recommended as the first-line procedure for diminutive polyps and to use CFP only when CSP is not possible.[14]

Small Polyps Less than or Equal to 10 mm: Cold Snare Polypectomy

Several studies have shown the superiority of CSP for the resection of colonic polyps less than or equal to 10 mm.[16,23–26] The superiority arises because of the decrease in adverse event rates compared with HSP and the improved CRR compared with CFP.[20]

Cold snare polypectomy versus cold forceps polypectomy

In 1 meta-analysis of 7 studies that compared the efficacy of various cold polypectomy techniques, it was shown that CSP was superior with regard to complete histologic eradication and had either faster or noninferior procedure times. This same meta-analysis also showed dedicated CSP to be superior to traditional CSP with regard to histologic eradication.[23] In a RCT, Kim and colleagues[16] showed that, for polyps 5 to

Table 2
Recommended techniques for polypectomy based on polyp size and morphology

Polyp Size/Morphology	Technique Recommended	Notes or Special Circumstances
Diminutive polyps 1–3 mm	CSP	CFP noninferior, use only if CSP not possible
Small polyps <10 mm	CSP	Dedicated cold snare superior to traditional snare
Pedunculated polyps 10–19 mm	HSP + mechanical hemostasis	± submucosal injection, watch for research on CSP
Sessile polyps 10–19 mm	HSP + submucosal injection	If high-risk lesion or patient → piecemeal CSP
Polyps 20–40 mm	Advanced endoscopic techniques	Surgery if evidence of deep invasion or aggressive histology
Polyps>40 mm	Appropriate staging work-up and surgery if appropriate	—

7 mm, there was a significant difference in the CRR for CSP versus CFP (93.8% vs 70.3%, $P = .013$), with CSP being superior to CFP.

Cold snare polypectomy versus hot snare polypectomy
The choice of CSP rather than HSP for lesions less than or equal to 10 mm arises because of its superior adverse event profile, shorter procedure times, and noninferiority with regard to CRR and retrieval rates.[24–26] It is generally accepted that HSP causes damage to the underlying submucosal vessels, and, although it can aid with immediate hemostasis, it can lead to delayed bleeding once the coagulated eschar sloughs off. In 1 meta-analysis of only RCTs, CSP was shown to have a retrieval rate similar to HSP (97% vs 97%, $P = .60$) and a similar CRR (94% vs 95%, $P = .31$). A higher delayed bleeding rate was found in the HSP group compared with CSP; however, this was not found to be statistically significant (0% vs 0.8%, $P = .06$).[24] In 1 RCT that compared CSP with HSP in 796 polypectomies, there was an increased risk of immediate bleeding with CSP versus HSP (7.1% vs 3.5%, $P = .02$); however, there were no incidences of delayed bleeding for CSP and the retrieval rates as well as CRR were similar between the 2 arms.[25] Notably, in most studies evaluated in the meta-analysis as well as in the aforementioned RCT, dedicated cold snares were not used; as such, it would be interesting to see how the results may be affected if this change were made. Regardless, it has been shown that CSP is not inferior to HSP, and had faster procedure times and decreased risk of delayed bleeding and perforation. However, it is possible that in these studies more care was taken than usual when completing resections, which could account for the lower than usual rates of delayed bleeding and perforation.

Pedunculated Polyps 10 to 19 mm: Hot Snare Polypectomy with Mechanical Hemostasis

Polyps greater than 10 mm have been associated with an increased risk of bleeding.[27] The stalks of pedunculated polyps are assumed to have penetrating vessels, which mandates some form of intentional hemostasis. The cautery associated with HSP is one means of preventing immediate bleeding; however, it is recommended to perform at least 1 form of prophylactic hemostasis to prevent delayed bleeding.[20] In 1 RCT, HSP of pedunculated polyps was completed with clipping plus or minus submucosal epinephrine injection, which showed that clipping alone was adequate to control immediate bleeding (12.0% vs 14.4%, $P = .64$). No cases of delayed bleeding were found in either group, which suggests that clipping is sufficient to prevent delayed bleeding.[28] An alternative to the endoscopic clip is the endoscopic loop; these 2 methods have been shown to be similar in efficacy for the prevention of both immediate and delayed bleeding.[29]

Sessile Polyps 10 to 19 mm: Hot Snare Polypectomy Plus Submucosal Injection

For sessile polyps of this size, HSP with submucosal injection is recommended. In general, HSP is considered standard of care for larger polyps because of its ability to remove lesions en bloc, which is theorized to decrease the risk of incomplete resection and recurrent adenoma formation.[20] In addition, HSP uses cautery, which damages the wound margins and theoretically serves 2 purposes: the prevention of immediate bleeding as well as damaging any residual microscopic dysplastic or malignant cells.[30,31] However, current European Society of Gastrointestinal Endoscopy (ESGE) guidelines recommend avoiding adjunctive ablative techniques whenever possible because of the risks of deep thermal injury. ESGE guidelines also recommend submucosal injection or mechanical hemostasis to prevent bleeding in this subpopulation.[20] A lesion not separating well with submucosal injection should also raise suspicion for invasion into the muscularis propria and there should be consideration for further workup.

In 1 large prospective study, the CARE study, incomplete resection rates were found to be as high as 47.6% for lesions 10 to 20 mm. The specific aspects of technique that were consistent in groups with better CRR included outlining and marking polyp margin before resection, use of advance imaging techniques, postresection marginal biopsies, and ablation of postresection margins.[31]

High-risk lesions or patients

Lesions that are high risk for an adverse event include location in the cecum or ascending colon. Patients are also at increased risk for bleeding if they are on anticoagulation or antiplatelet agents, even if they will be held for the procedure and restarted afterward. For these patients or high-risk lesions, piecemeal CSP with submucosal injection is recommended to decrease the risk of bleeding or perforation. CSP was shown in a meta-analysis to have a CRR of 99.3% and overall adverse event rate of 1.1%, both of which are comparable with HSP rates.[32] In a separate retrospective review of 4018 colonoscopies, CSP was shown to be noninferior to HSP for large sessile lesions with regard to CRR (89.4% vs 87.9%, $P = .33$). However, when subdivided for sessile serrated adenoma morphology, HSP was superior to CSP (88.7% vs 77.2%, $P<.05$), suggesting that HSP should be the technique of choice if no special circumstances exist. This same study also showed a trend toward increased adverse event rates for HSP compared with CSP; however, this study was not sufficiently powered to be statistically significant.[30] If piecemeal CSP is the selected technique, it is recommended to limit the size of resected pieces to less than 15 mm because this was shown to produce quicker and cleaner resections.[19]

Polyps Greater than or Equal to 20 mm: Advanced Endoscopic Techniques or Surgery

For larger lesions, patients require either advanced endoscopic techniques (lesions 20–40 mm) or surgical intervention (lesions greater than or equal to 40 mm).[14,20] Signs that the patient should be considered for surgical intervention include imaging consistent with lymph node spread or distant metastasis, deep invasion noted on advanced endoscopic imaging, or resection margins after polypectomy with advanced histologic features.[14,20,22] Advanced endoscopic techniques include EMR, UEMR, ESD, and EFTR, and these are discussed in detail in MacKenzie D. Landin and A. Daniel Guerrón's article, "Endoscopic Mucosal Resection and Endoscopic Submucosal Dissection"; and Christine Tat and colleagues' article, "Principles of Intramural Surgery," elsewhere in this issue.

PROCEDURAL APPROACH

In a large prospective study, CRRs were found to vary significantly among endoscopists.[31] This finding makes it even more salient to clarify the proper procedural steps for polypectomy and reinforce the care that must be taken to prevent interval development of colorectal cancer. Overarching principles in endoscopic polypectomy include choosing the correct technique for the correct polyp, minimizing residual polyp by taking a small margin of surrounding normal mucosa, tissue ablation at resection margins, closer surveillance after piecemeal resection, and applying proper technique (see **Table 2**).[22,24] The procedural steps of both CSP and HSP are discussed next.

Procedural Steps of Cold Snare Polypectomy

1. Place polyp in 5 to 7 o'clock position to match accessory channel of colonoscope[14,16,33] (**Fig. 2**)
   a. Maintain short distance to polyp
2. Capture polyp in snare
   a. Use dedicated CSP snare whenever available
   b. Take care to deliberately grasp a clear rim of normal tissue circumferentially around polyp
   c. Two ways to capture polyp
      i. Snare tip anchored to normal mucosa at the proximal edge of polyp; snare is slowly opened, capturing remainder of polyp
      ii. Snare fully opened above polyp and laid down flat against mucosa, flush against wall
3. Suction air to ease capture and close snare slowly to grasp and resect lesion
4. Retrieve lesion
5. Observe area of resection for at least 30 seconds to confirm hemostasis
   a. Consider use of advanced imaging to assist in determining completeness of resection (NBI [Narrow Band Imaging]); less likely to be helpful in HSP secondary to damage of tissues from cautery

Procedural Steps of Hot Snare Polypectomy

1. Submucosal injection to lift lesion[34] (**Fig. 3**)
   a. Optional for pedunculated polyps 10 to 19 mm
2. Optional: place hemostatic clips or endoloop around stalk of pedunculated lesion
3. Place polyp in 5 to 7 o'clock position to match accessory channel of colonoscope
   b. Maintain short distance to polyp

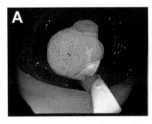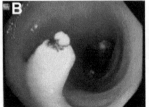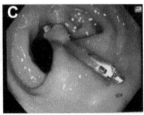

Fig. 3. Treatment of a pedunculated polyp by hot snare polypectomy technique. (*A*) Hot snare resection of the polyp, (*B*) postpolypectomy stalk with visible feeding vessel within stalk with high-risk stigmata for bleeding, (*C*) clip applied to stalk postpolypectomy.

4. Deploy snare and capture polyp in snare by placing snare directly over top of lesion and then approximating snare to mucosal surface
5. Apply current while simultaneously closing snare
6. Retrieve lesion
7. Observe area of resection for at least 30 seconds to confirm hemostasis and to inspect for gross completeness of resection

Retrieval Techniques

Some lesions are difficult to retrieve or are unretrievable. There are 4 different retrieval methods:

1. Conventional polyp trap placed at suction connector
2. Removal of suction valve and using a finger to apply suction
3. Roth net polyp retriever via the instrument channel
4. Connecting polyp trap to instrument channel

In 1 randomized controlled study, Barge and colleagues[35] showed that methods 1 and 2 had the highest rates of fragmentation, whereas methods 3 and 4 had the lowest rates (60.3%, 43%, 23.1%, 18.5% respectively). The decreased fragmentation rate was theorized to be secondary to either the lesion not passing by the suction channel causing shearing forces or the decreased length of tubing the lesion must travel to be retrieved.

Procedural Bleeding Maneuvers

The most efficacious time to control hemorrhage from a polypectomy is during the procedure. An increased immediate bleeding risk with CSP versus HSP is expected; however, it has been shown that dedicated cold snares have decreased bleeding risk compared with traditional snares used without cautery (4.1% vs 16%, $P = .009$).[33] This finding is consistent with our recommendation to use a dedicated cold snare when available. After polyp resection, it is important to inspect the site carefully to evaluate for bleeding as well as for deep muscular injury suggestive of perforation. Clinicians should also keep in mind that certain patients and polyp locations are at increased risk of bleeding, including patient age greater than 65 years, polyp size greater than 10 mm, stalk diameter greater than 5 mm, polyp location in the right colon, and presence of malignancy in polyp.[36] Once bleeding has been identified, there are 4 ways to address it: observation with lavage, tamponade techniques, thermal energy, and chemical hemostatic agents.

- Observation and lavage (conservative)

- o With minimal oozing, observation with water lavage often leads to spontaneous cessation
- Tamponade techniques
  - o Clipping
    - If brisk bleeding is encountered, continuous lavage can be used to identify the precise location of bleeding[36]
    - Through-the-scope clip application
    - Bleeding from a pedunculated stalk requires deploying clip perpendicular to stalk to properly ligate the feeding vessels
    - Bleeding from sessile polyp removal requires placing the clip such that it opposes mucosa from either side of resection defect to tamponade the site of bleeding[37]
    - For large sessile lesions where apposing mucosal edges is not possible, the clip should be closed over the area of suspected bleeding but not deployed until copious irrigation shows that closure of the clip has controlled the bleeding
  - o Endoloop
    - Can be use on pedunculated stalks of large lesions prophylactically[36]
  - o Over-the-scope clips
    - Can be used for difficult-to-control bleeding
- Thermal energy techniques
  - o A variety of thermal coagulation energy devices are currently on the market for hemostasis, which include gold probe/bipolar cautery, coagulation forceps, snare tip soft coagulation, and argon plasma coagulation[38]
  - o Argon plasma coagulation is recommended for refractory oozing as well as for ablation of residual polypoid tissue at resection margins[4]
  - o Procedural pearls
    - Extra care should be taken in the right colon/cecum because of thinner colon wall and increased risk of perforation
    - Thermal energy should be used cautiously in postpolypectomy sites to avoid risk of deep injury and further delayed bleeding
- Chemical hemostatic techniques: injections/powder
  - o Contact hemostasis powder spray: modified starch polymer
    - Not permanent and can be used as adjunct to more permanent hemostatic technique
  - o Fibrin glue
  - o Epinephrine
    - Should be used in dilution of 1:10,000 normal saline injected in 4 quadrants in aliquots of 0.5 to 2 mL with a 23-G or 25-G sclerotherapy needle

Procedural Pearls

- Define borders and size of polyp
  - o Tools to aid with this include use of a transparent cap, near focus imaging, or injection of contrast (methylene blue or indigo carmine)
- Snare getting stuck during CSP: despite closing snare tightly, the snare fails to completely cut through polyp[14,26]
  - o Keeping snare closed and placing device under mild tension while completely straightening the snare sheath and pulling snare partially into accessory channel can apply additional mechanical force
  - o Open snare slightly and close again, reorienting the snare to try to transect polyp

○ If the above fail, release lesion, and resection can be performed in a piecemeal fashion

COMPLICATIONS

Most studies evaluating endoscopic complications were performed in colonoscopy series, however these complications and their management can be extrapolated to apply to EGD as well.

Missed Lesions/Incomplete Resection

Missed lesions and/or incomplete resection of lesions raises concern for the development of interval cancer. Rates of incomplete resection have been reported as high as 23% in some studies.[31] If noted at time of procedure, the endoscopist can either resect more tissue or plan for a more advanced endoscopic intervention or surgery depending on circumstances. Not surprisingly, visual acuity has been shown to be inferior to microscopy for residual dysplastic or atypical tissue, which is why advanced imaging techniques such as NBI should be used when available.[16]

Immediate Bleeding

Techniques to manage intraprocedural bleeding include observation and lavage, tamponade techniques, thermal energy techniques, and chemical hemostatic techniques. A more detailed discussion was presented earlier in relation to procedural bleeding maneuvers.

Postprocedure Bleeding/Delayed Bleeding

Patients can present hours to days after a procedure with hematochezia, possibly acute blood loss anemia, and sometimes hemodynamic instability. Risk of delayed bleeding is greater following HSP, which is presumably secondary to sloughing of coagulated eschar created by thermal energy.[39] This risk is also increased in patients on anticoagulation and in larger lesions.[8,36] In a meta-analysis of management approaches to delayed bleeding, colonoscopy led to endoscopic resolution in 22.4% of cases, with a number needed to treat of 4.5 patients.[40] Because many patients resolve spontaneously without intervention, in hemodynamically stable patients the authors recommend a trial of expectant management followed by repeat endoscopy if the patient fails a conservative approach. If the patient is unstable or has persistent bleeding, repeat endoscopy with attempts at endoscopic hemostasis maneuver could be attempted, with embolization and surgical intervention considered as last measures.

Perforation

Perforation is the most feared complication of endoscopic polypectomy because it could turn a minimally invasive procedure into a major operation. The perforation risk is increased in patients with larger lesions, advanced resection techniques (EMR/ESD), and with the use of thermal energy.[39] In 1 prospective observational study of large colorectal lesions (≥20 mm), a perforation rate of 1% was reported.[37] Of these perforations, more than half were in lesions greater than or equal to 50 mm and 93.3% were from EMR or ESD procedures. However, in several large case series studying lesions less than or equal to 20 mm, there were no reported perforations.[24,25,39] The SCALP study reported that 86.6% of perforations were successfully treated with endoscopic clipping, whereas 13% required surgical intervention.[37] Ultimately, for simple endoscopic polypectomy the risks of perforation are low. The chances of identifying perforations intraprocedurally are higher if a submucosal injection that contains stain is used. In this case, if the transected surface displays a target sign, a white central circular disc surrounded by blue-stained submucosal tissue, this is typically suggestive of a perforation and/or significant damage to the muscular layer, which merits endoscopic clipping.[18] When discovered during the procedure, attempts at endoscopic closure with either clips or suturing are recommended to close the perforation. If discovered postprocedure, a stepwise approach is recommended, considering the patient's clinical presentation and hemodynamic status. In patients who are hemodynamically stable and without signs of peritonitis, a conservative approach can be taken. Initially this includes close monitoring and observation. This is followed by endoscopic attempts at repair should the patient's condition fail to improve or worsen.

Postpolypectomy Syndrome

Postpolypectomy syndrome is a term that encompasses nonspecific pain and discomfort following endoscopic polypectomy and more advanced endoscopic techniques. It has been found to likely represent a microperforation or full-thickness bowel injury without frank perforation. This condition can generally be managed with conservative treatment and clinical monitoring to be sure that it is not an early presentation of a more serious complication. Conservative management generally includes bowel rest, intravenous fluids, and broad-spectrum antibiotic administration. However, this is a diagnosis of exclusion in which most patients undergo computed tomography scanning to further evaluate the colon and rule out underlying perforation.[41]

RECOVERY AND REHABILITATION (INCLUDING POSTPROCEDURE CARE)

Patients undergoing endoscopic polypectomy should be closely monitored in a postprocedural care area following the procedure because early recognition and treatment of patients with discomfort or signs of complications is vital (**Fig. 4**).[38]

MANAGEMENT
Postprocedure/Pathology Surveillance

For upper endoscopy, the recommended surveillance following EGD with polypectomy varies based on pathology. For adenomatous polyps, the recommendation is repeat endoscopy within 1 year followed by long-term surveillance every 3 to 5 years. Because FGPs have minimal association with development of gastric cancer, there is no special follow-up endoscopy recommended at this time.[4]

Colonoscopy surveillance guidelines after polypectomy were recently updated and the current US Multi-Society Task Force guidelines are as follows:

- No special surveillance of hyperplastic colon polyps
  - Hyperplastic polyposis syndrome requires more intensive follow-up
- Resection of 1 to 2 small adenomas: return in 5 to 10 years
- Resection of 3 to 10 adenomas or any adenoma greater than or equal to 1 cm with villous features or high-grade dysplasia: return in 3 years
- More than 10 adenomas: return in less than 3 years
- Sessile adenomas removed in piecemeal fashion: 2 to 6 months to verify complete removal[42]

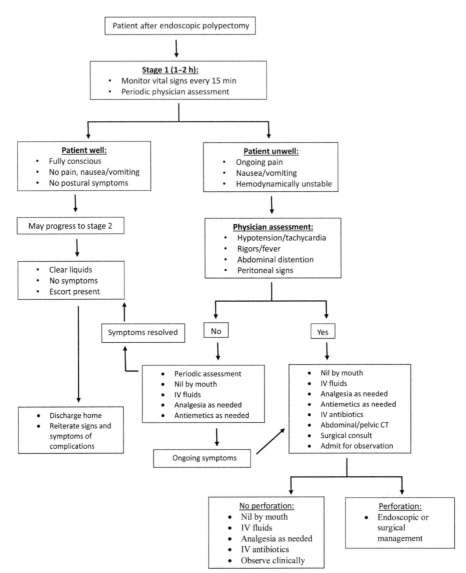

Fig. 4. Suggested recovery management scheme following polypectomy. CT, computed tomography; IV, intravenous.

For both upper and lower endoscopy, any lesions with positive margins or aggressive features, including lymphovascular invasion, should be considered for either more advanced endoscopic resection or surgical resection with lymph node sampling.

SUMMARY

Polypectomy is key for both the detection and treatment of premalignant and malignant lesions in the gastrointestinal tract to prevent the morbidity and mortality of malignancy. The management of polyps and polypectomy technique depend on size, morphology, and degree of invasion; these polypectomy techniques include the use of cold forceps, submucosal injection, dedicated cold snare, hot snare, and advanced endoscopic techniques. Complications from polypectomy include postprocedural bleeding, incomplete resection, perforation, and postpolypectomy syndrome. Patients should be monitored closely following polypectomy and complications should be managed expeditiously.

CLINICS CARE POINTS

- Endoscopic polypectomy of polyps up to 20mm in the gastrointestinal tract is the safest means to prevent the morbidity and mortality associated with gastrointestinal cancers
- Decisions regarding perioperative anticoagulation management are made on a case by case basis and should take both patient and procedural risks into account
- Use of dedicated cold snare is the recommended polypectomy technique for all polyps ≤10mm
- Lesions between 10 - 20mm should be resected with the hot snare polypectomy technique with adjunct procedures including mechanical hemostasis and submucosal injection
- Residual polyp can lead to recurrent or progressive disease and is avoided by adhering to the following principles: defining the borders of the lesion, including a margin of normal mucosa, tissue ablation at resection margins, closer surveillance after piecemeal resection, and employing the appropriate technique for any given polyp
- Extra care should be taken in the right colon due to thinner walls and increased risk of both bleeding and perforation
- Bleeding or perforation are potential serious complications which are most easily managed if discovered during the index procedure using thermal energy, clipping, or sewing as appropriate
- If discovered post procedure they should be managed in a stepwise fashion starting with observation and leaving surgical intervention as a last resort

REFERENCES

1. Zauber AG, Winawer SJ, O'Brien MJ, et al. Colonoscopic Polypectomy and Long-Term Prevention of Colorectal Cancer Deaths. N Engl J Med 2012;366:687–96.
2. Corral JE, Keihanian T, Diaz LI, et al. Management patterns of gastric polyps in the United States. Frontline Gastroenterol 2019;10:16–23.
3. Olmez S, Sayar S, Saritas B, et al. Evaluation of Patients with Gastric Polyps. North Clin Istanb 2018;5:41–6.
4. ASGE Standards of Practice Committee, Evans JA, Chandrasekhara V, Chathadi KV, et al. The Role of Endoscopy in the Management of Premalignant and Malignant Conditions of the Stomach. Gastrointest Endosc 2015;82:1–8.
5. Bray F, Ferlay J, Soerjomataram I, et al. Global cancer statistics 2018: GLOBOCAN estimates of incidence and mortality worldwide for 36 cancers in 185 countries. CA Cancer J Clin 2018;68:394–424.
6. Mattiuzzi C, Sanchis-Gomar F, Lippi G. Concise update on colorectal cancer epidemiology. Ann Transl Med 2019;7:609.
7. Stryker SJ, Wolff BG, Culp CE, et al. Natural History of Untreated Colonic Polyps. Gastroenterology 1987;93:1009–13.

8. Horiuchi A, Nakayama Y, Kajiyama M, et al. Removal of small colorectal polyps in anticoagulated patients: a prospective randomized comparison of cold snare and conventional polypectomy. Gastrointest Endosc 2014;79:417–23.

9. ASGE Standards of Practice Committee, Acosta RD, Abraham NS, Chandrasekhara V, et al. The management of antithrombotic agents for patients undergoing GI endoscopy. Gastrointest Endosc 2016;83:3–16.

10. ASGE Standards of Practice Committee, Saltzman JR, Cash BD, Pasha SF, et al. Bowel Preparation before Endoscopy. Gastrointest Endosc 2015;81:781–94.

11. Goudra B, Nuzat Z, Singh PM, et al. Association between Type of Sedation and the Adverse Events Associated with Gastrointestinal Endoscopy: An Analysis of 5 Years' Data from a Tertiary Center in the USA. Clin Endosc 2017;50:161–9.

12. ASGE Standards of Practice Committee, Early DS, Lightdale JR, Vargo JJ 2nd, et al. Guidelines for sedation and anesthesia in GI endoscopy. Gastrointest Endosc 2018;87:327–37.

13. Sturm MB, Wang TD. Emerging optical methods for surveillance of Barrett's oesophagus. Gut 2015;64:1816–23.

14. Moss A, Nalankilli K. Standardisation of Polypectomy Technique. Best Pract Res Clin Gastroenterol 2017;31:447–53.

15. van der Sommen F, Curvers WL, Nagengast WB. Novel developments in endoscopic mucosal imaging. Gastroenterology 2018;154:1876–86.

16. Kim JS, Lee BI, Choi H, et al. Cold Snare Polypectomy versus Cold Forceps Polypectomy for Diminutive and Small Colorectal Polyps: a Randomized Controlled Trial. Gastrointest Endosc 2015;81:741–7.

17. Panteris V, Vezakis A, Triantafillidis JK. Should Hot Biopsy Forceps Be Abandoned for Polypectomy of Diminutive Colorectal Polyps? World J Gastroenterol 2018;24:1579–82.

18. Castro R, Libanio D, Pita, et al. Solutions for Submucosal Injection: What to Choose and How to Do It. World J Gastroenterol 2019;25:777–88.

19. Choksi N, Elmunzer BJ, Stidham RW, et al. Cold snare piecemeal resection of colonic and duodenal polyps ≥1cm. Endosc Int Open 2015;3:E508–13.

20. Ferlitsch M, Moss A, Hassan C, et al. Colorectal Polypectomy and Endoscopic Mucosal Resection (EMR): European Society of Gastrointestinal Endoscopy (ESGE) Clinical Guideline. Endoscopy 2017;49:270–97.

21. Mahmud N, Tomizawa Y, Stashek K, et al. Endoscopic Resection of Duodenal Carcinoid Tumors: A Single-Center Comparison Between Simple Polypectomy and Endoscopic Mucosal Resection. Pancreas 2019;48:60–5.

22. ASGE Standards of Practice Committee, Fisher DA, Shergill AK, Early DS, et al. Role of Endoscopy in the Staging and Management of Colorectal Cancer. Gastrointest Endosc 2013;78:8–12.

23. Jung YS, Park CH, Nam E, et al. Comparative Efficacy of Cold Polypectomy Techniques for Diminutive Colorectal Polyps: a Systematic Review and Network Meta-Analysis. Surg Endosc 2018;32:1149–59.

24. Shinozaki S, Kobayashi Y, Hayashi Y, et al. Efficacy and Safety of Cold versus Hot Snare Polypectomy for Resecting Small Colorectal Polyps: Systematic Review and Meta-Analysis. Dig Endosc 2018;30:592–9.

25. Kawamura T, Takeuchi Y, Asai S, et al. A Comparison of the Resection Rate for Cold and Hot Snare Polypectomy for 4–9 Mm Colorectal Polyps: a Multicentre Randomised Controlled Trial (CRESCENT Study). Gut 2018;67:1950–7.

26. Keswani RN. Cold Snare Polypectomy: Techniques and Applications. Clin Gastroenterol Hepatol 2020;18:42–4.

27. Yamaguchi D, Yoshida H, Ikeda K, et al. Colorectal Endoscopic Mucosal Resection with Submucosal Injection of Epinephrine versus Hypertonic Saline in Patients Taking Antithrombotic Agents: Propensity-Score-Matching Analysis. BMC Gastroenterol 2019;19:192.
28. Park Y, Jeon TJ, Park JY, et al. Comparison of Clipping with and without Epinephrine Injection for the Prevention of Post-Polypectomy Bleeding in Pedunculated Colon Polyps. J Gastroenterol Hepatol 2015;30:1499–506.
29. Ji JS, Lee SW, Kim TH, et al. Comparison of Prophylactic Clip and Endoloop Application for the Prevention of Postpolypectomy Bleeding in Pedunculated Colonic Polyps: a Prospective, Randomized, Multicenter Study. Endoscopy 2014;46:598–604.
30. Gessl I, Waldmann E, Penz D, et al. Resection Rates and Safety Profile of Cold vs. Hot Snare Polypectomy in Polyps Sized 5–10 Mm and 11–20 Mm. Dig Liver Dis 2019;51:536–41.
31. Pohl H, Srivastava A, Bensen SP, et al. Incomplete Polyp Resection During Colonoscopy—Results of the Complete Adenoma Resection (CARE) Study. Gastroenterology 2013;144:74–80.
32. Chandrasekar VT, Spadaccini M, Aziz M, et al. Cold Snare Endoscopic Resection of Nonpedunculated Colorectal Polyps Larger Than 10 Mm: A Systematic Review and Pooled-Analysis. Gastrointest Endosc 2019;89:929–36.
33. Horiuchi A, Ikuse T, Tanaka N. Cold Snare Polypectomy: Indications, Devices, Techniques, Outcomes and Future. Dig Endosc 2019;31:372–7.
34. Kim HS, Jung HY, Park HJ, et al. Hot Snare Polypectomy with or without Saline Solution/Epinephrine Lift for the Complete Resection of Small Colorectal Polyps. Gastrointest Endosc 2018;87:1539–47.
35. Barge W, Kumar D, Giusto D, et al. Alternative Approaches to Polyp Extraction in Colonoscopy: a Proof of Principle Study. Gastrointest Endosc 2018;88:536–41.
36. Gutta A, Gromski MA. Endoscopic Management of Post-Polypectomy Bleeding. Clin Endosc 2019. https://doi.org/10.5946/ce.2019.062.
37. Amato A, Radaelli F, Correale L, et al. Intra-Procedural and Delayed Bleeding after Resection of Large Colorectal Lesions: The SCALP Study. United Eur Gastroenterol J 2019;7:1361–72.
38. Klein A, Bourke MJ. Advanced Polypectomy and Resection Techniques. Gastrointest Endosc Clin N Am 2015;25:303–33.
39. Horiuchi A, Hosoi K, Kajiyama M, et al. Prospective, Randomized Comparison of 2 Methods of Cold Snare Polypectomy for Small Colorectal Polyps. Gastrointest Endosc 2015;82:686–92.
40. Sonnenberg A. Management of Delayed Postpolypectomy Bleeding: A Decision Analysis. Am J Gastroenterol 2012;107:339–42.
41. Fung EC. Diagnostic lower endoscopy. In: Jones DB, Schwaitzberg SD, editors. Operative endoscopic & minimally invasive surgery. New York: CRC Press; 2019. p. 110–7.
42. Gupta S, Lieberman D, Anderson JC, et al. Recommendations for Follow-Up After Colonoscopy and Polypectomy: A Consensus Update by the US Multi-Society Task Force on Colorectal Cancer. Gastroenterology 2020;158:1131–53.

Endoscopic Mucosal Resection and Endoscopic Submucosal Dissection

MacKenzie D. Landin, MD, A. Daniel Guerrón, MD, FASMBS*

KEYWORDS

- Endoscopy • Endoscopic mucosal resection • Endoscopic submucosal dissection
- Therapeutic endoscopy

KEY POINTS

- Endoscopic mucosal resection (EMR)/endoscopic submucosal dissection are oncologically appropriate alternatives to surgery for polyps not amenable to traditional polypectomy.
- Endoscopic mucosal resection is technically easier to perform than endoscopic mucosal dissection, however EMR has a higher rate of piecemeal resection, which is correlated with a higher rate of recurrence.
- Additional studies need to be performed to identify the learning curve and potential improvements in training of therapeutic endoscopy.

INTRODUCTION/BACKGROUND

When people think of endoscopy, they typically think of a screening examination. Colonoscopy for cancer surveillance often comes to mind. Yet, endoscopies are performed for a variety of indications, like gastrointestinal bleeding and gastroesophageal reflux. In addition to diagnosis, the endoscopist must be prepared for an intervention when the examination shifts from diagnostic to therapeutic. For example, what to do when a polyp is seen (**Fig. 1**)? There was a time when polyps were either too large or too flat to be removed with an endoscope out of concern for inadequate resection or potential perforation.[1] Patients with these kinds of polyps were offered a surgical resection of the affected bowel to obtain tissue for diagnosis and to treat potential underlying malignancy. These polyps were often benign and the patient underwent an unnecessary operation.[2,3] Out of the desire to prevent overtreatment, the field of therapeutic endoscopy evolved. In this article, we review the history of therapeutic endoscopy and focus on 2 specific techniques and why they are

Division of Metabolic and Bariatric Surgery, Duke University, 407 Crutchfield Street, Durham, NC 27704, USA
* Corresponding author.
E-mail address: alfredo.guerron-cruz@duke.edu

Surg Clin N Am 100 (2020) 1069–1078
https://doi.org/10.1016/j.suc.2020.07.004
0039-6109/20/© 2020 Elsevier Inc. All rights reserved.

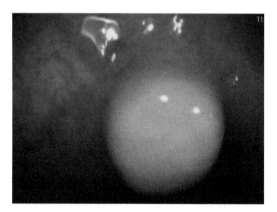

Fig. 1. Polyp.

used: endoscopic mucosal resection (EMR) and endoscopic submucosal dissection (ESD).

HISTORY

Therapeutic endoscopy has been in use since the 1950s. Rosenberg described submucosal injection to facilitate polypectomy of colon polyps in 1955.[4] As endoscopists became facile with this method, others were looking to expand its application. Compared with the West, Japan had and has a higher prevalence of gastric cancer.[5] As early as the 1990s, endoscopy was used to screen patients for potential disease and as a result of screening, a large population of patients with early-stage disease were diagnosed. Therapeutic endoscopy was used to treat early-stage lesions of gastric cancer in the 2000s.[1,5] By managing their disease endoscopically, patients were no longer exposed to the morbidity and mortality of partial or total gastrectomies. With time, therapeutic endoscopy has been studied and found to be an acceptable modality to treat Barrett disease and early-stage esophageal cancer, as well as benign and malignant polyps of the small and large intestine.[6–10] The minimally invasive potential of endoscopic tissue resection and the potential for organ preservation drove the innovation in this field.[5]

DEFINITIONS
What Is Endoscopic Submucosal Dissection?

ESD is a method of injecting the submucosal layer with fluid or gel to dissect the plane and lift a lesion. Once a lesion is raised, it can be resected, decreasing the risk of perforation of the underlying layers. Perforation rates are 2% to 3% and are usually identified and managed during the index endoscopic procedure.[5] ESD was created to address stomach lesions, as the mucosa is thicker within the stomach and difficult to resect with a snare.[1] ESD uses meticulous tissue dissection in the fluid-expanded submucosal space offering precise control over resection depth and lateral extent. Tissue margins can be predefined, the lesion excised en bloc, with adequate preselected margins achieving radical excision of the tumor without surgery.[5]

What Is Endoscopic Mucosal Resection?

EMR is a method of resecting a lesion using a variety of techniques (suction, lift, underwater). The division plane is within the submucosa and often is not as precise as

ESD. Typically, it is completed piecemeal. The indications have expanded to include the treatment of Barrett dysplasia, esophageal squamous dysplasia, small bowel and colorectal adenomas, and early cancers.[11]

Anatomy

To understand the difference between EMR and ESD, one must understand the division of the wall of the gastrointestinal tract. The mucosa, derived from the embryonic endoderm, and muscle arising from the embryonic mesoderm, are the principal layers existing in the wall of the gastrointestinal tract, and are attached by a loose connective tissue submucosa. Both EMR and ESD involve separation of these layers at their junction in the submucosa. ESD accomplishes a slightly deeper division of the tissues within the submucosal layer.[12]

EMR may be used for definitive therapy of premalignant and early-stage (T1N0) malignant lesions of the digestive tract if there is limited submucosal invasion.[13] Often esophagogastroduodenoscopy (EGD) and/or endoscopic ultrasound (EUS) are performed before EMR to confirm if the lesion of interest is appropriate for EMR resection (**Fig. 2**). When performing an EUS, the goal is to see that the lesion of interest does not penetrate into the submucosa or deeper layers, as an EMR resection would not be curative and attempts at resecting deeper parts of the lesion would likely cause a perforation.

Generally, EMR is indicated for any benign or precancerous lesion located throughout the gastrointestinal tract.[14] The limit of size for lesions amenable to EMR is at most 2 to 3 cm diameter and less than one-third the circumference of the esophageal lumen (**Fig. 3**). Beyond that size, the risk of perforation, incomplete resection, and later stricture are unacceptably high.[12] The recurrence rate of EMR is 6% to 10%, but can be higher if lesions are removed piecemeal.[12]

ESD is indicated for lesions of a similar size, occupying less than two-thirds of the esophageal lumen.[1] ESD has a recurrence rate of approximately 1%. It has a greater chance of en bloc resection because of clearly defined margins. However, it is associated with longer procedure times.[1,5,12]

EMR and ESD are indicated for treatment of superficial esophageal cancer and Barrett esophagus–associated neoplasia (high-grade dysplasia and intramucosal carcinoma) as well as resection of early-stage gastric cancer. EMR may be preferred in patients with severe comorbid conditions, such as liver cirrhosis or cardiovascular disease, because EMR is associated with shorter procedure times and fewer adverse events.[13] Data from Eastern groups demonstrate ESD to have significantly higher rates of en bloc resection and histologically complete resection as well as a lower

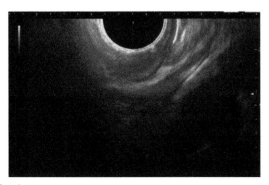

Fig. 2. Pre-EMR of polyp.

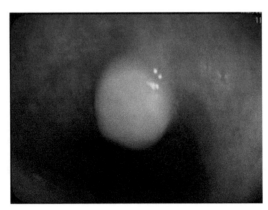

Fig. 3. Polyp seen on EUS.

recurrence frequency for ESD in comparison with EMR for resection of gastric cancer; however, it is unclear if this is applicable to the Western population.[5] There is low case volume and limited expertise in the West, as this disease is not as prevalent. There are reported rates of en bloc and R0 resection from 89% to 100% and 74% to 93%, as well as perforation rates of 4% and bleeding complications of 8%.[5] Duodenal lesions not involving the major duodenal papilla can be removed with a variety of EMR techniques, but carries an increased risk of bleeding and perforation because the duodenum has increased vascularity and a thin wall.[13] Reported success rates vary from 70% to 96% for nonampullary duodenal lesions.[13] Injection-assisted EMR is widely used for the resection of large or flat colonic lesions.[10,11,13]

Preoperative/Preprocedure Planning

The cornerstone of endoscopic management is accurate staging of lesions and patient selection[1]. The decision to perform polypectomy is determined by polyp size, bleeding, and perforation risk, and the inability to resect totally because of anatomic factors. Risks and benefits in the context of the endoscopist's experience and confidence must be evaluated in any type of polypectomy, especially when dealing with difficult polyps.[2] When polypectomy is not an option, EMR and ESD should be considered.

When considering if an endoscopic intervention can be performed, one must assess the depth of invasion of the polyp of interest. If there is a deep depression, expansive appearance, submucosal tumorlike margin, or defective extension is detected during ordinary or chromoendoscopic observation, deep submucosal invasion may be considered.[1]

The frequency of carcinomas increases as the tumor size increases. For large lesions with a size greater than half the circumference of the colorectal lumen, piecemeal EMR should be avoided and ESD should be performed by a skilled endoscopist. Only when ESD is not possible, surgery is considered as an alternative treatment.[1]

Patients should be NPO (nothing by mouth) before the procedure. For upper endoscopy, the American Society of Anesthesiologists[15] recommends 2 hours of fasting after the last clear liquid ingested, and 6 hours for solids. A bowel preparation should be complete before any colonoscopy, to allow for appropriate visualization of the lesion of interest and to identify any synchronous lesions. Anticoagulant and antiplatelet

agents are typically held per ACS guidelines.[16] As a general rule, written informed consent for performing endoscopic treatment should be obtained from the patient (31).

Depending on the organ of interest, patients are placed left lateral decubitus in a
semi-upright or flat position. Cardiac and pulmonary monitoring take place for the
duration of the procedure. Moderate sedation with versed, fentanyl, or propofol can
be used.[15] For longer procedure times or more complex lesions, general anesthesia
can be provided. Typically the anesthetic approach is discussed between the anesthesia team and the endoscopist based on the patient's comorbidities, expected procedure time, or anticipated events. Regardless of approach, an EGD and/or EUS
should be performed first to confirm the lesion is amenable to the intended therapeutic
intervention.

PROCEDURAL APPROACH
Endoscopic Mucosal Resection

There are multiple ways to complete an EMR of a sessile or flat polyp. One of the more
common ways is a saline lift or injection lift EMR. Saline or a different agent is injected
into the submucosa and the lesion becomes raised. This change in height allows the
endoscopist to remove the polyp with a snare and minimize the risk of perforation. The
ideal agent should be inexpensive, readily available, nontoxic, easy to inject, and provide a long-lasting submucosal cushion.[13] Addition of indigo carmine or methylene
blue can aid in the identification of the submucosal layer, and more importantly the
lateral margin of target lesions.[12] Of note, a cushion made with saline typically diffuses
into the tissues after a few minutes and therefore other agents are often used to avoid
this issue (eg, Hyaluronic acid).[17] The margins of the lesion are usually marked in
advance with cautery or dye before injection. An alternative method is using a suction
cap. Suction is applied to the lesion and a snare is fed through the cap to encircle and
amputate the lesion. A third method includes the use of a band, which is applied after a
suction cap retracts the lesion. A snare can then be placed above or below the band to
amputate the lesion (**Fig. 4**). A newer technique is underwater EMR. The intraluminal
air is suctioned and the lumen is filled with water, submerging the lesion. The idea
behind this technique is that by flooding the space, the lumen is not distended and
it actually brings the lesion closer to the scope and away from the muscularis propria
layer.[18,19] In doing so, the lesion can be resected without the risk of seeding the underlying tissue with saline lift injection. Once the lesion is removed, it is mounted,

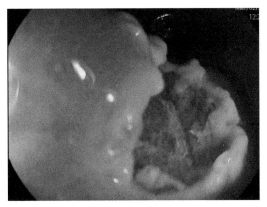

Fig. 4. Postendoscopic mucosal resection.

fixated, and examined by pathology. Goals of examination include whether or not the margins are involved, what the depth of invasion is, and for presence of malignant cells.

A technical issue for this procedure occurs when a lesion will not lift after injection. This may reflect fibrosis from prior biopsy or may be concerning for invasion of the lesion into deeper tissue. If a lesion does not lift well, this should give the provider pause to consider abandoning injection EMR or attempting a different approach (underwater EMR) if the concern for malignancy is low.[5]

Endoscopic Submucosal Dissection

For an ESD procedure to be successful, the lateral margins need to be identified first. The margins are marked with argon plasma coagulation (APC) or a needle knife at least 5 mm outside the edge of the lesion.[12] The mucosa is incised and the submucosa is injected and the dissection performed to the markings. A cap is used for the dissection. Careful hemostasis must be maintained or the planes can be obscured. In addition, dilute epinephrine (1:100,000–1:200,000) is often added to the submucosal injection fluid because of the theoretic effects of decreased bleeding and a sustained submucosal cushion. Submucosal injection of epinephrine can cause severe hypertension, ventricular tachycardia, and intestinal ischemia; however, these complications are rare.[13]

Recovery

Most of these procedures are completed in an endoscopy suite, although general anesthesia may require a more formal operating room setting. Patients can typically be discharged after a period of observation to ensure there are no cardiac or pulmonary complications. Complications from these procedures include complications related to the anesthesia, throat pain, abdominal distention, bleeding, and perforation.

The most concerning risk, perforation, is fortunately the most rare. EMR-associated perforations occur 0.5% to 1% of the time.[12] ESD has a perforation rate of 2% to 4%.[12] Depending on the method of dissection, if one uses a snare or a cautery knife, the size of the perforation varies. If a perforation is identified during the procedure, clips or sutures may be used to control the injury. If the injury cannot be controlled, then the patient should be taken for emergency surgery.

When adverse events do occur, bleeding is the most common adverse event. Bleeding occurs in between 11% and 22% of EMR cases in the colon.[13] Methods of obtaining hemostasis include using hot biopsy forceps, monopolar hemostatic forceps, bipolar electrocoagulation, APC, and endoscopic clips to obtain control. Risk factors for clinically significant postprocedural bleeding include a proximal colonic location, polyp size, and intraprocedural bleeding.[13] The vast majority of postprocedural bleeding presents within 24 hours; however, delayed bleeding may occur up to 5% of the time.[12] If bleeding is delayed, it is seen between 2 and 7 days post-ESD/EMR.[14] A US multicenter randomized controlled trial found that prophylactic placement of hemoclips after removal of large colon polyps does not influence the rate of important post endoscopic resection bleeding.[1] Other adjunctive measures used to augment bleeding include medications. A meta-analysis demonstrated that proton pump inhibitors are superior to histamine-type 2 receptor antagonists for the prevention of bleeding after gastric EMR.[13]

Occasionally, a patient may develop abdominal pain or fever after the procedure. These symptoms are concerning for postpolypectomy syndrome, or inflammation of the peritoneum due to electrocautery. Most patients do not require surgery. They can be treated nonoperatively with bowel rest, antibiotics, and close surveillance. If a patient fails nonoperative management, meaning the patient does not improve or develops hypotension, tachycardia, or fevers, the patient is typically taken for an emergency procedure to resect the affected bowel.

Outcomes/Surveillance

Large multicenter cohort studies demonstrate reduced morbidity and mortality and vastly superior cost efficacy of endoscopic treatment in comparison with surgery.[5] As a result, endoscopic therapy has become an accepted option of treating lower-stage lesions, without removing the option of future surgical intervention.

Curability is evaluated based on the tumor margin of the resected specimen and risk factors for lymph node/distant metastasis are considered for final diagnosis.[1] A meta-analysis comparing ESD and EMR for colorectal tumors demonstrated a higher en bloc resection rate and lower initial local recurrence rate with ESD. However, ESD was more time-consuming and generally required hospitalization for observation after the procedure.[16] Recurrence after colonic EMR ranges from 10% to 30% and is considered the greatest drawback of EMR, particularly piecemeal EMR.[20] Long-term data demonstrate that recurrences are usually small, unifocal, and easily treated during surveillance endoscopy.[20] Local recurrence after EMR (throughout the gastrointestinal tract) occurs in 3% of cases in which the lesion is removed en bloc and 20% in which the lesion is removed in piecemeal fashion. For recurrences that were treated with repeat endoscopic therapy, APC and/or EMR, the subsequent recurrence rate was 21% with successful eradication in 91% of cases.[13] ESD has a recurrence rate of approximately 1%.[12]

In EMR for colon polyps, if a large adenoma (>15 mm) is removed in piecemeal fashion, the patient should have a repeat colonoscopy in 6 to 12 months to evaluate for local recurrence.[13] One should be able to differentiate a normal-appearing scar from a scar with granulation tissue, or clip artifact, or a true adenomatous recurrence within the scar. Residual or recurrent tissue can be treated with hot snare resection or cold avulsion followed by thermal ablation.[20] A repeat endoscopy is performed at 12 months, and if findings are normal, the patient can resume a regular screening schedule. The aim for follow-up after colorectal ESR/EMR is early detection of local residual/recurrence, metastasis and metachronous lesions.[1]

FUTURE DIRECTIONS

Perhaps the most difficult aspect of EMR/ESD, is the achievement of technical proficiency. As discussed previously, lesions amenable to ESD/EMR are those meeting a specific size criterion as well as depth of invasion. The detection of these lesions depends on a robust screening program. Of those patients who meet the criteria for therapeutic endoscopy, they would need to be referred to a tertiary medical center where EMR/ESD is typically performed. Within these centers are commonly teams of specialists who perform these procedures; often they are physicians without surgical backgrounds. It is our position that this paradigm needs to change. Surgeons are ultimately the ones who would be called to manage the potential complications from these procedures. They would offer resections for bleeding or perforation, resections for recurrence not amenable to further therapeutic endoscopy. If they are so intimately involved with this anatomy and disease process, why then are they not involved in the stages of detection and therapy? This question is not to imply surgeons instead of gastroenterologists, but surgeons in addition to. Our choice of treatment should depend less on who touches the patient first and more on skill sets within an institution and what is the best treatment for this particular individual.[21]

To become a board-certified general surgeon, one must complete 35 endoscopies and 50 colonoscopies as well as pass the Fundamentals of Endoscopy examination. This skill set largely prepares the surgeon for diagnostic endoscopy. Surgeons can become credentialed for biopsies, polypectomy, tattooing, and occasionally dilation and stenting depending on their case volume and outcome record. As the world of therapeutic endoscopy becomes more complex, there needs to be an additional pathway of credentialing and supervision to add to the basic general surgery skill set. Part of this training pathway should include simulation as well as dedicated training time in both ex vivo and in vivo animal models. In addition, initial attempts at either EMR or ESD should be proctored by an experienced endoscopist. The issue that we as a surgical community will need to address is that of case volume.

There may not be substantial case volume to support technical proficiency in EMR, let alone ESD, unless a collaborative effort is made by the surgical and gastroenterological communities. Western endoscopists starting the field of ESD have not only a relatively low caseload of ESDs, their case mix will, even at the outset, consist of the larger and more complex lesions that are less suited to gain experience and where ESD is more challenging, potentially not appropriate, or, in inexperienced hands, unethical or dangerous.[5] A recent meta-analysis of EMR data concluded there is not enough literature to conclude what the learning curve is for EMR. The investigators discussed the learning curve for polypectomy as well as the available documented EMR learning curve. Rates of independent snare polypectomy were consistently greater than 90% after 300 colonoscopies.[4] Their analysis discussed a range from 50 to 300 EMR cases before attaining competency.[4] This is dramatically higher than the American College of Surgeons' minimum case volume for endoscopy. To go a step further, the literature suggests ESD procedural outcomes become similar to experts after more than 80 procedures.[12]

As these techniques were developed in Asia, there are several articles recommending training/experience in Asia while building one's technical skills.[5] This may be the most viable option until collaborative relationships form between gastrointestinal endoscopy and surgery to train individuals to achieve not only proficiency but excellence at therapeutic endoscopy. Training and competency for future surgeons is not merely to increase the usage of EMR and ESD, but to build translatable skills in future directions of therapeutic endoscopy. Control of an endoscopic knife in EMR is the same skill for endoscopic septotomy.[22–27] The field of intramural surgery will likely be populated by new deployable devices and new therapeutic techniques using a common tool, the endoscope, for diagnosis and treatment within a common anatomic location, the wall of the gastrointestinal tract. Intramural surgery will also usher in a new paradigm of surgical decision making and surgical thought.[14] As our technology evolves, so should our methods of education. We aim to promote a culture of innovators, collaborators and guardians; for the sole purpose of innovating and collaborating is to enhance the quality of care we provide.

SUMMARY

There are defined criteria for which lesions are amenable to EMR and ESD. These criteria are based on multiple studies evaluating outcomes that include bleeding, perforation, and recurrence. EMR/ESD help minimize morbidity and mortality that patients would otherwise face with a surgical resection. Surgeons, along with gastrointestinal endoscopists, should collaborate to ensure appropriate training, credentialing, and mentoring of these modalities with the goal of improving quality and patient safety.

CLINICS CARE POINTS

- EMR is technically easier to perform than endoscopic mucosal dissection
- EMR has a higher rate of piecemeal resection, which is correlated with a higher rate of recurrence
- Before performing EMR or ESD, the proceduralist should evaluate if the lesion is resectable with EGD and/or EUS
- Patients should be monitored for postprocedural bleeding or perforation
- Additional studies need to be performed to identify the learning curve and potential improvements in the training of therapeutic endoscopy

DISCLOSURE

Nothing to disclose.

REFERENCES

1. Thota PN, Sada A, Sanaka MR, et al. Correlation between endoscopic forceps biopsies and endo- scopic mucosal resection with endoscopic ultrasound in patients with Barrett's esophagus with high-grade dysplasia and early cancer. Surg Endosc 2016;31(3):1336–41.
2. Hammond JS, Watson NFS, Lund JN, et al. Surgical endoscopy training: the joint advisory group on gastrointestinal endoscopy national review. Frontline Gastroenterol 2012;4(1):20–4.
3. Holmes I, Hing T, Friedland S, et al. Combining endoscopic submucosal dissection and endoscopic mucosal resection to treat neoplasia in Barrett's esophagus. Surg Endosc 2016;30(12):5330–7.
4. Rosenberg N. Submucosal saline wheal as safety factor in fulguration of rectal and sigmoidal polypi. Arch Surg 1955;70(1):120.
5. Chandrasekhara V, Sigmon JC, Surti VC, et al. A novel gel provides durable submucosal cushion for endoscopic mucosal resection and endoscopic submucosal dissection. Surg Endosc 2013;27(8):3039–42.
6. Anderson J, Lockett M. Training in therapeutic endoscopy: meeting present and future challenges. Frontline Gastroenterol 2019;10(2):135–40.
7. Bourke MJ, Neuhaus H, Bergman JJ, et al. Endoscopic submucosal dissection: indications and application in western endoscopy practice. Gastroenterology 2018;154(7). https://doi.org/10.1053/j.gastro.2018.01.068.
8. Hornor MA, et al. American College of Surgeons guidelines for the perioperative management of antithrombotic medication. J Am Coll Surg 2018;227(5). https://doi.org/10.1016/j.jamcollsurg.2018.08.183.
9. Lee W-H, Kim S-W, Lim C-H, et al. Efficacy of endoscopic mucosal resection using a dual-channel endoscope compared with endoscopic submucosal dissection in the treatment of rectal neuroendocrine tumors. Surg Endosc 2013;27(11):4313–8.
10. Mannath J, Ragunath K. Endoscopic mucosal resection: who and how? Ther Adv Gastroenterol 2011;4(5):275–82.
11. Morino M. The impact of technology on surgery. Ann Surg 2018;268(5):709–11.

12. Tanaka S, Kashida H, Saito Y, et al. Japan gastroenterological endoscopy society guidelines for colorectal endoscopic submucosal dissection/endoscopic mucosal resection. Dig Endosc 2019;32(2):219–39.

13. Klein A, Bourke MJ. How to perform high-quality endoscopic mucosal resection during colonoscopy. Gastroenterology 2017;152(3):466–71.

14. Strong AT, Ponsky JL. Review: endoscopic submucosal dissection (ESD) and endoscopic mucosal resection (EMR). Ann Laparosc Endosc Surg 2016;1:44.

15. Rajendran A, Pannick S, Thomas-Gibson S, et al. PTH-141 The learning curve for polypectomy and endoscopic mucosal resection (EMR): a systematic review. Gut 2018;67:A276–9.

16. Hwang JH, Konda V, Abu Dayyeh BK, et al. Endoscopic mucosal resection. Gastrointest Endosc 2015;82(2):215–26.

17. Chang KJ. Endoscopic foregut surgery and interventions: the future is now. The state-of-the-art and my personal journey. World J Gastroenterol 2019;25(1):1–41.

18. Siau K, Ishaq S, Cadoni S, et al. Feasibility and outcomes of underwater endoscopic mucosal resection for ≥ 10 mm colorectal polyps. Surg Endosc 2017; 32(6):2656–63.

19. Strong AT, Rodriguez J, Kroh M, et al. Intramural surgery: a new vista in minimally invasive therapy. J Am Coll Surg 2017;225(2):339–42.

20. Kozarek RA. The Society for Gastrointestinal Intervention. Are we, as an organization of disparate disciplines, cooperative or competitive? Gut Liver 2010; 4(Suppl.1). https://doi.org/10.5009/gnl.2010.4.s1.s1.

21. Lee E-J, Lee JB, Lee SH, et al. Endoscopic treatment of large colorectal tumors: comparison of endoscopic mucosal resection, endoscopic mucosal resection–precutting, and endoscopic submucosal dissection. Surg Endosc 2012;26(8): 2220–30.

22. Diaz R, Welsh LK, Perez JE, et al. Endoscopic septotomy as a treatment for leaks after sleeve gastrectomy. Endosc Int 2020;8:E70–5.

23. Gardner AK, Marks JM, Pauli EM, et al. Changing attitudes and improving skills: demonstrating the value of the SAGES Flexible Endoscopy Course for Fellows. Surg Endosc 2016;31(1):147–52.

24. Gorgun E, Benlice C, Church J, et al. Does cancer risk in colonic polyps unsuitable for polypectomy support the need for advanced endoscopic resections? J Am Coll Surg 2016;223(3):478–84.

25. Guerrón AD, Ortega CB, Portenier D, et al. Endoscopic abscess septotomy for management of sleeve gastrectomy leak. Obes Surg 2017. https://doi.org/10.1007/s11695-017-2809-0.

26. Ortega CB. Endoscopic abscess septotomy: a less invasive approach for the treatment of sleeve gastrectomy leaks. J Laparoendosc Adv Surg Tech 2017; 00(No 0):105.

27. Practice guidelines for moderate procedural sedation and analgesia 2018. Anesthesiology 2018;128(3):437–79.

Advanced Colonic Polypectomy

Ipek Sapci, MD, Emre Gorgun, MD*

KEYWORDS

- Advanced colonic polypectomy • Endoscopic submucosal dissection • Endoclips

KEY POINTS

- Advanced colonic polypectomy techniques are endoscopic mucosal resection (EMR) and endoscopic submucosal dissection (ESD), and they aim at organ preservation with low complication rates.
- Main goal of endoscopic submucosal dissection (ESD) is to accomplish en-bloc resection that will subsequently allow accurate histopathological evaluation.
- It consists of injection, circumferential incision, and dissection of lesion. Injection is a vital step and it aims to elevate the mucosa and create a submucosal cushion.
- Snaring (EMR) and dissection (ESD) should be performed by achieving clear surgical margins.
- Different platforms that facilitate ESD are available and can be used to assist with dissection, especially for large lesions. These platforms aim at stabilizing the field and providing tools for retraction.

INTRODUCTION

Value and effectiveness of colonoscopic evaluation and polypectomy in preventing colorectal cancer is widely recognized.[1] Most polyps that are found during a routine colonoscopic examination are less than 10 mm in size and can be removed with simple snaring. For polyps that are larger than 10 mm and have advanced morphologic features and are not amenable for conventional removal, surgical resections are common; however, as reported in one of our studies, in greater than 92% of these surgical resections the final pathology does not reveal any malignancy.[2]

Advanced polypectomy techniques such as endoscopic mucosal resection (EMR) and endoscopic submucosal dissection (ESD) have been developed to remove these advanced lesions and attain organ preservation. ESD was initially popularized for the upper gastrointestinal system and stomach.[3] Advanced polypectomy techniques initially became popular in Asia and has recently become more popular in the United

Department of Colorectal Surgery, Digestive Disease Institute, Cleveland Clinic, 9500 Euclid Avenue, Cleveland, OH 44195, USA
* Corresponding author.
E-mail address: gorgune@ccf.org

Surg Clin N Am 100 (2020) 1079–1089
https://doi.org/10.1016/j.suc.2020.08.014
0039-6109/20/© 2020 Elsevier Inc. All rights reserved.

surgical.theclinics.com

States.[4] Although anatomy and physiology of the lower gastrointestinal system limited widespread use of this method in colon and rectum, nowadays it is being performed more frequently.

EMR and ESD consist of injection, resection/dissection, and removal of the lesion. Elevating the lesion by using an injectate creates a submucosal cushion and ensures safe resection. Steps of each procedure are explained in detail in this article.

Choosing between different polypectomy techniques depends on the lesion characteristics such as the surface morphology as well as the experience of the endoscopist.[5] It must be noted that ESD of colonic lesions can be technically challenging compared with upper gastrointestinal ESD, as colon has a thinner wall, and folds and flexures/corners make it more difficult to maintain a stable scope position for ideal dissection[6,7] (**Fig. 1**). Goal of the procedure should be to remove the lesion en-bloc with minimal complications.

Indications for Advanced Polypectomy

Both Japanese and US Guidelines recommend advanced polypectomy techniques to be reserved for lesions that are larger than 20 mm. US Multi-Society Task Force on Colorectal Cancer recommends snare polypectomy for lesions smaller than 10 mm. For lesions larger than 20 mm advanced polypectomy is recommended and for these lesions to be managed by an advanced endoscopist.[5]

Recommendations favor ESD to be reserved for more advanced lesions with possible invasion to the submucosa. When compared with EMR, ESD was found to have a higher rate of en-bloc resection rate and lower recurrence rate with comparable complication rates.[8] In addition, en-bloc resection rate of 96% was reported in a systematic review.[9] Performing an ESD with en-bloc resection has certain advantages such as increased accuracy on histopathologic evaluation and decreased risk of recurrence.[6,10,11]

Periprocedural Management

Previous colonoscopy reports should be obtained before the procedure, and colored images of the colonoscopies should be assessed. This gives the endoscopist the opportunity to evaluate the lesion in detail and decide if any additional equipment might be beneficial during the procedure. Endoscopist can use the advanced endoscopic imaging techniques such as focal interrogation with narrow-band imaging to predict risk of invasion. These methods where available are helpful to evaluate the surface

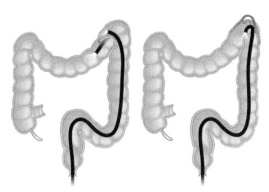

Fig. 1. Colonoscope manipulation in flexures. (Reprinted with permission, Cleveland Clinic Center for Medical Art & Photography ©2020. All Rights Reserved.)

morphology in detail and pit patterns that are related to submucosal invasion risk.[6,11–13] Perioperative evaluation of patients is critical for successful results.

- Patients' medical history and medication use should be questioned in detail. Information about anticoagulant use and dosage is crucial. Typically stopping anticoagulants for 5 days before procedure is necessary.
- Endoscopy suites or operating room settings can be used for performing ESD. Operating room setting can be preferred for patients who have comorbidities and/or high risk lesions. In addition, combined endolaparoscopy can be used for cases that are performed in the operating room. Operating room is also recommended if additional endolumenal platforms are planning to be used.
- A follow-up colonoscopy at 6 months for surveillance to rule out recurrence is recommended for standard evaluation.
- It is preferred to position the lesion at 6 o'clock; however, specific position changes can be necessary for lesions in particular locations such as the ileocecal valve.

Injectate Types and Injection Techniques

Injectate introduction to the submucosal space is the first crucial step of both EMR and ESD. There are various injectates available for use during advanced polypectomy. ORISE Gel Submucosal Lifting Agent (Boston Scientific) and Eleview are FDA approved and are readily available injectates that do not require mixing before injection.[9] They are premixed solutions that involve dye and colloid agents. They can help decrease the procedure time by cutting down on preparation step. Repeat injections increase the total case time; therefore solutions that stay in the submucosal plane for long durations are preferred.

In addition to these solutions, diluted adrenalin (1 mL of 0.1% adrenalin) and hydroxyethyl starch solution mixed with methylene blue or other dyes can be used.[14] Saline is not a preferred injectate, as its stay in tissue is limited and it disperses quickly.[15]

- Goal of the injection step is to achieve balanced and adequate lift of the lesion. Injection needle should be advanced tangentially to the mucosa. Endoscopist positions and inserts the needle and the assistant starts the injection. After starting the injection if tissue elevation is not observed this could be due to entry into an incorrect plane. Injection needle should be adjusted slightly and realigned before continuing the injection (**Fig. 2**).

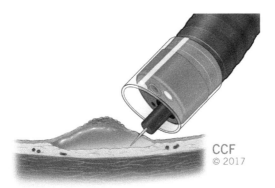

CCF
© 2017

Fig. 2. Injection step for EMR and ESD. (Reprinted with permission, Cleveland Clinic Center for Medical Art & Photography ©2020. All Rights Reserved.)

- For lesions that are located on a fold, it is advantageous to start the injection along the far aspect of the lesion. If the injection is started from the distal side (anal side), lesion may fall away from the view.
- If the correct plane is ensured but adequate lift cannot be achieved (non-lifting sign), this could be a sign of deep invasion into the submucosa or fibrosis due to previous resection/biopsy. When deep invasion is suspected procedure should be stopped. However, we recently reported our institution's results that non-lifting may be also from previous attempts of tissue resection. In those cases the procedure can proceed.

Endoscopic Mucosal Resection

EMR consists of snaring the lesion piecemeal or en-bloc after injection step. The goal should be en-bloc lesion removal but when not practical, repeating the snaring as few times as possible is favored. Increasing the number of pieces snared will decrease the adequacy of the histopathological examination.

- Many different shapes and sizes of snares are available. First step should be to choose the snare shape/size that is the best fit for the lesion.
- A 2 to 3 mm normal mucosal margin should be aimed while snaring. Snare should be opened and aligned right above the lesion. Following this, the lesion is included fully in the snare and snare is closed tightly.
- If lesion will be removed in a piecemeal fashion, snare should be aligned at the resected margin edge and snaring should be repeated until lesion removal is completed.

Endoscopic Submucosal Dissection

ESD is a unique method that allows applying surgical principles to endoscopic lesion removal. Endoscopic knives are crucial instruments for ESD, and there are different knives that can be used for this step of the procedure.[16] Different knives available for commercial use in ESD are FlexKnife Electrosurgical Knife (Olympus, Tokyo, Japan), HookKnife (Olympus America Inc., Center Valley, PA), the DualKnife (Olympus America Inc., Center Valley, PA), and the HybridKnife (ERBE, Tübingen, Germany).[17–19] HybridKnife aims to decrease the instrument change time by integrating the injection needle and knife functions into one instrument. In terms of safety and postprocedural complications all were found to be comparable and are adequate to achieve the cutting step of the procedure.[7,10]

Decision of which instrument to use should be based on the availability and endoscopists' comfort level with the instrument.

- First step after injection and tissue elevation is marking the borders of the lesion circumferentially with the knife before dissection. This should be done considering the 2 to 3 mm normal mucosal margin. Although this step is not critical, it can be helpful for visualizing the borders. A distal disposable cap can be helpful to achieve additional traction.
- Once dissection along the borders is started and continued along the first half of the lesion, it is continued deep into the submucosa. Submucosal plane should be visualized clearly during this step. If there is difficulty continuing the dissection due to elevation loss, injections should be repeated as necessary (**Fig. 3**).
- These steps should be continued until complete resection is achieved. En-bloc resection should be the main goal. During dissection, retraction can be helpful, and in some cases necessary and different platforms can be used. These will be explained in detail (**Figs. 4** and **5**).

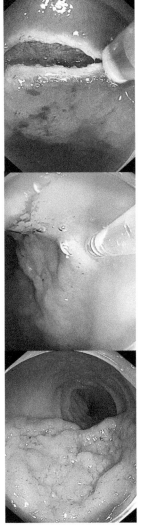

Fig. 3. Injection and dissection steps of ESD with visualization of submucosal entry.

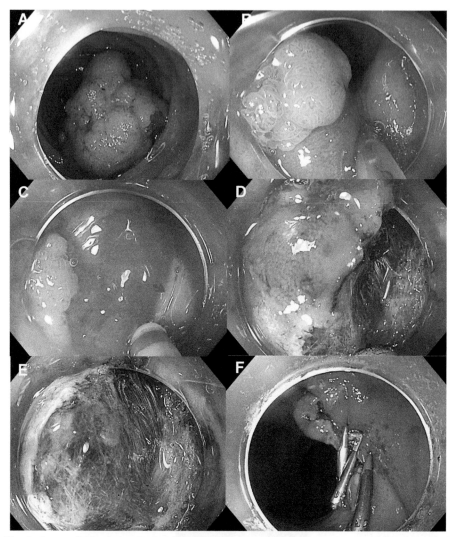

Fig. 4. Steps of ESD: lesion is visualized (*A*); injection (*B*); dissection is pointed with the red arrow (*C*); submucosal entry (*D*); dissection continued in submucosal plane (*E*), and defect is closed with endoclips (*F*).

- It is important to clean the field after dissection and clearly visualize the resected area and inspect for any defects.
- Hemostasis can be achieved using coagulation forceps. During the procedure, submucosal defects can be caused by thermal injury. If any submucosal defects are observed they should be closed with endoscopic hemoclips, as this may help prevent delayed bleeding.
- If necessary, multiple clips can be applied for closure and for large defects over-the-scope clips can be applied.[20] Success rate of over-the-scope clips for acute perforation was reported as high as 90%.[21]

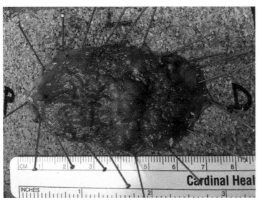

Fig. 5. En-bloc removed specimen via ESD.

In our center we have been performing advanced polypectomy since 2011, and we have performed more than 500 cases. We started our experience in the operating room, and after the learning curve is achieved our practice transitions to the endoscopy suite. By performing the polypectomy in the endoscopy suite, general anesthesia is avoided and the patients can be discharged the same day. When novel endoluminal platforms are used, we prefer to do the cases in the operating room under general anesthesia.

Recent Developments and Novel Endolumenal Platforms

Required skills for ESD are hard to acquire, and thus adaption of the technique in the Western countries has been slow. Consequently, enabling technologies have been developed to overcome some of the difficulties and the steep learning curve of the technique. Because ESD is becoming more popular in North America, these platforms have been introduced in few centers to facilitate the advance endoscopic resection techniques. They aim to help the endoscopist to stabilize the procedure field and incorporate surgical principles such as traction-countertraction.

ORISE Tissue Retractor System consists of a cagelike structure that has 2 instrument channels, and it can be inserted over a standard colonoscope. This platform stabilizes the intraluminal space, and endoscopic instruments can be introduced to retract the lesion. After starting the dissection, this platform can be introduced with the colonoscope, and after positioning the platform on the lesion the cage-like structure is opened. Similar to other platforms, this provides stability of the dissection field, and separate instrument channels allow forceps to be introduced for precise and active real-time retraction (**Fig. 6**).[22,23]

Dilumen Endolumenal Interventional Platform consists of an overtube that has 2 balloons and aims to stabilize the colonoscope, therefore aiding with ESD. In our practice, after completing the dissection on the first half of the lesion, using an endoclip, we deflate the balloon in front of the scope and clip it to the lesion. This method helps the endoscopist to retract the dissected portion and achieve better exposure of the submucosa, facilitating dissection (**Fig. 7**). One of the recent developments is Lumendi C platform. It can fit over the colonoscope, and in addition to the balloons for stabilization, it consists of two 6-mm working channels to introduce graspers and scissors. These instruments can be used for retraction and cutting. We performed first 6 cases using this platform and showed the feasibility and safety of the platform.

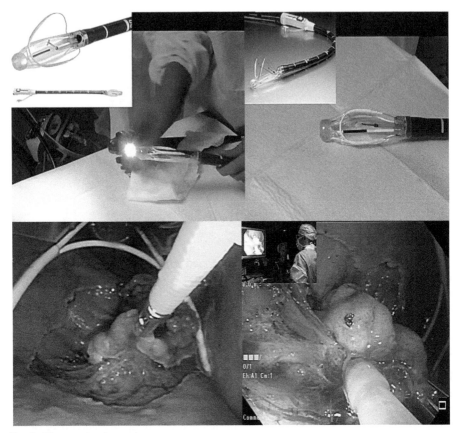

Fig. 6. Tissue retractor system.

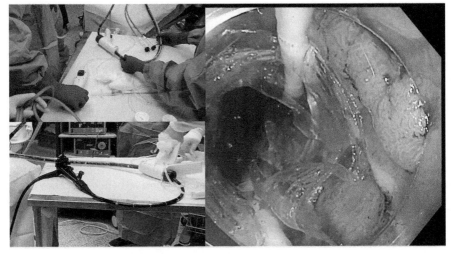

Fig. 7. Endolumenal Interventional Platform.

These platforms may help overcome the challenges of ESD by applying surgical principals and possibly increase the efficiency.

Complications of Advanced Polypectomy

Complications can occur during or after the procedure, with most common ones being perforation and bleeding. Perforation is diagnosed based on the clinical presentation of the patient and commonly presents with abdominal pain and fever. Immediate perforation rates were reported to be higher than delayed perforation rates, with the latter being less than 0.5%.[4] Immediate perforation may warrant surgical intervention if the defect cannot be managed with clipping.

Minimal bleeding may occur during the procedure and should not be alarming. Endoscopic clips and snare coagulation can be used to control bleeding. Cleaning the resection field frequently is important, as it will allow the endoscopist to detect any bleeding immediately and intervene.

Delayed bleeding rates have been reported to be 2%, and these may require exploration and resections if they cannot be controlled.[4] Delayed bleeding rates and perforation rates were 3.6% and 2.7% in our early experience with 110 patients.[2]

Learning Curve and Optimal Procedure Location

ESD can be performed in the endoscopy suite or in the operating room. This decision should be made based on the expertise of the endoscopist. Initially during the learning curve phase it is useful to perform ESD in the operating room, as this enables immediate intervention if a complication occurs. This can also help facilitate Combined Endoscopic-Laparoscopic Surgery for difficult lesions if the ESD attempt cannot be completed successfully.

Learning curve for EMR and ESD has not been widely investigated. A recent systematic review of more than 25 studies showed that for EMR competency was achieved between 50 and 300 procedures. For ESD this was reported to be 20 to 200 cases.[23] Goal for EMR and ESD should be to achieve en-bloc resection and minimal complications, and endoscopists should start performing these on small lesions on locations that are easy to reach to perfect their skills.

SUMMARY

EMR and ESD are valuable advanced polypectomy techniques. These techniques are moving the practice forward in terms of organ preservation and are becoming more widely accepted and practiced.

With the help of new instruments and platforms, the challenges of these techniques are being overcome, and they have evolved from a truly endoscopic procedure to a combined endolumenal surgery technique. Increased education and research in addition to availability of the tools to perform will help more endoscopists be adept in this procedure in the future.

CLINICS CARE POINTS

- Aim of endoscopic submucosal dissection (ESD) is to accomplish en-bloc resection that will subsequently allow accurate histopathological evaluation with organ preservation.
- Steps of the procedure are in the following order: injection, circumferential incision, and dissection of lesion.
- Injection is a vital step and it aims to elevate the mucosa and create a submucosal cushion.

- Macroscopic clear margins should be obtained when resecting the lesion.
- Resection field should be examined carefully and hemostasis should be obtained.

DISCLOSURES

Ipek Sapci, MD has no financial disclosures. Emre Gorgun, MD has financial disclosures with Boston Scientific and DiLumen as honoraria.

REFERENCES

1. Zauber AG, Winawer SJ, O'Brien MJ, et al. Colonoscopic polypectomy and long-term prevention of colorectal-cancer deaths. N Engl J Med 2012;366(8):687–96.
2. Gorgun E, Benlice C, Abbas MA, et al. Experience in colon sparing surgery in North America: advanced endoscopic approaches for complex colorectal lesions. Surg Endosc 2018;32(7):3114–21. Available at: http://orcid. org/000.-0001-7725-3522.
3. Oyama T, Tomori A, Hotta K, et al. Endoscopic submucosal dissection of early esophageal cancer. Clin Gastroenterol Hepatol 2005. https://doi.org/10.1016/S1542-3565(05)00291-0.
4. Akintoye E, Kumar N, Aihara H, et al. Colorectal endoscopic submucosal dissection: a systematic review and meta-analysis. Endosc Int Open 2016. https://doi.org/10.1055/s-0042-114774.
5. Kaltenbach T, Anderson JC, Burke CA, et al. Endoscopic removal of colorectal lesions—recommendations by the US multi-society task force on colorectal cancer. Gastroenterology 2020;158(4):1095–129.
6. Klein A, Bourke MJ. Advanced polypectomy and resection techniques. Gastrointest Endosc Clin N Am 2015. https://doi.org/10.1016/j.giec.2014.11.005.
7. Tanaka S, Oka S, Kaneko I, et al. Endoscopic submucosal dissection for colorectal neoplasia: possibility of standardization. Gastrointest Endosc 2007. https://doi.org/10.1016/j.gie.2007.02.032.
8. Wang J, Zhang XH, Ge J, et al. Endoscopic submucosal dissection vs endoscopic mucosal resection for colorectal tumors: a meta-analysis. World J Gastroenterol 2014. https://doi.org/10.3748/wjg.v20.i25.8282.
9. Repici A, Hassan C, De Paula Pessoa D, et al. Efficacy and safety of endoscopic submucosal dissection for colorectal neoplasia: a systematic review. Endoscopy 2012. https://doi.org/10.1055/s-0031-1291448.
10. Saito Y, Uraoka T, Yamaguchi Y, et al. A prospective, multicenter study of 1111 colorectal endoscopic submucosal dissections (with video). Gastrointest Endosc 2010. https://doi.org/10.1016/j.gie.2010.08.004.
11. Moss A, Bourke MJ, Williams SJ, et al. Endoscopic mucosal resection outcomes and prediction of submucosal cancer from advanced colonic mucosal neoplasia. Gastroenterology 2011;140(7):1909–18.
12. Hayashi N, Tanaka S, Hewett DG, et al. Endoscopic prediction of deep submucosal invasive carcinoma: validation of the narrow-band imaging international colorectal endoscopic (NICE) classification. Gastrointest Endosc 2013. https://doi.org/10.1016/j.gie.2013.04.185.
13. Kudo S, Hirota S, Nakajima T, et al. Colorectal tumours and pit pattern. J Clin Pathol 1994. https://doi.org/10.1136/jcp.47.10.880.
14. Sapci I, Gorgun E. Endoscopic submucosal dissection. In: Bardakcioglu O, ed. Advanced techniques in minimally invasive and robotic colorectal surgery. Springer; :9-16.

15. Sanchez-Yague A, Kaltenbach T, Raju G, et al. Advanced endoscopic resection of colorectal lesions. Gastroenterol Clin North Am 2013. https://doi.org/10.1016/j.gtc.2013.05.012.
16. Maple JT, Abu Dayyeh BK, Chauhan SS, et al. Endoscopic submucosal dissection. Gastrointest Endosc 2015. https://doi.org/10.1016/j.gie.2014.12.010.
17. Choi HS, Chun HJ. Accessory devices frequently used for endoscopic submucosal dissection. Clin Endosc 2017. https://doi.org/10.5946/ce.2017.070.
18. Ciocîrlan M, Pioche M, Lepilliez V, et al. The ENKI-2 water-jet system versus dual knife for endoscopic submucosal dissection of colorectal lesions: a randomized comparative animal study. Endoscopy 2014. https://doi.org/10.1055/s-0033-1344892.
19. Benlice C, Gorgun E. Endoscopic mucosal dissection. In: Lee S, Ross HM, Rivadeneira D, Steele SR, Feingold D, editors. Advanced colonoscopy and endoluminal surgery. Springer International Publishing; 2017. p. 159–68.
20. Morgan SA, Sapci I, Hrabe JE, et al. Endoscopic submucosal dissection with closure of colonic perforation using over-the-scope clip system. Dis Colon Rectum 2019;62(3):379.
21. Honegger C, Valli PV, Wiegand N, et al. Establishment of over-the-scope-clips (OTSC®) in daily endoscopic routine. United European Gastroenterol J 2017. https://doi.org/10.1177/2050640616657273.
22. Sapci I, Gorgun E. Removal of a large rectal lesion with endoscopic submucosal dissection using a new endolumenal platform. Dis Colon Rectum 2020;63(5):710.
23. Rajendran A, Pannick S, Thomas-Gibson S, et al. Systematic literature review of learning curves for colorectal polyp resection techniques in lower gastrointestinal endoscopy. Colorectal Dis 2020. https://doi.org/10.1111/codi.14960.

Endoscopic Enteral Access

Nabil Tariq, MD[a],*, Aman Ali, MD[b], Chen Chen, MD[b]

KEYWORDS

- Percutaneous endoscopic gastrostomy • Percutaneous endoscopic jejunostomy
- Endoscopic feeding access • Nasoenteric feeding catheters

KEY POINTS

- With the importance of adequate nutrition being realized in multiple disease states, clinicians have to be familiar with the various options available to provide it. Timing and route of optimal feeding-tube placement greatly depends on the underlying clinical condition.
- There also are increasing numbers of patients with altered anatomy in the overall patient population and though there are challenges, endoscopic options are available for enteral access in the altered anatomy. It is important to fully assess such altered anatomy with preprocedural imaging.
- With more than 200,000 PEGs being done per year in the United States alone and many other types of feeding tubes being used beyond that, complications are also increasingly encountered that range from minor to life threatening. It is important to have a high degree of suspicion for complications and to follow up with imaging studies if suspected.
- Tube dislodgment should be addressed immediately. When it occurs within 1 or 2 weeks it is a true emergency, and when it occurs late it still needs to be rescued urgently because the tract can start closing within 24 hours.

INTRODUCTION

Enteral access has been reported as far back as 3500 years ago but was mostly confined to rectal access and feeding.[1] Surgical access had been reported by Stamm and Witzel in the 1890s but needed laparotomies.[2] The Levin tube, a large-bore gastric tube, was developed in 1921 and used for decompression or feeding, and the current polyvinylchloride nasogastric tubes became more common after the 1960s.[1]

The history of endoscopic enteral access started to take off after a culmination of out-of-the-box thinking and endoscopic skills came together in Case Western Reserve's University Hospitals in Cleveland.[2] In June of 1979, a 4.5-month-old infant with neurologic difficulties was referred to Dr Michael Gauderer, a pediatric surgeon. He had been thinking about less invasive ways of permitting gastrostomies in children and had the

[a] General Surgery Residency, Weill Cornell Medical College, Department of Surgery, Houston Methodist Hospital, 6550 Fannin Street, Smith Tower 1661, Houston, TX 77030, USA; [b] General Surgery, Department of Surgery, Houston Methodist Hospital, 6550 Fannin Street, Smith Tower 1661, Houston, TX 77030, USA
* Corresponding author.
E-mail address: NTariq@HoustonMethodist.org

Surg Clin N Am 100 (2020) 1091–1113
https://doi.org/10.1016/j.suc.2020.08.009
0039-6109/20/© 2020 Elsevier Inc. All rights reserved.

surgical.theclinics.com

general concept in mind. At University Hospitals he met a young surgeon and skilled endoscopist named Dr Jeffrey Ponsky. On June 12, 1979, Dr Ponsky performed insertion of the first percutaneous endoscopic gastrostomy (PEG) tube. The initial experience, though successful in general, also illustrated what they learned from the procedure and what complications or difficulties can occur with this technique. They had initial challenges with external migration of the tube and the initial small mushroom catheter they used, so they adapted the approach by decreasing tension on it and increasing the size of the catheter and mushroom. On encountering some initial wound infections, they added antibiotics and increased the size of the skin incision for the tube to allow egress of fluid.[2] Thus began the era of more widespread use of endoscopy for enteral access. By the year 2000, it was estimated that around 200,000 PEGs were done per year in the United States alone with only 4% of them being in children.[2,3] Around 260,000 PEG kits were being sold by the medical device industry.[2,4] This has likely increased with time and the increasing elderly adult population.

Malnutrition or the risk of developing malnutrition, observed in up to one-third of hospitalized patients, is associated with increased morbidity and mortality that may be decreased by improvement of nutritional status.[5] Adequate nutrition can be critical in decreasing adverse effects such as decreased immune function, poor wound healing, and tissue breakdown.[6] Even psychological well-being can be improved because malnutrition may be associated with apathy, fatigue, and decreased morale.[7]

Enteral access can be easier to administer than parenteral access and requires less specialist training, and is usually cheaper to administer and more consistent with our natural physiology.[5,8–10] Compared with parenteral nutrition, the enteral route may better preserve gut integrity and function and decrease inflammation.[8] The parenteral route may expose the patient to higher levels of metabolic, infectious, and liver dysfunction risks. This can all add to increased cost of care.

Outcomes in the critically ill, acute or chronic pancreatitis, severe trauma, or burns favor enteral nutrition when possible.[5,9–13] These patients have a hypermetabolic but preserved gut function. Other conditions in which the oropharyngeal tract is functionally or anatomically defective, or whereby global neurologic conditions prevent any or adequate oral intake, also benefit from enteral access and feeding. This article discusses the various methods of enteral access, the pitfalls and management of complications that can occur, and options for access to surgically altered anatomy, which exists in an increasing proportion of the population.

PREREQUISITES BEFORE OBTAINING ENTERAL ACCESS
Skills

Basic upper endoscopy skills are needed before being trained in enteral access and performing them. The ASGE (American Society of Gastrointestinal Endoscopy) has published that trainees should have a minimum of 20 supervised endoscopic gastrostomy procedures, but this is merely expert opinion.[14] ASGE does state that moving to a competency-based curriculum rather than a numbers-based one is desired, and suggests that competency should be demonstrated in both the traditional 2-provider method and the 1-provider method whereby the percutaneous portion is assisted by a gastrointestinal (GI) technician or nurse.[14] Placement in altered anatomy will require much more experience.

Patient Assessment

A thorough history and physical examination is necessary to evaluate the patient. These patients can be critically ill and have airway or hemodynamic issues.

Sedation-related concerns in terms of the setting in which to perform the procedure (intensive care unit [ICU] vs endoscopy suite), the provider administering sedation (endoscopist or anesthetist), and type of sedation should all be addressed, for which the provider should have adequate training and credentialing. If operating in altered anatomy, preprocedural imaging for anatomic assessment can be very useful. Use of anticoagulation, as well as its periprocedural management including when to resume, should be reviewed and discussed with the care team and plans communicated.

Ethics

The endoscopist's role is not only technical; he or she must also determine, as with any other intervention, whether endoscopy will be beneficial to the patient. This may involve discussions with the care team, family, and the patient regarding goals, expectations, and aftercare. There is controversy regarding whether endoscopy can improve survival and functional status or decrease aspiration in certain patient populations.[14,15]

Indications

It is very important to be familiar with the indications and contraindications of the procedure being performed. Many prior contraindications for a PEG are now relative contraindications such as obesity, ascites, peritoneal metastasis, or surgically altered anatomy.[14] Options and alternatives should be discussed. If shorter-term access is needed, potentially less than 4 to 6 weeks, nasoenteric options can be evaluated. Gastric outlet and function also needs to be kept in mind to discover whether postpyloric feeding will be needed. **Tables 1** and **2** describe common indications and contraindications for PEG. Some of the anatomic concerns may be contraindications for

Table 1 Indications for PEG insertion	
Cerebro-vascular Accidents	Hemorrhagic stroke Ischemic stroke
Traumatic Brain Injury	Blunt trauma Penetrating trauma
Neurologic impairment	Motor neuron disease (ALS, LMN, Kennedy disease) Alzheimer's disease Parkinson's disease Chronic coma
Malignancy	Esophageal cancer Head & Neck cancer (pharynx, thyroid, etc.) Brain tumor
Infection	HIV encephalopathy
Other	Esophageal stricture Pharyngeal dysphagia Congenital gastrointestinal conditions (CF, TEF) Gastric decompression (GOO, refractory gastroparesis) History of recurrent aspirations Chronic dysphagia Polytrauma Burns

Abbreviations: ALS, amyotrophic lateral sclerosis; CF, cystic fibrosis; GOO, gastric outlet obstruction; LMN, lower motor neuron syndrome; TEF, Tracheo-esophageal fistula.

Table 2
Contraindications for PEG insertion

Coagulopathy	ESLD (eg, Cirrhosis)
	DIC
	Plt Dysfunction (eg, VWD, Glanzmann disease, WAS)
	Active coagulopathy (INR > 1.5, PTT > 50 s, Plt < 50,000/mm3)
Cardiac illness	Unstable angina
	Recent myocardial infarction
Anatomic variations	History of gastrectomy (eg, total, partial)
	Hepatosplenomegaly
	Ascites
	Peritoneal carcinomatosis
	Organ Interposition (eg, spleen, liver, colon)
	Complete pharyngeal or esophageal obstruction
Gastric mucosal abnormalities	Gastric varices
	Portal hypertensive gastropathy
Infection	Abdominal wall skin infection
	Open abdominal wound at skin site
	Sepsis
Other	Morbid obesity
	Hemodynamic instability

Abbreviations: DIC, disseminated intravascular coagulation; ESLD, end stage liver disease; INR, international normalized ratio; Plt, platelets; PTT, partial thromboplastin time; VWD, Von Willebrand disease; WAS, Wiskott-Aldrich syndrome.

*Many of these are relative contraindications for PEG insertion and are not absolute contraindications. If the indication for PEG insertion is strong, then proper expertise and diligent preprocedural planning may result in successful PEG insertion.

PEG but not necessarily for percutaneous endoscopic jejunostomy (PEJ) or PEG with jejunal extension (see later discussion).

ENDOSCOPIC PLACEMENT OF NASOGASTRIC TUBE OR NASOJEJUNAL TUBE

In a clinical setting, when it is deemed that the patient needs enteral access it is important to decide whether the patient would benefit from prepyloric or postpyloric feeding access. In general when comparing the two, prepyloric gastric feeding is less invasive and less technically challenging. Often prepyloric gastric feeding is contraindicated if the patient has severe reflux, repeated regurgitative events, risk of aspiration, significant gastroparesis, or any gastric outlet obstruction. When selecting the type of enteral access, it is also important to predict the duration of enteral access needed for the patient. In general, 30 days of use is frequently used as the cutoff to decide between a temporary or more semipermanent route of enteral feeding access.[5,16,17] If the patient requires less than 30 days of enteral access, a nasoenteric catheter may be selected. If longer duration of enteral access is needed in the patient's clinical course, the nasoenteric catheter can be exchanged for a gastrostomy or jejunostomy. There may be clinical situations when nasoenteric catheters are used for longer than 30 days. One such situation is often seen in the surgical liver ICU, where cirrhotic patients with high Model for End-stage Liver Disease scores are often waiting for their liver transplant. These cirrhotic patients are at high risk for endoscopic or surgical enteral feeding access because of their end-stage liver disease, coagulopathy, esophageal varices, gastric varices, and ascites.[5]

In the clinical setting, the most widely used method is blind placement of a nasogastric tube (NGT) at the bedside with postprocedural radiographic confirmation. The NGT can be used for gastric decompression to decrease the risk of aspiration of gastric contents. If the patient has no contraindications for prepyloric gastric feeds, the NGT also offers an option for enteral feeding access until the patient can tolerate a peroral diet. If there is a contraindication for prepyloric gastric feeding, blind placement of a softer, thinner, longer, weighted-tip nasojejunal catheter can be used for temporary enteral feeding access. Nasojejunal feeding catheters have a high failure rate of successful placement in a postpyloric anatomic location. Various solutions have been devised to compensate for this high failure rate, such as repeated insertion attempts, administration of pharmacologic promotility agents including metoclopramide, use of wire stylets to stiffen the catheters, and use of electromagnetic stylets. In their surgical ICU, the authors use COR-TRAK*, which uses electromagnetic stylets to provide real-time location of the nasojejunal catheter tip. Even after all of these various solutions, approximately 30% of nasojejunal catheters successfully migrate into a postpyloric anatomic position.[5] Malposition of the nasojejunal catheters into the bronchus, pleura, mediastinum, or cranium can present complications with an estimated reported incidence of 0.5% to 16% for blindly placed nasoenteric feeding catheters.[8] To prevent complications from blind placement of nasoenteric catheters, there has been an emergence of the endoscopic approach for nasoenteric catheters. With the use of endoscopy, the success rate of correct postpyloric placement greatly increases, although there are also potential risks such as anesthetic risks, perforation of gastrointestinal tract with the endoscope, bleeding, infection, catheter malfunction, reflux, aspiration from stenting opening the lower esophageal sphincter with the catheter, sinusitis, and ulceration of the nares.[5] Even though initial correct placement of the nasojejunal catheters may be achieved, these catheters are notorious for being prematurely dislodged or accidently retracted back to a prepyloric position. Several solutions to prevent early dislodgments have been used, including the nasal bridle (**Fig. 1**). As depicted in **Fig. 1**, in the nasal bridle a tube with magnets is passed through one nare and returned externally from the contralateral nare to form a loop around the nasal septum. This loop is then tied to the catheter to secure it and prevent dislodgment. The next sections explore the various options used by clinicians and the various techniques used by endoscopists to place these catheters.

Guide-Wire Technique

The guide-wire technique follows the concept of the Seldinger technique whereby a guide wire is inserted to allow safe access to hollow luminal structures with a subsequent catheter being introduced over the wire. In this technique, first an oronasal transfer tube is placed and clamped, then a standard upper endoscope is passed through the esophagus, stomach, and into the small intestine until the ligament of Treitz. A guide wire is then passed through the endoscope; often, fluoroscopy can be used to confirm the placement. After correct placement is confirmed, a guide-wire exchange is done over the scope, meaning that the endoscope is retracted while the guide wire remains in place. Often, intermittent fluoroscopy can be used to confirm that the tip of the guide wire is in a stable position and not being retracted. After the endoscope has been removed, the guide wire is secured and the feeding catheter is passed over the guide wire down the entire length. During this technique, one of the most challenging aspects is the wire exchange over the endoscope. It is imperative to remove the endoscope while leaving the guide wire in a stable position without

Safe Placement

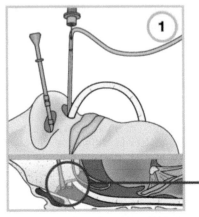

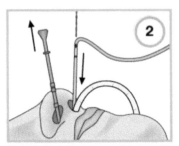

Slowly remove probe, drawing the bridle catheter around the vomer bone and out the patient's nare.

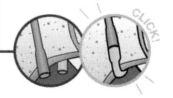

Advance probe in nare opposite the nasal tube, then safety stylet with bridle catheter in the other nare until magnets connect (you may hear an audible 'click'). Remove safety stylet from the bridle catheter.

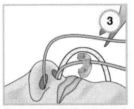

Cut the excess bridle catheter off, leaving enough length to tie a knot, and then discard.

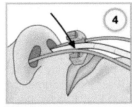

For the Range Clip place loose strand of bridle catheter between the clear flats below the circular region of the clip.*

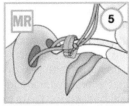

Secure clip 1cm below nose. Below the clip, tie both strands of the bridle catheter in a simple knot and cut excess catheter.

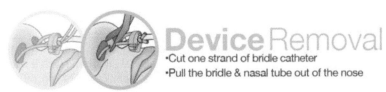

Device Removal
•Cut one strand of bridle catheter
•Pull the bridle & nasal tube out of the nose

Fig. 1. The AMT Bridle Pro is easily placed using magnets to draw bridle tubing through the nasopharynx; in one nare, around the vomer bone, and out the other nare, then securing it to the nasal tube with a French-size–specific clip. (Images courtesy of Applied Medical Technology, Inc.)

displacing the tip of the guide wire; fluoroscopy helps to monitor the tip. A nasopharyngeal exchange tube can be used to allow the feeding tube to exit from the nares. Many techniques can be used, such as finger sweep maneuvers or McGill forceps, although the authors prefer to visualize the posterior pharynx with the endoscope and use the endoscopic grasper to pull it through.

Drag-and-Pull Technique

Multiple methods for the drag-and-pull nasoenteric catheter placement technique with the use of an endoscope have been described. The specific technique used will depend on the endoscopist, in terms of his or her individualized training, experience, and comfort with the given approach. All of the methods described herein share similar procedure times and similar rates of successful placement.

Chang and colleagues[18] described a method of securing the tip of the catheter with nylon sutures, then blindly cannulating the stomach with the catheter and grasping the sutures with endoscopic graspers before pulling the catheter into the small bowel under direct vision. The group reported a 97% rate of successful placement (n = 86) with a procedure time ranging from 5 to 14 minutes. The main limitation of this approach occurs when retracting the endoscope from the small bowel into the stomach, because often the catheter is displaced simultaneously during the retraction of the endoscope. To prevent this from occurring, many endoscopists use endoscopic mucosal clips to anchor the nasoenteric catheter in place. With any additional intervention with mucosal clips, there are always inherent risks such as bleeding, erosion of the clip, or migration of the clips associated with inadequate deployment. The authors consider a mucosal clip to be a useful tool and an appropriate way to secure the catheter in place so it does not migrate back.

Hudspeth and colleagues[19] described a slight modification of this approach by not placing a suture on the catheter tip but rather stiffening the catheter with 2 guide wires that remain fully within the catheter. In this approach, there is also blind placement of the catheter into the stomach before advancing the stiffened catheter with the endoscope and placing it in the small bowel. With this approach, if the catheter is dislodged when retracting the endoscope, the wires will still remain in the correct position. Therefore, the catheter can be fed over the guide wire back into the jejunum.

Wiggins and DeLegge[20] described a method of stiffening a 12-french (12F) nasoenteric feeding catheter with multiple wires and also blindly cannulating the stomach with the feeding tube, then using the endoscope to push the nasoenteric catheter past the pylorus, advancing the endoscope to visually confirm the position, then removing the endoscope followed by the stiff wires. The rate of successful placement with this approach was 97.6% (n = 42) with an average procedure time of 11 minutes.

Bosco and colleagues[21] described a different approach by using a longer and smaller-caliber nasoenteric feeding catheter, typically 250 cm in length and 8F to 10F gauge, fed directly into the working channel of an endoscope. Under direct vision, the upper endoscope is advanced all the way to the small bowel, and the thin nasoenteric catheter is fed through the working channel of the endoscope into the correct position under direct vision. The endoscope is then retracted while simultaneously advancing on the nasoenteric feeding catheter, making sure not to dislodge it proximally into the prepyloric space. An oronasal transfer is then performed, similar to the aforementioned guide-wire technique. With this approach there was a 90% rate of successful placement and a mean procedure time of 19 minutes. The authors currently prefer this approach for the placement of nasoenteric feeding catheters. The larger-caliber catheter (10F) clogs less than the 8F catheter (Cook NJFT 10 and 8; Wilson-Cook Medical, Winston-Salem, NC). The authors recommend placing a wire through the feeding catheter to allow for easier passage of the feeding catheter through the working channel of the endoscope. The catheter should be well lubricated to allow for easier transit through the working channel; a spray lubricant can be helpful. This procedure is often performed at the bedside in the ICU. A therapeutic scope, with its larger working channel, is needed for this technique.

Transnasal Technique

A transnasal approach for placing a nasoenteric catheter has been proposed after Johnson and colleagues[22] described esophagogastroscopy through nasal intubation in 1987. The main advantage of this approach is the decrease or lack of sedation, making it attractive in certain high-risk patient populations. With this approach there is also no need for oronasal transfer as is necessary in the other peroral techniques already described. As described by Wildi and colleagues,[23] a small-caliber (5.3 mm diameter) gastroscope is passed through the nares into the stomach and ultimately the small bowel. A guide wire is passed through the working channel of the endoscope and a wire is left in place in the jejunum while the endoscope is removed. The catheter is then placed over the wire. One of the main limitations of this approach is the difficulty of cannulating the small bowel compared with traditional larger endoscopes; however, their rate of successful placement is similar at 90%, with a slightly longer average procedure time of 19 minutes.

PERCUTANEOUS ENDOSCOPIC GASTROSTOMY TUBE

When enteral access is likely required for significantly longer than a month, the clinician may elect to place a PEG. Typically, a patient with cerebrovascular disorder requires a PEG placement because these patients have a functional GI tract but lack the ability to consume peroral intake safely. Other patients suffering from gastroparesis, intractable nausea, or malignant gastric outlet obstruction may also require a PEG, but mostly for gastric decompression.

The first successful creation of a surgically placed gastrocutaneous stoma in humans was described in 1876 by Verneuil.[24] Various modifications were then made such as a serosal tunnel described by Witzel in 1891[25] and invagination of the serosa around a tube by Stamm in 1894,[26] ultimately leading to the use of a percutaneous approach via endoscopy by Gauderer and Ponsky at University Hospital of Cleveland, Case Western Reserve University in 1979.[27] The PEG approach revolutionized the placement of gastrostomies, as stomas could now be placed without a major abdominal incision such as a laparotomy or laparoscopy. Bankhead and colleagues[28] showed that a percutaneous endoscopic approach not only was quicker (procedure time 30 minutes endoscopic [Ponsky method]) compared with laparoscopic approach (procedure time 48 minutes) and laparotomy approach (procedure time 68 minutes). Compared with the other approaches, the PEG approach also had the lowest cost and morbidity, and least time until initiation of feeds (n = 91). After insertion of the PEG, feedings can be generally initiated within 4 hours. McCarter and colleagues[29] demonstrated in a randomized prospective trial that early feeding with 4 hours of PEG insertion was just as safe as the historical late feeding regimen (24 hours post PEG).

Contraindications for PEG placement include anatomic status hindering the safe passage of an endoscope into the stomach, prior gastric surgery, coagulopathy, gastric varices, and neoplastic or inflammatory disease of the gastric or abdominal wall. Reports of metastases to the stoma and abdominal wall from a primary oropharyngeal or esophagogastric neoplastic disease[30] have been described in the literature as well as candidal stomal infections from esophageal candidiasis,[31] which represent relative contraindications of PEG placement. With the increasing obese population in the Western world, it is important to realize that obesity is not a contraindication for PEG placement. In fact, PEG in obese patients has been shown to have outcomes similar to those for PEG placement in nonobese patients.[32] The percutaneous endoscopic approach for gastrostomy tube placement is the safest, quickest, and cheapest option for long-term gastric feeding access. There is a small subset of patients with ascites or peritoneal dialysis for whom percutaneous radiologic gastrostomy can offer superior outcomes and benefits; however, this is not the focus of discussion of this article.[33,34]

Techniques

Various techniques have been developed to insert the PEG tube since its introduction by Gauderer and colleagues.[35] All of these various techniques, however, share a common principle of inserting the gastrostomy tube through the abdominal wall where the stomach and the abdominal wall are at closest proximity.

The Ponsky Pull and the Sachs-Vine Push techniques require two operators, one for the surgical portion on the abdominal wall and one to guide and manage the endoscope. Preprocedural prophylactic antibiotics are administered, and the patient's abdomen is prepped and draped in sterile fashion. The endoscope is passed down into the stomach, which is insufflated with carbon dioxide. The surgeon who is scrubbed palpates the abdominal wall in the left upper quadrant while the endoscopist transilluminates the abdominal wall by pushing the endoscope along the anterior surface of the stomach and increasing the light-source intensity on the endoscope. A safe access site is selected and a small incision is made below the costal margin. The "safe-track" technique, pioneered by Foutch and colleagues[36] and subsequently verified by Stewart and Hagan,[37] is performed, which can help in defining the optimal site for gastrostomy. A safe-track maneuver helps confirm that there are no loops of bowel, usually transverse colon, between the abdominal wall and the stomach. The technique is performed by insertion of a 21-gauge needle on a syringe filled with saline, while continuously aspirating the syringe as the needle advances through the abdominal wall and into the stomach. Close attention is required on the endoscopic view as the needle is being advanced to ensure that no gas or bubbles are encountered in the syringe until the needle is visualized entering the anterior stomach wall. If this occurs, one can have a high degree of certainty that the needle did not cannulate an interposing lumen of intestine, thus obtaining a safe track. After the needle is safely inserted, a wire is passed through the needle in the Push technique or a double-stranded wire loop in the Pull technique, which is then grasped by an endoscopic snare or grasper. The endoscope is then retracted and removed from the mouth, which allows the wire or wire loop to exit from the mouth as well. The gastrostomy tube is attached to the wire or wire loop depending on the Push or Pull technique, and advanced down the esophagus, into the stomach, and either pushed or pulled through the abdominal wall. The lead point is cut off from the gastrostomy tube and an external bumper is applied to the external portion of the gastrostomy tube. The internal bumper of the gastrostomy tube is then visualized with the endoscope to ensure that the bumper is snug but not too tight. As the patient gains considerable weight and has expansion of the abdominal wall, it is important to adjust the fit of the gastrostomy tube to prevent significant pressure from a tight fit to avoid pressure necrosis.

GASTROJEJUNOSTOMY AND JEJUNOSTOMY INSERTION TECHNIQUES
Percutaneous Endoscopic Gastrojejunostomy

Various methods for distal enteral access are described in the literature. Banshodani and colleagues[38] reported PEG with jejunal extension (PEG-JET) as palliative enteric decompression. This allows for postpyloric feeding while simultaneously decompressing the stomach for patients with significant gastroesophageal reflux, gastroparesis, history of inability to tolerate gastric feeds, recurrent aspiration events, or malignant gastric outlet obstruction not amenable to resection. However, this method has a high failure rate of up to 84% because the catheter frequently becomes malpositioned into the stomach.[39–43] The JET catheter is also thin and easily clogged or kinked. Limited success is achieved in anchoring the distal tip of the JET catheter with endoscopic clips. Nevertheless, this method of enteric access is most ideal for patients requiring gastric decompression and enteral feeding. These various types of tubes are illustrated in **Fig. 2**.

Wire and Snare

After traditional PEG placement, an air-retention valve is placed on the gastrostomy tube to allow gastric insufflation. A guide wire is passed through the PEG and an endoscope is passed from the oral cavity into the stomach. The guide wire is grasped by endoscopic graspers under direct vision and both are advanced into the small intestine beyond the ligament of Treitz. Once appropriate distance has been reached, the endoscopic graspers are advanced as the endoscope is pulled back into the gastrum. The jejunal extension catheter is then fed over the guide wire until it reaches the endoscopic graspers at the distal guide wire. The endoscopic forceps are then released and retracted back into the endoscope followed by complete removal.

Trans-Percutaneous Endoscopic Gastrostomy

A small-caliber endoscope (<6 mm) is passed through a PEG tube and advanced into the jejunum, ideally beyond the ligament of Treitz. A guide wire is passed through the working channel of the endoscope and light resistance is met. The endoscope is then retracted and removed while the guide wire is simultaneously advanced to keep it in the same position in the jejunum. A jejunal feeding catheter is advanced over the wire into its final position and attached to the PEG. Fluoroscopy can be used for placement assistance.

To prevent malpositioning of JET catheters, the authors prefer a suture and clip technique to secure the catheter in the jejunum. A 2-0 nylon or Prolene suture is used at the tip of the JET catheter to create a loop. The JET catheter is lubricated and fed through the PEG. Once it reaches the stomach, the looped suture is grasped with a clip and the tip is dragged with the endoscope to at least the fourth portion of the duodenum. The clip with the looped suture is clipped to a mucosal fold and the endoscope is then withdrawn. The JET catheter should stay in the jejunum affixed to the mucosal fold. Despite this technique, the tube often malfunctions in a few

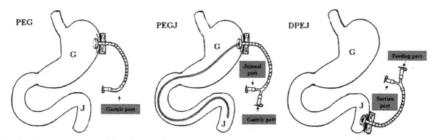

Fig. 2. Various types of feeding tubes. Percutaneous gastrostomy tube (PEG, *left*); PEG with jejunal extension (PEG-JET, *middle*); direct percutaneous endoscopic jejunostomy (DPEJ, *right*). (*From* Zhu Y, Shi L, Tang H, et al. Current considerations of direct percutaneous endoscopic jejunostomy. Can J Gastroenterol. 2012;26(2):92–96; with permission.)

weeks. Usual practice is to exchange the PEG-JET to a gastrojejunal (GJ) tube placed by interventional radiology (IR) once the tract is mature. IR-placed GJ tubes are larger in diameter, can be guided well beyond the ligament of Treitz, and usually last longer because they do not tend to flip back as often.

Direct Percutaneous Endoscopic Jejunostomy

This technique involves direct puncture of a jejunal loop to establish access. Direct percutaneous endoscopic jejunostomy (DPEJ) catheters are made with sturdier materials and the lumen is larger in comparison with PEG/PEJ, so they are less likely to clog or dislodge back into the stomach. They are ideal for patients with altered postsurgical anatomy, such as patients without a stomach (eg, postgastrectomy) or those without direct access to the stomach (eg, postesophagectomy or post–gastric bypass surgery).

DPEJ was first described in 1987 by Shike and colleagues[44] in postgastrectomy patients. The method was based on the Ponsky Pull technique but there are many variations.

DPEJs are technically more difficult than PEGs and PEG-JETs, especially in patients without prior upper GI surgery. The length for access is usually shorter and more direct in patients who have had an esophagectomy, partial or complete gastrectomy, or gastric bypass. Even with the safe-track method and finger indentation, finding the appropriate jejunal loop is difficult because the thin wall of the small bowel can easily be transilluminated through an intervening loop of small bowel. In addition, the small bowel is very mobile. The ideal position for tube placement can be found with a seeker needle, although this can be quickly lost with minor changes in movement of the scope or introducer needle trajectory.

DPEJ placement involves accessing the proximal jejunal loop with an enteroscope or pediatric colonoscope. Similar to essential techniques of PEG placement, good transillumination and finger indention are key to a successful procedure. The safe-track method is used by using a seeker needle (21- or 22-gauge, 1.5-inch needle or spinal needle) to access the jejunal loop. The seeker needle can be snared intraluminally to prevent the small bowel from slipping away.[45] A guide wire is threaded into the seeker needle—the wire from a usual PEG kit will suffice. The snare can then be placed around the trocar/angiocatheter with the wire once the wire is in place with guidance from the seeker needle. A 20F PEG is placed with a Pull technique; however, a 14F PEG kit has been used when the patient's small bowel appeared to be of small caliber. The 14F PEG tube has a slightly smaller mushroom bumper.

Srinivasa and colleagues[46] described a similar snare technique whereby the snare is advanced into the jejunum and an ultrasonic probe is used to locate the snare in the bowel lumen, followed by passage of the seeker needle. A wire is passed through the needle and grasped by the snare. Endoscopic snares to grasp the smaller finder needle during initial percutaneous access have also been described. This allows a larger needle to be placed next to the smaller finder needle for jejunal access. The snare releases the smaller finder needle and snares the larger needle.[47]

Yang and colleagues[48] indicated failure of DPEJ insertion caused by inadequate abdominal wall transillumination, with a success rate of ~39% in patients with abdominal wall thickness >3 cm. These investigators advocate for an alternative method of locating the access site when transillumination, finger indentation, and safe-track methods have failed. A balloon dilation catheter is passed through the working channel of the endoscope, positioned in the jejunum, and filled up with water until maximal contact is made with the bowel lumen. An ultrasound probe is used to visualize the hypoechoic structure corresponding to the fluid-filled balloon, as shown in **Fig. 3**, and a jejunostomy (J) tube is placed using the introducer technique.

The success rate of DPEJ is higher in patients with prior upper GI surgery because the route to the jejunum tends to be shorter. Fluoroscopy can be used at the same time to confirm the position of the tube, and air/CO_2 insufflation can be helpful to outline the bowel lumen. Water-soluble contrast can be injected to delineate the small bowel segment of interest. Fluoroscopy can also recognize T-fasteners if they were previously used.

Lim and colleagues[49] reported 90% success rates in 83 patients in DPEJ placement with a pediatric colonoscope. Successful DPEJ placement with regular endoscopes has also been reported.[47,49] Other endoscopic approaches such as single-balloon (SBE) or double-balloon (DBE) endoscopy have been reported in the literature. Using SBE, Velázquez-Aviña and colleagues[50] reported 96% success in 25 patients, and Aktas and colleagues[51] reported 92% success rate in 12 patients. Technical success rates of 93% to 100% have been reported with DBE. The disadvantage of balloon enteroscopy is that appropriately trained personnel are required, which is not available

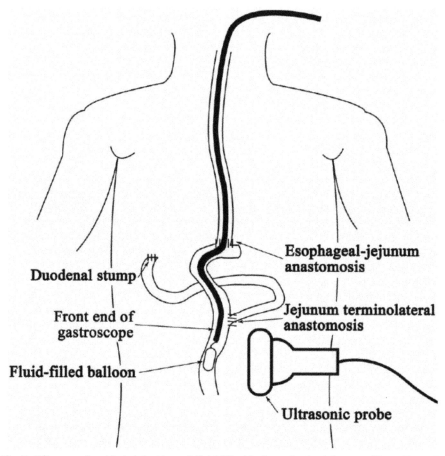

Fig. 3. Ultrasound-guided detection of fluid-filled balloon in the jejunum. (*From* Yang, Z., Wei, J., Zhuang, Z. et al. Balloon-assisted ultrasonic localization: a novel technique for direct percutaneous endoscopic jejunostomy. Eur J Clin Nutr. 2028;72(4):618–622; with permission.)

in all hospitals. These procedures can be performed in the endoscopy suite or operating room. Strong and colleagues[47] reported in a series of 59 patients that 50.8% of the procedures were done in the endoscopy suite and 47.5% in the operating room. The endoscopists in the study were all surgeons who indicated that the advantage of being in the operating room allowed them to proceed with laparoscopic J-tube placement if DPEJ was unsuccessful.

Direct Percutaneous Endoscopic Jejunostomy in Patients with Altered Anatomy

Roux-en-Y gastric bypass

Patients who have undergone gastric bypass may require enteral access for nutrition after neurologic insults or critical illness. Upper GI tract illnesses such as a leak, non-healing ulcers, and strictures causing persistent nausea and vomiting, as well as protein calorie malnutrition, often require enteral nutrition support. The first technical consideration is to understand whether an antecolic or retrocolic Roux limb was created. Roux limb/jejunum anterior to the colon is much easier to access and suitable for transillumination. Access can be found about 15 to 20 cm past the gastrojejunostomy with a regular upper endoscope. This is a reliable area of access because of its proximity to the anastomosis and decreased mobility of the Roux limb from adherence to the mesentery and adhesions from surgery. In practice, the authors routinely obtain a computed tomogram of the abdomen and pelvis even with access to the prior operative notes. The imaging helps the planning of access to the abdomen, in addition to evaluation of the altered anatomy. Successful placement of a DPEJ in the Roux limb theoretically has less chance of a significant leak because the biliopancreatic secretions are bypassed. If a DPEJ is placed for acute leaks in the Roux limb, it is usually appropriate to place a JET, similar to a PEG-jejunostomy tube, to feed further down the limb. This minimizes reflux of contents back to the gastrojejunostomy leak, as the access point is only 15 to 20 cm from the gastrojejunostomy. It is difficult to primarily access the distal Roux limb because the transverse colon and omentum drape over it. It is also difficult to get a distal small bowel loop to come up to the abdominal wall endoscopically with good transillumination and finger indentation. This same principle can be applied to patients with total or subtotal gastrectomy.

DBE has been used to access the excluded stomach for placement of PEG.[52] This is easier to perform on shorter Roux limbs that are 75 to 100 cm, commonly carried out in the past. Currently Roux limbs are frequently 150 cm, making access to the remnant very challenging. Recently there has been interest in using endoscopic ultrasound (EUS) for guidance to the excluded stomach. A combined approach with fluoroscopy has been described by Attam and colleagues,[53] whereby 9 out of 10 patients had successful outcomes in their case series. The position of the Roux limb to the gastric remnant was confirmed and EUS was used to find the gastric remnant from the proximal Roux limb or gastric pouch. The excluded stomach was then accessed with a 19-gauge EUS biopsy needle and a guide wire was passed. This allowed the gastric remnant to be insufflated with 300 to 600 mL of air and distended against the anterior abdominal wall. A PEG tube was placed using the introducer technique, and T-fasteners were used as anchoring sutures. Fluoroscopy was used during the procedure for guidance.[53]

Endoscopic access to the remnant stomach to perform endoscopic retrograde cholangiopancreatography has also been described using a lumen-apposing metal stent. Under EUS guidance, an anastomosis is created between the remnant and pouch or proximal Roux limb with a stent. In a case series of 13 patients, Ngamruengphong and colleagues[54] reported 92% fistula closure after removal of the stent several weeks later. To our knowledge, this method has not been reported for feeding access.

Duodenal switch

A similar approach can be applied to patients using duodenal switch if the alimentary limb is antecolic. However, most duodenal-switch patients will benefit from placement of the feeding tube in the biliopancreatic limb (BPL) for better absorption. Endoscopic access to the BPL is theoretically possible with EUS, as is using a lumen-apposing stent such as Axios to create a fistula between the stomach or alimentary/Roux limb and duodenum, but to our knowledge this technique has not yet been reported.

Esophagectomy

These patents have a gastric conduit, but there usually has also been a previous J-tube placement in the small bowel about 15 to 20 cm from the ligament of Treitz. This segment of small bowel is adhered to the anterior abdominal wall and makes it easier and safe to access. Occasionally, a divot or mucosal scar can be seen intraluminally to identify the spot.

The skin scar does not always correlate to prior jejunal entry because of weight loss. DPEJs are placed with the previously described Pull technique, and fluoroscopic assistance is essential.

Whipple, Billroth II

DPEJ can be tried using techniques previously mentioned if the gastrojejunostomy is created in an antecolic fashion. Alternatively, a PEG can be placed using the standard push-and-pull technique because these patients have a partial gastrectomy, and there may be enough gastric body that will be available for access. A JET catheter can be placed through the PEG to access the distal efferent limb. This can be complicated by the angle of the efferent limb or if there is a stenosis. Often, the limb is away from the direction of the stomach, and cannulating deep into the efferent limb in a backward direction is difficult. IR can try to access the efferent limb via a gastrostomy tube. Other endoscopic solutions have been described, including the triangulation method by Chennat and colleagues.[55] The case report involved a post-Whipple gastric outlet obstruction and need for gastric decompression as well as distal feeding access. A 5-mm ultraslim endoscope was used to go through a 24F PEG tube. This allows for visualization of the efferent limb for cannulation and wire-guided placement of the JET. Chick and colleagues[56] also described a similar transgastric approach by using a 24F sheath such as a PEG tube and using a slim endoscope to access the efferent limb under visual guidance, as shown in **Fig. 4**.

COMPLICATIONS OF GASTROSTOMY AND JEJUNOSTOMY
Major Complications

Dislodgement

Early dislodgment of a gastrostomy (G) or J tube results in separation from the abdominal wall, whereby gastric or enteric contents can leak into the sterile abdominal cavity causing peritonitis. If the feeding tube is dislodged within 1 week, blind reinsertion is not recommended. Immediate exploration in the operating room is indicated if the patient develops peritonitis or signs of sepsis. In the absence of peritonitis or sepsis, an NGT should be inserted for gastric decompression and broad-spectrum antibiotics initiated. Endoscopic reinsertion can be attempted 5 to 7 days later. If retention sutures were used, such as T-fasteners, replacement endoscopically may be attempted as early as 24 hours.[57]

The authors' view is that the stomal tract matures in 4 to 6 weeks for most endoscopic tubes. If gastropexy sutures are used (retention sutures or T-fasteners) or it was a surgically placed G or J tube whereby the stomach or small bowel is sutured

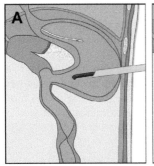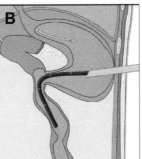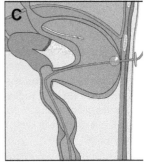

Fig. 4. Gastrojejunoscopy-facilitated placement of a percutaneous transgastric jejunostomy in a patient status post pancreaticoduodenectomy. (*A*) Nasogastric tube insufflation of the stomach. (*B*) Advancement of the endoscope into the efferent limb and placement of an Amplatz super-stiff guide wire. (*C*) Removal of the endoscope followed by jejunostomy tube placement. (*From* Chick JFB, Shields J, Gemmete JJ, et al. Gastrojejunoscopy facilitates placement of a percutaneous transgastric jejunostomy in a patient with a pancreaticoduodenectomy and multiple-failed feeding tube placements. Radiol Case Rep. 2018;13(1):142–145; with permission.)

up to the abdominal wall, it may be accessible sooner. In these types of cases, endoscopic rescue is possible.

A temporary tube such as a deflated Foley catheter or red rubber urethral catheter should be gently placed into the stoma tract to prevent tract narrowing and closure, which occurs within a few hours after tube dislodgment. Care should be taken to avoid going too far into the abdomen, thus creating a false tract or separating the stomach or small bowel from the abdominal wall. The tube should not be used until the G or J tube is replaced by a trained clinician.

In their practice, the authors proceed with G- or J-tube exchange by IR if the feeding tube has been in place for at least 4 weeks. G tubes with T-fasteners can be exchanged as early as 2 weeks. Bedside feeding-tube exchange for G or J tubes less than 4 weeks old is generally not recommended except perhaps for a surgically placed G tube whereby the stomach is sutured to the abdominal wall.

Feeding-tube replacement in mature tracts can be performed at bedside. The replacement tube should be the same size. After the tube is replaced, placement is confirmed by aspiration fluid and flushing the tube to ensure there is no resistance or pain. G tubes should be able to rotate 360°, although this should be avoided in GJ and J tubes because it may cause malposition. If there are any concerns with the replacement tube, a confirmation radiograph should be obtained in the case of G tubes, and a tube study is recommended for all J-tube replacements.

Buried bumper syndrome

This syndrome results from excessive external traction causing the internal retention device to become buried within the gastric/enteric wall or abdominal wall tissue; this usually occurs slowly over time. Patients experience pain at the stoma site, which is worsened with infusions, resistance to infusions, and inability to rotate the G tube 360°.

Treatment depends on the depth of the buried bumper. The tube can be pushed from the outside to push the bumper into the lumen. If the bumper is superficial in the mucosa or granulation tissue, various techniques have been described including argon coagulation, needle knife cautery, or just pulling the tube out externally.[58–63]

One technique involves threading the looped blue wire from a PEG kit through the old PEG tube. Loop the blue wire through a new PEG tube similar to traditional PEG insertion and use the Pull technique. As the new tube is being pulled out, it will push the old bumper and tube out externally.

Buried bumper syndrome can be prevented by evaluating the external retention device daily and loosening the bumper if it is too tight to the skin, placing a mesentery tape on the tube and taping it on the skin to prevent accidental pulling of the tube, and rotating the G tube 360° daily.[6] The patient should self-administer this action, otherwise a caregiver will have to be trained to perform this as part of daily tube maintenance.

Necrotizing soft-tissue infection

Necrotizing soft-tissue infection is a morbid and even fatal condition that can result after feeding-tube insertion. Immunocompromise, type 2 diabetes mellitus, excessive pressure and traction to the feeding tube, and incorrectly sized skin incisions for tube insertion are risk factors for this feared complication. It is important to correctly size the skin incision for the PEG tube to avoid this complication. If a necrotizing infection is suspected, it is a surgical emergency and immediate sharp debridement and broad-spectrum antibiotics are indicated with close monitoring in an intensive care setting. Loosely fitting the PEG tube following insertion, making sure the skin incision is larger than the tube diameter to allow egress of fluid, and frequent follow-up to monitor the pressure on the external and internal bumpers as the patient may gain weight can help prevent this complication. Educating the patient and caregiver to only use a thin piece of gauze between the skin and external bolster can prevent excessive pressure and skin necrosis.

Gastrocutaneous fistula

After G-tube removal, the tract closes between 3 days and 1 week but rarely can take longer. Risk factors for persistent fistulas include infection at the site, a short and wide tract in a thin patient, and very-long-standing G tubes. In the pediatrics population, G tubes placed for longer than 8 months were reported to be associated with persistent fistula.[64]

Initial management includes silver nitrate chemical cauterization of the tract and any granulation tissue, placing patients on twice-daily proton-pump inhibitors, and addition of prokinetic agents. If this is not successful, patients may need to be placed on nothing by mouth with or without an NGT. Alternatively, endoscopic approaches can be pursued such as "roughing" up the tract to disrupt the epithelialization lining, and clips can be placed endoscopically to close the tract. Endoscopic suturing devices such as the Apollo Overstitch have also been used.[27] If all of the aforementioned fails, definitive treatment with laparoscopic surgical approach is undertaken. The fistula is taken down and the stomach wall is closed by stapling or suturing.

Gastrocolocutaneous fistula

Gastrocolocutaneous fistula occurs when the PEG is inadvertently placed through the colon and into the stomach. Patients are usually asymptomatic, but some may develop an ileus. Diagnosis is confirmed by gastrograffin study, or the condition may not be discovered until weeks or months later when the tube is exchanged. Diarrhea can be a delayed presentation of colonic access. The internal bumper pulls away from the stomach into the colon as the tract matures and the feeding goes directly into the colon. The safe-track technique decreases the risk. Aspiration of stool or air without visualization of the needle indicates that another hollow viscus is accessed. In the early postprocedural period, the tube should not be removed because this will cause leakage of stool and peritonitis. An exception to this rule is a large bowel obstruction caused by the feeding tube, which will require removal in the operating room for surgical repair of colonic injury. If no obstruction is encountered, the tract should be given time to mature, and the gastrostomy tube can be used for gastric access during this time. The G tube is removed once the tract is mature (approximately 4 weeks) to allow spontaneous closure. The patient should be monitored closely for signs of peritonitis.[65]

Tumor seeding
The transoral approach to feeding-tube insertion can seed oropharyngeal cancer to the abdominal wall and feeding-tube site. Tumor cells are transferred from the primary lesion to the feeding tube itself as it passes the upper GI tract. In one study of 218 patients with head and neck cancer, 2 patients (0.92%) had PEG-site metastasis.[30] Alternative techniques by which the oropharynx and esophagus are bypassed, such as the transabdominal approach or Russell introducer technique, should reduce the risk.

Minor Complications

Bleeding
Hemorrhage can occur intra-abdominally or intraluminally. Gastric or splenic arteries, mesenteric veins, rectus sheath hematoma, and mesentery are all potential culprits. Tightening the external retention device to provide pressure for hemostasis is the main treatment; however, it must be loosened in 24 to 48 hours to avoid skin necrosis or buried bumper syndrome. If intraluminal bleeding is not controlled with pressure, an endoscopy is warranted for usual endoscopic techniques such as injection and clips; surgical exploration for intra-abdominal bleeding is very rare. For PEGs, placement should be on the anterior body of the antrum, halfway between lesser and greater curves if possible, to avoid vessels on the lesser and greater curvature.

Wound infection
Stoma wound infection has prevalence from 5% to 25%.[66,67] Routine use of prophylactic antibiotics within the hour of skin incision is well established to reduce local wound-infection rates.[68] Cleaning the mouths of patients scheduled for feeding-tube insertion with antiseptic rinse or mouthwash has also been shown to decrease contamination.[69] Mild erythema around the stoma is common. Redness in addition to induration, edema, pain, and sometimes fever may indicate stomal site infection. Treatment includes obtaining cultures and targeted antibiotics.

Stoma leakage
Leakage from gastric or enteric contents around the tube and externally can cause severe skin irritation. The tube should be evaluated for any underlying causes of leak such as tube displacement/malfunction, external bumper separating too far, balloon fluid volume, or problems with gastric emptying. The authors do not recommend replacing the tube for a larger diameter because this can exacerbate leaking and result in a larger gastrocutaneous fistula. If the balloon volume is low, replacing the fluid or increasing the volume of the balloon may decrease the leakage. For G tubes, a J-tube extension can be placed to instill liquids distally while allowing the G-tube site to heal by placing it to drainage.[6] In extreme cases with a mature PEG-tube tract, the PEG is removed to allow the tract to heal and close completely.

Zinc-based products such as ointments or powders can be applied to the feeding-tube site and covered with gauze to provide a moisture barrier. Excessive leakage may require dressing with greater absorptive capacity, nonalcohol skin-barrier films, or skin-barrier wafer.[70]

Granulation tissue
Beefy red, lumpy, moist, and shiny tissue growth growing from the stoma is due to moisture and tube movement, which in turn exacerbates further drainage and moisture for granulation tissue growth.[6] Interventions include silver nitrate cauterization, steroids, and even surgical excision. Most granulation tissue will resolve with application of silver nitrate, although multiple applications are required for larger tissue. Clinicians should be aware of the characteristics of granuloma formation and should not misdiagnose it as gastric prolapse, which can have a similar appearance. Tube stabilization to avoid excessive tube movement at the stoma can help decrease this.

Clogging
Medications and tube feedings can clog feeding tubes up to 35%.[71] Good education on tube-feeding maintenance is the key to decrease clogging. The tube should be flushed routinely with 30 to 60 mL of water before and after each bolus feeding, periodically if feeding is continuous, and after administration of all medications.

    If the tube becomes clogged, several options are available to unclog the tube. Nicholson[72] compared multiple substances including pancreatic enzymes, bromelain, papain, Coca-Cola, cranberry juice, pork pancreatin, chymotrypsin, and distilled water to unclog a feeding tube, and discovered that papain (meat tenderizer) and chymotrypsin were the most successful decloggers. Commercial declogging devices are also available, such as the cleaning brush or Clog Zapper (CORPAK MedSystems, Buffalo Grove, IL).[73]

Pneumoperitoneum
Pneumoperitoneum is a common finding in the postprocedural period after PEG or PEJ tube placement. In the absence of peritoneal signs, it can be safely ignored as a benign finding.[74] Pneumoperitoneum that persists beyond 72 hours and/or associated with significant abdominal pain, peritoneal signs, or sepsis should raise suspicion of occult bowel injury. Usually a computed tomography scan will clarify the diagnosis. The pneumoperitoneum should dissipate more quickly with the use of carbon dioxide gas, instead of atmospheric air, during endoscopy.

Rare Complications

Splenic avulsion
Splenic avulsion has been reported as a complication of PEG placement with intra-abdominal bleeding and may require splenectomy. Splenic injury from stress placed on the spleen, splenic vessels, or gastrosplenic ligament by air insufflation of the stomach or curvature of the endoscope in the stomach was reported as the culprit.[75]

Gastric outlet obstruction
Migration of the PEG beyond the pylorus can lead to a gastric outlet obstruction. This has been observed in Foley catheters used as feeding access.[76] Securing the external bumper no further than 1 cm from the skin can prevent internal migration of the feeding tube.

Internal hernia and small bowel volvulus in direct percutaneous endoscopic jejunostomy
Perhaps one of the most rare but lethal complications after DPEJ insertion is an internal hernia caused by small bowel volvulus. In their case report, Potter and colleagues[77] reported that the technique of anchoring the small bowel to the abdominal wall causes a redundancy of small bowel resulting in freely mobile small bowel near a point of fixation. This redundancy places patients at risk of volvulus.

Awareness of this complication and early diagnosis is key in preventing potentially disastrous outcomes.

CLINICS CARE POINTS

- Route of optimal feeding-tube placement greatly depends on the underlying clinical condition and duration of feeding tube access.
- In patients with altered anatomy, it is important to obtain preprocedural imaging before performing endoscopic enteral access.
- It is important to be familiar with the indications and contraindications of the procedure being performed (**Table 1**, **Table 2**).
- It is important to be familiar with the complications of feeding tubes and how to manage the complications.
- Feeding tube dislodgment within 1-2 weeks of insertion should be addressed immediately. Blind reinsertion is not recommended in early dislodgement.

DISCLOSURE

The authors have nothing to disclose.

REFERENCES

1. Pash E. Enteral nutrition: options for short-term access. Nutr Clin Pract 2018; 33(2):170–6.
2. Gauderer MW. Gastrointestinal feeding access—from idea to application. J Pediatr Surg 2019;54:1099–103.
3. Gauderer MW. Percutaneous endoscopic gastrostomy: 20 years later: a historical perspective. J Pediatr Surg 2001;36:217–9.
4. Gauderer MW. Percutaneous endoscopic gastrostomy and the evolution of contemporary long- term enteral access. Clin Nutr 2002;21:103–10.
5. Gramlich L, Kichian K, Pinilla J, et al. Does enteral nutrition compared to parenteral nutrition result in better outcomes in critically ill adult patients? A systematic review of the literature. Nutrition 2004;20(10):843–8.
6. Lord LM. Enteral access device: types, function, care, and challenges. Nutr Clin Pract 2018;33(1):16–38.
7. Pennington CR. Artificial nutritional support for improved patient care. Aliment Pharmacol Ther 1995;9:471–81.
8. DiSario JA. Endoscopic approaches to enteral nutritional support. Best Pract Res Clin Gastroenterol 2006;20(03):605–30.
9. McClave SA, Martindale RG, Rice TW, et al. Feeding the critically ill patient. Crit Care Med 2014;42(12):2600–10.
10. Moore FA, Feliciano DV, Andrassy RJ, et al. Early enteral feeding, compared with parenteral, reduces postoperative septic complications. The results of a meta-analysis. Ann Surg 1992;216(02):172–83.
11. Windsor AC, Kanwar S, Li AG, et al. Compared with parenteral nutrition, enteral feeding attenuates the acute phase response and improves disease severity in acute pancreatitis. Gut 1998;42(03):431–5.
12. Marik PE, Zaloga GP. Early enteral nutrition in acutely ill patients: a systematic review. Crit Care Med 2001;29(12):2264–70.
13. Iqbal S, Babich JP, Grendell JH, et al. Endoscopist's approach to nutrition in the patient with pancreatitis. World J Gastrointest Endosc 2012;4(12):526–31.

14. ASGE Training Committee, Enestvedt BK, Jorgensen J, Sedlack RE, et al. Endoscopic approaches to enteral feeding and nutrition core curriculum. Gastrointest Endosc 2014;80(1):34–41.
15. Finucane TE, Bynum JP. Use of tube feeding to prevent aspiration pneumonia. Lancet 1996;348:1421–4.
16. Stellato TA. Endoscopic intervention for enteral access. World J Surg 1992; 16(06):1042–7.
17. Applied Medical. The AMT Bridle nasal tube retaining system. Available at: https://www.appliedmedical.net/enteral/bridle/. Accessed February 29, 2020.
18. Chang W-K, McClave SA, Chao Y-C. Simplify the technique of nasoenteric feeding tube placement with a modified suture tie. J Clin Gastroenterol 2005; 39(01):47–9.
19. Hudspeth DA, Thorne MT, Meredith JW. A simple endoscopic technique for nasoenteric feeding tube placement. J Am Coll Surg 1995;180(02):229–30.
20. Wiggins TF, DeLegge MH. Evaluation of a new technique for endoscopic nasojejunal feeding-tube placement. Gastrointest Endosc 2006;63(04):590–5.
21. Bosco JJ, Gordon F, Zelig MP, et al. A reliable method for the endoscopic placement of a nasoenteric feeding tube. Gastrointest Endosc 1994;40(06):740–3.
22. Johnson DA, Cattau EL Jr, Khan A, et al. Fiberoptic esophagogastroscopy via nasal intubation. Gastrointest Endosc 1987;33(01):32–3.
23. Wildi SM, Gubler C, Vavricka SR, et al. Transnasal endoscopy for the placement of nasoenteral feeding tubes: does the working length of the endoscope matter? Gastrointest Endosc 2007;66(02):225–9.
24. Verneuilh A. Observation de gastrostomie pratique avec succes pour un retrecessement cicatriciel infranchissable de l'oesophage. Bull Acad Med 1876;25: 1023–38.
25. Witzel O. Zur Technik der Magenfistelanlegung. Zentralbl Chir 1891;18:601–4.
26. Stamm M. Gastrostomy by a new method. Med News 1894;65:324–6.
27. Gauderer MW, Ponsky JL, Izant RJ Jr. Gastrostomy without laparotomy: a percutaneous endoscopic technique. J Pediatr Surg 1980;15(06):872–5.
28. Bankhead RR, Fisher CA, Rolandelli RH. Gastrostomy tube placement outcomes: comparison of surgical, endoscopic, and laparoscopic methods. Nutr Clin Pract 2005;20(06):607–12.
29. McCarter TL, Condon SC, Aguilar RC, et al. Randomized prospective trial of early versus delayed feeding after percutaneous endoscopic gastrostomy placement. Am J Gastroenterol 1998;93(03):419–21.
30. Cruz I, Mamel JJ, Brady PG, et al. Incidence of abdominal wall metastasis complicating PEG tube placement in untreated head and neck cancer. Gastrointest Endosc 2005;62(05):708–11 [quiz: 752, 753].
31. Trevisani L, Sartori S, Rossi MR, et al. Degradation of polyurethane gastrostomy devices: what is the role of fungal colonization? Dig Dis Sci 2005;50(03):463–9.
32. Wiggins TF, Garrow DA, DeLegge MH. Evaluation of percutaneous endoscopic feeding tube placement in obese patients. Nutr Clin Pract 2009;24(06):723–7.
33. Albrecht H, Hagel AF, Schlechtweg P, et al. Computed tomography-guided percutaneous gastrostomy/jejunostomy for feeding and decompression. Nutr Clin Pract 2017;32(02):212–8.
34. Lyon SM, Haslam PJ, Duke DM, et al. De novo placement of button gastrostomy catheters in an adult population: experience in 53 patients. J Vasc Interv Radiol 2003;14(10):1283–9.
35. Gauderer MW, Ponsky JL, Izant RJ Jr. Gastrostomy without laparotomy: a percutaneous endoscopic technique. J Pediatr Surg 1980;15(6):872–5.

36. Foutch PG, Talbert GA, Waring JP, et al. Percutaneous endoscopic gastrostomy in patients with prior abdominal surgery: virtues of the safe tract. Am J Gastroenterol 1998;83:147–50.

37. Stewart JAD, Hagan P. Failure to transluminate the stomach is not an absolute contraindication to PEG placement. Endoscopy 1998;30:621–2.

38. Banshodani M, Kawanishi H, Moriishi M, et al. Percutaneous endoscopic gastrostomy with jejunal extention for an encapsulating peritoneal sclerosis refractory to surgical enterolysis. Perit Dial Int 2016;36(05):562–3.

39. Fortunato JE, Darbari A, Mitchell SE, et al. The limitations of gastro-jejunal (G-J) feeding tubes in children: a 9- year pediatric hospital database analysis. Am J Gastroenterol 2005;100(01):186–9.

40. Doede T, Faiss S, Schier F. Jejunal feeding tubes via gastrostomy in children. Endoscopy 2002;34(07):539–42.

41. Teasell R, Foley N, McRae M, et al. Use of percutaneous gastrojejunostomy feeding tubes in the rehabilitation of stroke patients. Arch Phys Med Rehabil 2001;82(10):1412–5.

42. Simon T, Fink AS. Recent experience with percutaneous endoscopic gastrostomy/jejunostomy (PEG/J) for enteral nutrition. Surg Endosc 2000;14(05):436–8.

43. Mathus-Vliegen LM, Koning H. Percutaneous endoscopic gastrostomy and gastrojejunostomy: a critical reappraisal of patient selection, tube function and the feasibility of nutritional support during extended follow-up. Gastrointest Endosc 1999;50(06):746–54.

44. Shike M, Schroy P, Ritchie MA, et al. Percutaneous endoscopic jejunostomy in cancer patients with previous gastric resection. Gastrointest Endosc 1987;33(05):372–4.

45. DeLegge MH. Enteral access and associated complications. Gastroenterol Clin North Am 2018;47(1):23–37.

46. Srinivasa RN, Sherk WM, Chick JFB, et al. Transgastric jejunal snare technique facilitates primary jejunostomy placement. Radiol Case Rep 2017;13(1):150–2.

47. Strong AT, Sharma G, Davis M, et al. Direct percutaneous endoscopic jejunostomy (DPEJ) tube placement: a single institution experience and outcomes to 30 days and beyond. J Gastrointest Surg 2017;21(03):446–52.

48. Yang Z, Wei J, Zhuang Z, et al. Balloon-assisted ultrasonic localization: a novel technique for direct percutaneous endoscopic jejunostomy. Eur J Clin Nutr 2018;72:618–22.

49. Lim AH, Schoeman MN, Nguyen NQ. Long-term outcomes of direct percutaneous endoscopic jejunostomy: a 10-year cohort. Endosc Int Open 2015;3(06):E610–4.

50. Velázquez-Aviña J, Beyer R, Díaz-Tobar CP, et al. New method of direct percutaneous endoscopic jejunostomy tube placement using balloon-assisted enteroscopy with fluoroscopy. Dig Endosc 2015;27(03):317–22.

51. Aktas H, Mensink PB, Kuipers EJ, et al. Single-balloon enteroscopy-assisted direct percutaneous endoscopic jejunostomy. Endoscopy 2012;44(02):210–2.

52. Ross AS, Semrad C, Alverdy J, et al. Use of double balloon enteroscopy to perform PEG in the excluded stomach after Roux-en-Y gastric bypass. Gastrointest Endosc 2006;64(05):797–800.

53. Attam R, Leslie D, Freeman M, et al. EUS-assisted, fluoroscopically guided gastrostomy tube placement in patients with Roux-en-Y gastric bypass: a novel

technique for access to the gastric remnant. Gastrointest Endosc 2011;74(03): 677–82.

54. Ngamruengphong S, Nieto J, Kunda R, et al. Endoscopic ultrasound-guided creation of a transgastric fistula for the management of hepatobiliary disease in patients with Roux-en-Y gastric bypass. Endoscopy 2017;49(06):549–52.

55. Chennat J, Khan N, Waxman I, et al. Novel endoscopic triangulation approach to percutaneous transgastric placement of jejunal extension feeding tube. South Med J 2010;103(12):1243–5.

56. Chick JFB, Shields J, Gemmete JJ, et al. Gastrojejunoscopy facilitates placement of a percutaneous transgastric jejunostomy in a patient with a pancreaticoduodenectomy and multiple-failed feeding tube placements. Radiol Case Rep 2018; 13(1):142–5.

57. Timratana P, El-Hayek K, Shimizu H, et al. Percutaneous endoscopic gastrostomy (PEG) with T-fasteners obviates the need for emergent replacement after early tube dislodgement. Surg Endosc 2012;26:3541–7.

58. Hucl T, Spicak J. Complications of percutaneous endoscopic gastrostomy. Best Pract Res Clin Gastroenterol 2016;30(05):769–81.

59. Gençosmanoğlu R, Koç D, Tözün N. The buried bumper syndrome: migration of internal bumper of percutaneous endoscopic gastrostomy tube into the abdominal wall. J Gastroenterol 2003;38(11):1077–80.

60. Kejariwal D, Aravinthan A, Bromley D, et al. Buried bumper syndrome: cut and leave it alone! Nutr Clin Pract 2008;23(03):322–4.

61. Venu RP, Brown RD, Pastika BJ, et al. The buried bumper syndrome: a simple management approach in two patients. Gastrointest Endosc 2002;56(04):582–4.

62. Boyd JW, DeLegge MH, Shamburek RD, et al. The buried bumper syndrome: a new technique for safe, endoscopic PEG removal. Gastrointest Endosc 1995; 41(05):508–11.

63. Ma MM, Semlacher EA, Fedorak RN, et al. The buried gastrostomy bumper syndrome: prevention and endoscopic approaches to removal. Gastrointest Endosc 1995;41(05):505–8.

64. Janik TA, Hendrickson RJ, Janik JS, et al. Analysis of factors affecting the spontaneous closure of a gastrocutaneous fistula. J Pediatr Surg 2004;39(08):1197–9.

65. Bechtold ML, Mir FA, Boumitri C, et al. Long-term nutrition. Nutr Clin Pract 2016; 31(6):737–47.

66. Vanis N, Saray A, Gornjakovic S, et al. Percutaneous endoscopic gastrostomy (PEG): retrospective analysis of a 7- year clinical experience. Acta Inform Med 2012;20(04):235–7.

67. Preclik G, Grüne S, Leser HG, et al. Prospective, randomised, double blind trial of prophylaxis with single dose of co-amoxiclav before percutaneous endoscopic gastrostomy. BMJ 1999;319(7214):881–4.

68. Lipp A, Lusardi G. A systematic review of prophylactic antimicrobials in PEG placement. J Clin Nurs 2009;18(07):938–48.

69. Akkersdijk WL, van Bergeijk JD, van Egmond T, et al. Percutaneous endoscopic gastrostomy (PEG): comparison of push and pull methods and evaluation of antibiotic prophylaxis. Endoscopy 1995;27:313–6.

70. WOCN Society Clinical Practice Ostomy Subcommittee. Management of gastrostomy tube complications for the pediatric and adult patient. Laurel (NJ): Wound Ostomy and Continence Nurses Society; 2008.

71. Bourgault AM, Heyland DK, Drover JW, et al. Prophylactic pancreatic enzymes to reduce feeding tube occlusions. Nutr Clin Pract 2003;18:398–401.

72. Nicholson LJ. Declogging small-bore feeding tubes. JPEN J Parenter Enteral Nutr 1987;11:594–7.
73. Heinzelmann EJ, Wong S. Obstructed PEG tubes. Gastrointest Endosc 1993;39: 600–1.
74. Wojtowycz M, Arata JA Jr, Nicklos TJ, et al. CT findings after uncomplicated percutaneous gastrostomy. AJR Am J Roentgenol 1988;151:307–9.
75. Patel BB, Andrade C, Doraiswamy V, et al. Splenic avulsion following PEG tube placement: a rare but serious complication. ACG Case Rep J 2014;2:21–3.
76. Barosa R, Santos C, Fonseca J. Gastric outlet obstruction: an unusual adverse event of percutaneous endoscopic gastrostomy. Rev Esp Enferm Dig 2016; 108:53–4.
77. Potter MB, Bowers SB, Pruitt A. Internal hernia with small bowel volvulus in a patient with altered gut motility: a complication of direct percutaneous endoscopic jejunostomy. Dig Dis Sci 2007;52:1910–3.

Endoscopic Management of Postoperative Complications

Steve R. Siegal, MD, Eric M. Pauli, MD*

KEYWORDS

- Flexible endoscopy • Surgical complications • Gastrointestinal defects
- Gastrointestinal bleed • Gastrointestinal fistulae

KEY POINTS

- Surgical complications of the gastrointestinal tract are uncommon events; however, they can lead to great morbidity.
- With the advent for more and newer flexible endoscopy tools, many complications can be managed in an endolumenal fashion.
- Gastrointestinal bleeding, leaks, and fistula can be successfully addressed with flexible endoscopy.
- The authors detail technical aspects and outcomes of these procedures.

INTRODUCTION

In 2009, there were more than 6 million operations performed on the gastrointestinal (GI) tract in the United States. Over the subsequent decade, that number has continued to increase.[1] Despite continued advances of surgical technique, technology and devices as well as a revolution in perioperative care pathways, postoperative complications remain an unavoidable part of modern GI surgical practice. Traditional management of these issues often requires a return to the operating room, at times necessitating a laparotomy to safely address the pathology underlying the complication.

Advances in the last 15 years have ushered in a modern era of flexible endoscopic interventions. Although many of these interventions are designed to avoid surgical procedures, endoscopists now routinely use lumenal-based, nonsurgical interventions to negate the need for repeat operations in the management of postoperative complications.[2] Continuous technologic advancement has expanded the toolbox

Division of Minimally Invasive and Bariatric Surgery, Department of Surgery, Penn State Health, 500 University Drive, PO Box 850, Hershey, PA 17033, USA
* Corresponding author.
E-mail address: epauli@pennstatehealth.psu.edu
Twitter: @ericpauliMD (E.M.P.)

Surg Clin N Am 100 (2020) 1115–1131
https://doi.org/10.1016/j.suc.2020.08.007
0039-6109/20/© 2020 Elsevier Inc. All rights reserved.

available for therapeutic endoscopists, allowing them to address increasingly more complex postoperative issues. This article reviews the endoscopic management of a variety of common postoperative complications with a particular focus on the management of full-thickness GI tract defects.

ACUTE POSTOPERATIVE BLEEDING

GI bleeding related to a surgical intervention is much less common than de novo bleeding (eg, ulcers, diverticular bleed). Postoperative bleeding can be a consequence of a recently performed intestinal transection, bowel anastomosis, or after polypectomy or tissue sampling. Rates of bleeding range from 0.6% to 2.0% for sleeve gastrectomy, 1.0% to 3.0% for post polypectomy, and less than 5% for intestinal anastomosis creation.[2–8] Although GI bleeding can be managed with both thermal and nonthermal methods, we generally prefer to avoid the use of electrosurgical energy when working around fresh staple lines or areas of tissue transection and resection to obviate the risk of a delayed full-thickness injury resulting from energy use. Nonthermal techniques include clip application, injection therapy, and hemostatic sprays.

Through-the-Scope Clips

Endoscopic clips that are passed through the endoscopic working channel and are deployed within the lumen of the GI tract were initially designed for hemostasis and endolumenal marking (**Fig. 1**A). Although these devices go by many colloquial names (endoclips, hemoclips), we prefer to refer to them as through-the-scope (TTS) clips to differentiate them from the more recently developed over-the-scope (OTS) clips. Clips can be used to achieve hemostasis in actively bleeding tissue, or prophylactically (as in after polypectomy). Trials have demonstrated that clip closure following endoscopic mucosal resection of large polyps can decrease the rate of bleeding from 4% to 10% down to less than 2%.[9,10]

TTS clips work through focal mechanical compression of bleeding vessels and the surrounding tissue. This makes them ideal for an anastomotic or staple line bleed where this is generally a ridge of healthy tissue with a solitary area of bleeding (**Fig. 1**B). Once the target tissue is identified, the field of view should be maximized by irrigating and suctioning the tissue and orienting the bleed head-on with the endoscope (ideally at the 7 o'clock position) because the jaws of TTS clips are forward

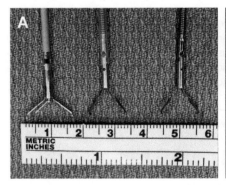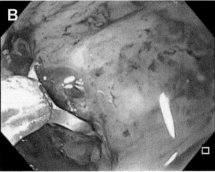

Fig. 1. (*A*) Comparison of commercially available endoscopic through-the-scope (TTS) clips, including rotatable and not-rotatable varieties. (*B*) TTS clip being applied to an acutely bleeding gastrojejunal anastomosis.

facing. Most modern TTS clips are capable of rotation to maximize the deployment angle of the clip. Nonrotatable clips can be repositioned through a variety of endoscopic maneuvers to achieve the same result. Before clip deployment, accurate placement and cessation of bleeding should be confirmed. These clips are easily removable in the event of misdeployment or if needed to remove to permit a surgical intervention, such as a staple load to be fired. Additionally, clips can be easily placed around previously deployed clips in the event that bleeding persists or a second bleeding focus is identified.

Over-the-Scope Clips

OTS clips are large nitinol devices loaded on a distal cap deployment device in an open position and are attached to the endoscope. There are presently 2 devices approved in the United States by the Food and Drug Administration (FDA): OTSC (Ovesco Endoscopy, Tubingen, Germany) and Padlock (US Endoscopy, Mentor, OH) (**Fig. 2**). These clips have a variety of endoscopic applications (see the

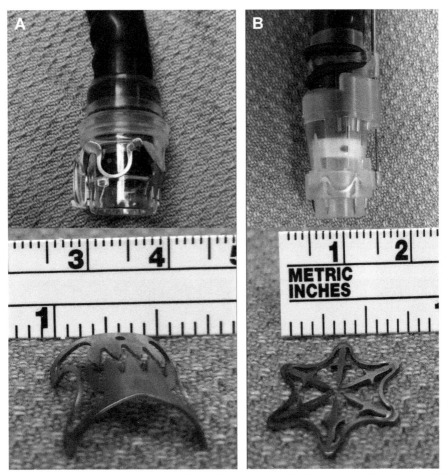

Fig. 2. Commercially available OTS clips. (*A*) Curvilinear closing, removable clip, and (*B*) circumferential closing, nonremovable clip.

Gastrointestinal Tract Defect section), including the management of GI bleeding. Because they are capable of grasping large amounts of tissue (potentially the full thickness of portions of the GI tract), they may have a role in larger postoperative bleeds or those that are difficult to localize or capture within a TTS clip (**Fig. 3**). The OTSC is able to be removed using a commercially available device, although removal can be a painstaking endeavor at times. The Padlock clip has no available removal device. Placing 1 OTS clip adjacent to another is also difficult, because the first clip often prevents the proper deployment of a second clip. As such, although OTS clips have a larger deployment footprint in the area of bleeding, the consequences of a misdeployment are much higher than those for a TTS clip.

Injection Therapy

Needle injection is performed with administration of epinephrine in a 1:10,000 concentration in normal saline, causing vasoconstriction of the local vessels and tissue. Injection is carried out through a 23-G or 25-G needle tip catheter, generally in a 3 or 5 mm length tip. The catheter is advanced through the working channel and once the area of bleed is identified, 4 quadrants around the bleed are injected with approximately 0.5 mL of solution in the submucosal space. The correct tissue plane is achieved when a submucosal bleb is noted and there is mild resistance in the injection syringe. A lack of resistance may indicate leakage or inadequate positioning. The mucosa should blanch as the epinephrine is instilled. Injection as a monotherapy may be ineffective for control of GI bleeding and consideration should be given to applying an endoscopic clip to the area of concern. Because it decreased local blood flow to a staple line or anastomosis, we reserve the use of epinephrine to situations where the bleeding cannot be completely localized for TTS clip application owing to the brisk nature of the bleeding.

Hemostatic Sprays

Despite their longstanding use in surgical applications, hemostatic sprays and powders to address GI tract bleeding have only recently been approved by the FDA. Hemospray (Cook Medical, Winston-Salem, NC) is a proprietary mineral of bentonite-absorbent aluminum phyllosilicate clay that adheres to and congeals on bleeding tissue (**Fig. 4**A). The powder then absorbs moisture from the tissue which produces tamponade while concentrating native hemostatic factors to promote

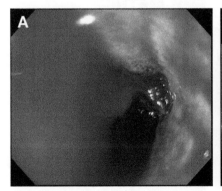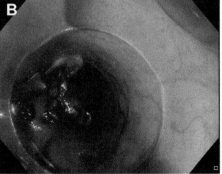

Fig. 3. OTSC application for a severe upper GI bleed from an aortic graft erosion into the esophagus. (*A*) Actively bleeding esophageal lesion. (*B*) OTSC deployed with cessation of bleeding.

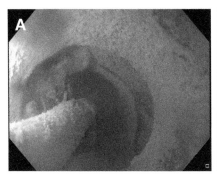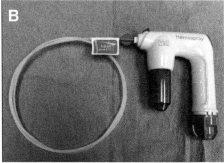

Fig. 4. (*A*) Endoscopic view of hemostatic powder application. (*B*) Hemostatic powder applicator with pressurized carbon dioxide within the handle.

thrombus formation. The spray is deployed using pressurized carbon dioxide (**Fig. 4**B).[11] Hemospray is indicated for nonvariceal GI bleeding and may be used for extensive diffuse bleeding or when visualization of localized bleeding is challenging. Although there are limited data in postoperative applications, diffuse oozing from a staple line or anastomosis can be treated with wide application of these topical agents.

POSTPROCEDURAL STRICTURE

Stricturing of the GI tract is a well-documented consequence of surgical and endoscopic interventions. Bowel anastomosis can stricture over time as a consequence of reduced blood flow, tension, poor technique, leak, and patient factors (eg, immunosuppression, smoking). Strictures can be noted in as many as 40% of patients after esophagectomy with gastric conduit, 27% after gastric bypass, and 30% after colorectal resections.[12–16] Strictures after endoscopic mucosal resection become increasingly common as the resection increases in length and hemicircumference. Series have reported strictures in up to 6% of esophageal mucosal resections.[17] In addition to postanastomotic stricturing, symptomatic narrowing can follow tight fundoplications. Stricture management options depend on the stricture location and characteristics. Before dilation, the location and diameter of the stricture should be documented.[18]

Dilation is the most common endoscopic tool used to manage benign strictures.[19] There are 3 main types of dilation: weighted bougie dilators, wire-guided dilators, and balloon dilators. The 2 forms of bougie dilators include tapered tips (Maloney) and rounded tips (Hurst). Bougie dilators are almost exclusively used for esophageal strictures, such as those found after esophagectomy with gastric conduit. These dilators are passed down the esophagus without endoscopic guidance or visualization, by carefully feeling for resistance as it is passed. Because of this limitation, wire-guided dilators offer the ability to pass a dilator in a Seldinger technique. Hurst dilators are available in a wire-guided format, as are Savary-Gilliary dilators. With this technique, a wire can be advanced beyond the stricture under endoscopic or fluoroscopic guidance. Then an appropriately sized wire-guided dilator is passed over the wire and through the stricture. Generally, the dilator is held in place along the stricture for 1 minute. With both bougie dilators, increasingly larger sizes are passed. It is generally accepted that bougies are not passed greater than 3 sizes (or 6 Fr) above the first felt resistance.[20,21] The origin of this "rule of 3s" is the subject of much debate, and the recent literature seems to contradict the rule.[22]

Balloon dilators are available as TTS or over-the-wire (OTW) delivery systems. Because TTS dilators are passed down the working channel of the endoscope, almost any stricture that is reached by the scope can be dilated, with or without a guidewire. Modern TTS balloon dilators have a controlled radial expansion mechanism whereby the balloon dilates in three 1.0 to 1.5 mm intervals over the 5.5 to 8 cm balloon length providing pure radial force.[2] After identification and sizing of the stricture, an appropriate balloon (6–20 mm) is selected and passed through the working channel and across the stricture (**Fig. 5**). A 0.035″ guidewire can be passed across the stricture in difficult to traverse anatomy. The midportion of the balloon should remain at the level of the stricture and the balloon is held tightly against the scope during dilation to prevent prograde or retrograde motion. Balloons inflate to their nominal diameter based on certain pressures, which are displayed on the package insert. Each controlled radial expansion balloons can be serially dilated to 3 increasing sizes.

Although it does not prevent complications, fluoroscopy can be a valuable adjunct during dilation. An inability to pass a stricture with the endoscope may be circumvented with wire passage across the stricture under fluoroscopic guidance. Additionally, strictures can be dilated under fluoroscopy whereby the waist on the balloon created by the stricture is observed as the dilation obliterates the stricture. Fluoroscopy should be used in OTW balloon dilation to determine the location of stricture and appropriate placement of balloon during dilation.

Endoscopic balloon dilation of benign strictures is generally successful. Gastrojejunal anastomotic strictures after gastric bypass procedures have an 80% success rate after one dilation, and more than 90% success with 2 or more dilations.[23] Benign gastric strictures can also follow sleeve gastrectomy procedures and similar outcomes have been demonstrated with greater than 70% success after balloon dilation.[24] Although dilation of malignant lesions is not recommended, benign anastomotic strictures after GI resection for cancer may be approached in this manner. Strictures in these settings often require multiple sessions, but at least 90% symptomatic improvement has been reported.[25]

One adjunct to mechanical dilation is the concurrent use of steroid injection of strictures, which has shown benefit in benign strictures related to colorectal resections, anastomotic strictures in Crohn's disease, bariatric surgery, and esophagogastric anastomosis.[26–28] We use triamcinolone acetonide (Kenalog, Bristol-Myers Quibb,

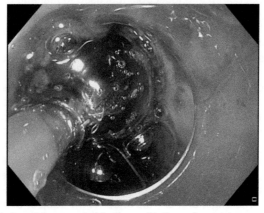

Fig. 5. TTS controlled radial expansion balloon dilation of a stricture.

Princeton, NJ) in a 10 mg/mL concentration. The solution is injected in 0.25 to 1.0 mL aliquots via 23-G sclerotherapy needle in 4 to 6 locations within the stricture before or after mechanical dilation.

Another form of mechanical dilation of GI strictures is the use of self-expanding metal stents made of nitinol. When used for a benign indication, the more commonly used self-expanding metal stents are covered (fully or partially) with polyester or silicone to prevent tissue ingrowth. It is important to note that only 1 stent is approved by the FDA for benign strictures (Polyflex Self Expanding Plastic Stent, Boston Scientific, Natick, MA) and that all other stents for benign strictures are used off-label; this use should be disclosed to patients. Similar to balloons, stents can be deployed TTS or OTW and initial setup and evaluation is equivalent. After localizing the stricture, a TTS stent guidewire is passed under endoscopic vision if the scope can traverse the lesion. If not, the guidewire can be passed under fluoroscopic guidance. A biliary catheter preloaded with a wire may assist in passing through very tight lesions. The stent is then deployed, ideally with 2 cm of stent length on either side of the stricture. For OTW deployment, the endoscope is withdrawn over the wire and fluoroscopy confirms appropriate wire location. Under fluoroscopic guidance, the stent system is advanced over the wire. As desired, the endoscope can be passed parallel to the stent delivery system to directly observe the stent deployment. Using radiopaque markers, the stent is centered about the stricture and deployed under fluoroscopic control (**Fig. 6**). After deployment, patency can be ensured either visually with the endoscope or contrast injection and fluoroscopy.

Although outcome data are varied, the success rate in treating benign strictures is as high as 50%. The most common complication is migration of the stent, which can be seen in up to 20% of cases.[29] Antimigratory steps may include clipping the proximal aspect of the stent to the underlying mucosa with TTS clips, endoscopic suturing, the use of an OTS stent fixation clip, or the use of a long suture positioned as a nasal bridal. Other complications of stent use include perforation and bleeding.

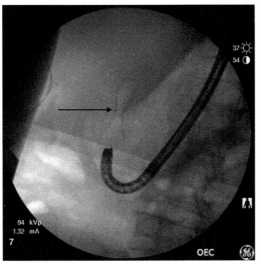

Fig. 6. Fluoroscopy image of stent deployment (*arrow* demonstrating stent deploying across the stenosis).

GASTROINTESTINAL TRACT DEFECTS

Full-thickness defects can be found anywhere along the GI tract. The size of leaks can range from asymptomatic microperforations to large defects leading to peritonitis and sepsis. Overall, the rate of endoscopic-associated perforations are low, approximately 0.03% in upper endoscopy and 1:1400 and 1:1000 during diagnostic and therapeutic colonoscopy, respectively.[30,31] Acute leaks after GI resections and anastomosis have a higher incidence, although they are still rare. For example, there is an approximate 1.5% to 7.0% leak rate after sleeve gastrectomy and 1.7% to 2.5% after Roux-en-Y gastric bypass.[32–34] The timing can be immediate, as with endoscopic perforations; acute (within 1 week of a surgical procedure); or chronic (fistulae). Evidence shows that there is greater success with endoscopic management of acute perforations, followed by leaks and then fistulae.[35]

Traditionally, full-thickness GI defects are managed with surgery and drainage. With the advancement of flexible endoscopy, the endoscopist has increasing numbers of accessories to assist in managing defects via a luminal approach. Given the wide array of defect presentation, we adhere to a treatment algorithm applied to all patients that includes (1) diagnostic endoscopy to identify anatomy and the defect; (2) evaluation and management of extraluminal fluid collections/abscesses; (3) management of distal obstruction (if present); (4) management of the defect; and (5) consideration of feeding access (if unable to take oral nutrition).

Identify the Anatomy and the Defect

As with any flexible endoscopy case, preprocedure preparation is essential to procedural success; this is never truer than in a patient with a suspected (or documented) GI tract defect. A clear understanding of the patient's specific GI tract anatomy can be obtained by reviewing operative records, prior endoscopies, and available imaging.[36] Finally, and possibly most important, discussion with the operating surgeon can provide valuable information. All these resources can provide necessary information to build a mental roadmap of the GI tract before intervention.

Most patients with GI defects will have been evaluated with some form of contrast-enhanced imaging. Computed tomography scans are easy to obtain and have the benefit of showing the entire abdominal cavity and elucidating other pathology or localized abscesses. Despite this advantage, computed tomography scans are taken at a moment in time and poorly timed contrast administration may miss a GI leak. Real-time fluoroscopic images (eg, upper GI series, gastrograffin enema) are useful modalities to diagnose a leak, but unlike computed tomography scans, do not show surrounding structures and pathologies. With the limitations of the previous aside, pre-endoscopic imaging helps as a road map before therapy.

As a matter of routine, we perform these procedures in the operating room using carbon dioxide insufflation and endotracheal intubation. We prefer to use carbon dioxide for insufflation owing to its rapid reabsorption rate and the low pressure of insufflation. Unregulated insufflation of room air can lead to hemodynamic changes from pneumoperitoneum, pneumothorax, or pneumomediastinum. To help with evaluating leaks as well as guiding placement of wires, stents, and so on, we frequently use C-arm fluoroscopy.

The endoscope is driven to the known (or presumed) area of pathology with careful evaluation along the way. The endoscopist should evaluate the GI tract distally to rule out a distal obstruction. If the defect is not appreciated on the initial passage, the following maneuvers can be attempted. A distal cap can be attached to the end of the scope to help move mucosal folds outward to better evaluate for a hidden defect ostium (**Fig. 7**). Generous use of fluoroscopy with contrast administration through a fistula, wound, drain (sinogram), or endoscope can help to define defects and their associated tracts (or abscess pockets).

Extraluminal Fluid Collections

Preprocedural imaging or fluoroscopy can help asses for undrained extraluminal cavities. This step is mandatory as closing a GI defect will orphan an extraluminal cavity, preventing it from draining, potentially resulting in abscess formation. Extraluminal cavities can be copiously irrigated by the endoscope through the GI defect. For defects smaller than 1 cm, we often use a 4.9-mm ultraslim transnasal endoscope (with a 2-mm working channel) to traverse the defect and debride the cavity. Previously placed drains should be flushed to visually ensure their functionality and can be endoscopically repositioned by using endoscopic grasping forceps to manipulate the drain location. This process may require moving the drain closer to the leak to permit better drainage or farther from the leak if the drain is eroding in to the lumen or at risk of being captured during a subsequent attempt at endoscopic defect closure. Large, undrained collections can be drained externally or internally as indicated. External drainage is done percutaneously (placed with combined radiographic or endoscopic guidance). Extraluminal cavities may be drained internally into the GI tract with catheters (double-j, biliary) or vacuum therapy (as discussed elsewhere in this article).

Distal Obstruction

Evaluating for distal obstruction is paramount, as a distally obstructed GI tract creates back-pressurization within the lumen, perpetuating the leak. Physiologic obstructions can include the lower esophageal sphincter, pylorus, or ileocecal valve. Postsurgical and pathologic obstructions are often from anastomosis (bowel resections, gastric bypass), but may be a sequalae of tight angulation of the stomach after sleeve gastrectomy or a fundoplication. Obstructions can be managed with botulinum toxin injections (native sphincters), dilation, or stenting.

Management of the Defect

The management of the defect itself requires careful assessment and planning. Once the previous steps have been accomplished, it is important to understand multiple

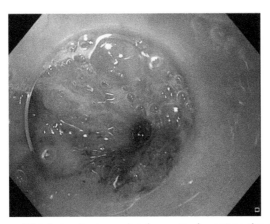

Fig. 7. Identification of fistula tract using a distal cap attachment on the endoscope to push away surrounding folds of tissue.

characteristics of the defect, including its acuity or chronicity, the number and size of defects, attempts at previous closure, and the clinical acuity of the patient's condition. The local availability of endoscopic and surgical equipment also needs to be considered.

We typically define defect management attempts as definitive (planned full closure of the defect endoscopically) or nondefinitive (planned control of leak and contamination but without formal defect closure). Definitive therapy for closing defects includes clipping or suturing, whereas nondefinitive therapy includes stents, internal drainage, and endolumenal vacuum therapy.

As discussed elsewhere in this article, endoscopic clipping can be performed with TTS or OTS clips. Despite their small size and low grasping forces, TTS clips have been shown to reliably close GI perforation.[37,38] TTS clips are best used on smaller defects with straight, clean edges (eg, small perforation occurring during the course of an endoscopic submucosal dissection) rather than large holes with irregular, devitalized tissue margins (eg, several day old staple line leak with ischemia). Although they are not our go-to clip for managing defects, TTS clips have a clear role in the algorithm for endoscopic management. Owing to length and diameter constraints, some defects may not be reachable by an endoscope with a dedicated closure device affixed to the end. In these scenarios, TTS clips represent an acceptable alternative if clips can be used to sequentially closure the defect.

OTS clips allow for full-thickness defect closures of up to 2 cm in diameter.[39] Once the defect has been identified, the diagnostic scope is removed and an endoscope with an OTS clip affixed to the end is navigated into position. The defect should be approached head on (if possible) and centered in the cap. Suction is used to bring the defect and surrounding tissue fully into the cap. Tissue acquiring tools, including a grasper with independently functional jaws and a tripronged spike grasper, can be passed through the working channel to manually draw tissue into the cap. Once a circumferential purchase of tissue is in the cap, the OTS clip is deployed. Advantages of OTS clips include full-thickness tissue coaptation with up to 2 cm of closure. Limitations to the use of OTS clips include working retroflexed endoscope position as well as the need for a large cap that may hinder the ability to reach the defect. Our group has demonstrated successful closure of 80% of enteric leaks and 55% of chronic fistulae with OTSC application.[40]

Definitive closure of GI defects can also be accomplished with endoscopic suturing devices. Suturing offers the advantage of more control over defect closure at the expense of a device that is substantially more complex to work with than OTS clips. The endoscopist can choose the suture material (permanent vs absorbable), closure pattern (simple, running, figure-of-8, purse string) and has full of bite depth while not being limited by the size of the defect that is potentially closable.

Multiple devices have been trialed for this purpose, but there are currently only 2 FDA-approved devices for endoscopic suturing. The Overstitch (Apollo Endosurgery, Austin, TX) is a disposable device that affixes to the end of a double channel endoscope and allows for safe and effective suture placement (**Fig. 8**). The more recently released Overstitch Sx (Apollo Endosurgery) offers the same suturing capabilities with the added benefit of compatibility with a standard single lumen endoscope, because the working mechanism of the device travels parallel to the exterior of the scope rather than through the working channel.

We use endoscopic suturing for defects larger than 2 cm and for those unable to be approached by clipping. These defects, however, must be amenable to an endoscope position that is not under much torque and in a location that allows the suturing arm of the device to fully open and close to acquire tissue bites. Small proximal staple line

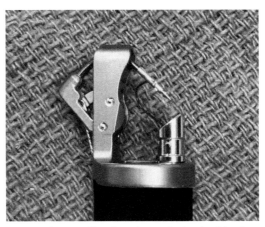

Fig. 8. Endoscopic suturing device affixed to the end of a double channel endoscope.

leaks from sleeve gastrectomy (for example) are challenging to close via suturing because the location of the defect requires the scope to be torqued and retroflexed, and the defect occurs in a small corner that may not allow the suturing arm to fully open. This device requires multiple intricate steps, so adequate training and practice is mandatory. Defect closure with both suturing and OTS clips has been demonstrated with the Ovesco over Overstitch method, whereby suturing narrows the defect size to one amenable to complete closure with the Ovesco.[41]

There are various forms of nondefinitive therapies for GI defect management. One of the most common is endolumenal stenting with self-expanding metal stents. Stenting allows for diversion of enteric contents distally, while minimizing the amount flowing through the defect. Stents must be at least partially (or fully) covered to prevent fluid through the interstices of the stent. Greater success is achieved in straighter areas of the GI tract, because stents tend to migrate away from bent areas to assume their straight structure. Similarly, stents are designed to oppose strictures that hold them in place, so migration in the treatment of GI defects should be considered. Clips can be used to secure the stent to prevent against migration (as discussed elsewhere in this article).

The authors emphasize a few important points of managing GI defects with endolumenal stents. First, in the United States this is an off-label use of stents and this information must be disclosed to the patients. Second, enteric contents may continue to pass around the stent, which means that complete diversion is difficult to achieve. And last, stents provide a radial force (by design to open strictures) that can lead to tissue ischemia, breakdown, and erosion. Despite this limitation, success has been documented with closure of GI defects.[34,42,43] Higher rates of defect closure, however, are accomplished when additional therapies are added to stenting, such as cyanoacrylate glue.[34,44]

With the previously mentioned shortcomings of stent use for the management of defects, new attention has turned to internal drainage techniques. Small diameter internal drains (eg, biliary drains, pigtail drains, pancreatic drains) can be deployed across small GI defects to traverse the leak and enter the extraluminal cavity (**Fig. 9**). In doing so, the pressure differential allows for extraluminal cavity to drain into the GI tract so it can collapse as it heals. The advantages of this technique include the avoidance of cumbersome external percutaneous drains, as well as the pitfalls of endolumenal

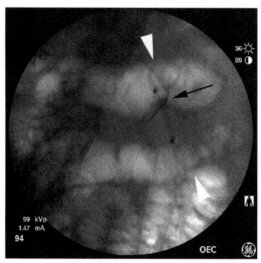

Fig. 9. Fluoroscopic image of a deployed double pigtail stent (*white arrowheads*) to manage a sleeve leak that has failed a previously closure attempt with an OTS clip (*black arrow*).

stents (migration, etc). The majority of recent data analyzing this technique comes from patients with leaks after sleeve gastrectomy. Donatelli and colleagues[45] demonstrated a high success rate (98.5%) of closure with multiple endoscopic sessions (average = 3). We advocate for this approach in appropriately selected patients, namely, those with small defects able to be traversed by the stent deployment system and an extraluminal cavity requiring drainage.

Other adjuncts to manage defects in a nondefinitive manner include fibrin glue, fistula plugs, and tissue sealants. Borrowed from the management of fistula-in-ano disease, bioprosthetic collagen matrix products designed for tissue ingrowth have been used and studied to manage GI defects. Multiple sessions were used; however, successful closure of gastrocutaneous fistulae after gastric bypass with acellular fibrogenic matrix biomaterial was achieved in a series by Maluf-Filho's group.[46] Use of both fibrin and cyanoacrylate glue products has been reported, though often requires multiple sessions for durable closure of GI defects.[47–49] Rather, improved outcomes have been noted when glue products have been used as an adjunct to other closure techniques.[50–52]

More recently, great success has been demonstrated with endolumenal vacuum therapy for GI defects. First reported in 2008, this technique involves the attachment of a piece of open pore surgical vacuum sponge to the end of a nasogastric tube, which is then placed endoscopically into the defect and/or extraluminal cavity **(Fig. 10)**.[53] Prepackaged, commercial devices are available internationally, though none are approved for use in the United States as of yet.

After the defect size has been measured endoscopically, a nasogastric tube is passed through the nares and retrieved through the mouth. A custom shape and size portion of black vacuum foam created including a channel created in the center. The nasogastric tube tip can also be cut to size and the foam is slid onto the nasogastric tube (like a lollipop is on the end of a stick) ensuring that all the side holes of the nasogastric tube are covered with foam. To prevent slippage, a 2-0 Prolene suture is passed through the proximal end of the foam and the tubing material and suture ligated in place. To permit endoscopic delivery, a second 2-0 Prolene suture is passed

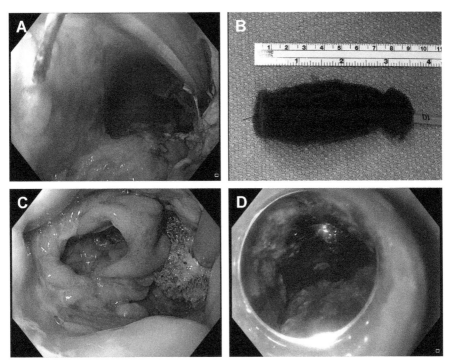

Fig. 10. Endolumenal vacuum (EVAC) therapy for a gastrojejunal anastomotic leak. (*A*) heavily contaminated cavity adjacent to the anastomosis. (*B*) Assembled EVAC foam. (*C*) EVAC positioned in leak cavity adjacent to the partial anastomotic disruption. (*D*) Smaller cavity with less contamination and granulation tissue after 16 days of EVAC therapy.

through the foam and tubing at the distal tip and loosely tied to form a suture loop handle. The foam is then carefully dragged into position endoscopically and placed on continuous suction. The sump tubing of the NT tube needs to be disabled, and this maneuver is easily accomplished by tying it in a tight knot. The therapy is repeated 1 to 2 times a week with the foam being decreased in size as the defect and cavity collapse.

Advantages of this therapy include the ability to promote cavity debridement, effluent control, defect contracture, granulation, and eventual healing. Limitations of this therapy include having to assemble the pieces manually (in the United States). Additionally, this therapy is labor intensive because it requires inpatient hospitalization for maintenance of suction as well as frequent sponge changes (ranging from every 2–3 days to weekly). This process may be challenging in centers with limited experienced endoscopists. However, data are very promising; successful closure has been detailed in 78% to 100% of reports.[2,54]

Feeding Access

After addressing the defect in either a definitive or nondefinitive manner, it is important to consider the patient's nutritional status to allow for adequate healing. Confidence in defect closure is imperative before allowing the patient to take enteral nutrition. However, without defect closure or in a sick or healing patient, feeding access distal to the defect should be considered. Feeding access can be placed at the time of or after endoscopic defect management; however, in acutely ill patients, management of the defect and associated extraluminal collections should be addressed promptly. In patients with foregut defects, a nasojejunal tube can be placed distally if short-term tube feeding is required. Longer term feeding access can be provided via a percutaneous endoscopic gastrostomy or percutaneous endoscopic jejunostomy tube to obviate a transnasal tube. For details on technique, refer to the Enteral Access Nabil Tariq and colleagues' article, "Endoscopic Enteral Access," in this issue. For patients undergoing per-oral endolumenal vacuum therapy, we prefer to use total parental nutrition; feeding tubes are dislodged frequently with endolumenal vacuum therapy changes, patients need to have a tube in each nare, and feedings are held several times a week to permit general anesthesia to be delivered. For these reasons, parenteral nutrition is preferred.

SUMMARY

Although technical refinements and quality improvement studies have helped to decrease postoperative GI surgical complications, there will remain a subset of patients who experience problems. Operative repair remains the gold standard of addressing most issues, but comes with a notable morbidity and in some cases mortality. Flexible endoscopy provides a platform for endolumenal management of postoperative complications in an incisionless manner that obviates much of the risk of an operation. New technology, devices and techniques in flexible endoscopy opened the doors for flexible endoscopists to address increasingly more postsurgical pathology in a safe and reliable manner. The future of flexible endoscopy is broad and will be a key component in the toolbox of management of GI surgical patients.

CLINICS CARE POINTS

- Postoperative complications remain an unavoidable part of modern GI surgical practice.
- Continuous technologic advancement has expanded the toolbox available for therapeutic endoscopists, allowing them to address increasingly more complex postoperative issues.
- Postsurgical GI bleeding can be successfully managed with endoscopic clips, injection therapy, and hemostatic sprays.
- GI tract strictures can be approached with various dilation therapies as well as stenting under certain circumstances.
- Full-thickness GI tract defects range from acute leaks to chronic fistulae.
- Defects can be managed in either a definitive or nondefinitive manner with multiple endoscopic tools available.

DISCLOSURE

S.R. Siegal has nothing to disclose. E.M. Pauli has relationships with the following commercial companies: Bard, Cook, Boston Scientific, Baxter, Wells-Fargo, Actuated Biomedical, Springer, and UpToDate.com. These relationships have no direct financial interest in subject matter or materials discussed in article or with a company making a competing product.

REFERENCES

1. Prevention CDCa. National Hospital Discharge Survey: 2010 Table, Procedures by selected patient characteristics. Available at: https://wwwcdcgov/nchs/nhds/nhds_tableshtm. Accessed February 6, 2020.

2. Witte SR, Pauli EM. Endoscopic management of gastrointestinal complications. Dig Dis Interv 2018;02(04):346–58.
3. Gupta A, Shah MM, Kalaskar SN, et al. Late postoperative bleeding after Roux-en-Y gastric bypass: management and review of literature. BMJ Case Rep 2018; 11:e226271.
4. Golda T, Zerpa C, Kreisler E, et al. Incidence and management of anastomotic bleeding after ileocolic anastomosis. Colorectal Dis 2013;15:1301–8.
5. Consolo P, Luigiano C, Strangio G, et al. Efficacy, risk factors and complications of endoscopic polypectomy: ten year experience at a single center. World J Gastroenterol 2008;14:2364–9.
6. Kim HS, Kim TI, Kim WH, et al. Risk factors for immediate postpolypectomy bleeding of the colon: a multicenter study. Am J Gastroenterol 2006;101:1333–41.
7. Iannelli A, Treacy P, Sebastianelli L, et al. Perioperative complications of sleeve gastrectomy: review of the literature. J Minim Access Surg 2019;15:1–7.
8. Mocanu V, Dang J, Ladak F, et al. Predictors and outcomes of bleed after sleeve gastrectomy: an analysis of the MBSAQIP data registry. Surg Obes Relat Dis 2019;15:1675–81.
9. Zhang QS, Han B, Xu JH, et al. Clip closure of defect after endoscopic resection in patients with larger colorectal tumors decreased the adverse events. Gastrointest Endosc 2015;82:904–9.
10. Liaquat H, Rohn E, Rex DK. Prophylactic clip closure reduced the risk of delayed postpolypectomy hemorrhage: experience in 277 clipped large sessile or flat colorectal lesions and 247 control lesions. Gastrointest Endosc 2013;77:401–7.
11. Holster IL, Kuipers EJ, Tjwa ET. Hemospray in the treatment of upper gastrointestinal hemorrhage in patients on antithrombotic therapy. Endoscopy 2013;45:63–6.
12. Schlegel RD, Dehni N, Parc R, et al. Results of reoperations in colorectal anastomotic strictures. Dis Colon Rectum 2001;44:1464–8.
13. Luchtefeld MA, Milsom JW, Senagore A, et al. Colorectal anastomotic stenosis. Results of a survey of the ASCRS membership. Dis Colon Rectum 1989;32:733–6.
14. Hanyu T, Kosugi S, Ishikawa T, et al. Incidence and Risk Factors for Anastomotic Stricture after Esophagectomy with Gastric Tube Reconstruction. Hepatogastroenterology 2015;62:892–7.
15. Go MR, Muscarella P, Needleman BJ, et al. Endoscopic management of stomal stenosis after Roux-en-Y gastric bypass. Surg Endosc 2004;18:56–9.
16. Blackstone RP, Rivera LA. Predicting stricture in morbidly obese patients undergoing laparoscopic Roux-en-Y gastric bypass: a logistic regression analysis. J Gastrointest Surg 2007;11:403–9.
17. Katada C, Muto M, Manabe T, et al. Esophageal stenosis after endoscopic mucosal resection of superficial esophageal lesions. Gastrointest Endosc 2003; 57:165–9.
18. Morrell DJ, Pauli EM, Juza RM. Endoscopy in Surgically Altered Anatomy. Ann Laparosc Endosc Surg 2019;4:11.
19. Pauli EM, Marks JM. Endoscopic tools and techniques for strictures and stenoses. In: Principles of flexible endoscopy for surgeons. New York: Springer; 2013. p. 105–18.
20. Langdon DF. The rule of three in esophageal dilation. Gastrointest Endosc 1997; 45:111.
21. Tulman AB, Boyce HW Jr. Complications of esophageal dilation and guidelines for their prevention. Gastrointest Endosc 1981;27:229–34.

22. Grooteman KV, Wong Kee Song LM, Vleggaar FP, et al. Non-adherence to the rule of 3 does not increase the risk of adverse events in esophageal dilation. Gastrointest Endosc 2017;85:332–7.e1.

23. Peifer KJ, Shiels AJ, Azar R, et al. Successful endoscopic management of gastro-jejunal anastomotic strictures after Roux-en-Y gastric bypass. Gastrointest Endosc 2007;66:248–52.

24. Agnihotri A, Barola S, Hill C, et al. An Algorithmic Approach to the Management of Gastric Stenosis Following Laparoscopic Sleeve Gastrectomy. Obes Surg 2017; 27:2628–36.

25. Fukagawa T, Gotoda T, Oda I, et al. Stenosis of esophago-jejuno anastomosis after gastric surgery. World J Surg 2010;34:1859–63.

26. Brooker JC, Beckett CG, Saunders BP, et al. Long-acting steroid injection after endoscopic dilation of anastomotic Crohn's strictures may improve the outcome: a retrospective case series. Endoscopy 2003;35:333–7.

27. Kochhar R, Poornachandra KS. Intralesional steroid injection therapy in the management of resistant gastrointestinal strictures. World J Gastrointest Endosc 2010;2:61–8.

28. Lucha PA Jr, Fticsar JE, Francis MJ. The strictured anastomosis: successful treatment by corticosteroid injections–report of three cases and review of the literature. Dis Colon Rectum 2005;48:862–5.

29. Repici A, Hassan C, Sharma P, et al. Systematic review: the role of self-expanding plastic stents for benign oesophageal strictures. Aliment Pharmacol Ther 2010; 31:1268–75.

30. Panteris V, Haringsma J, Kuipers EJ. Colonoscopy perforation rate, mechanisms and outcome: from diagnostic to therapeutic colonoscopy. Endoscopy 2009;41: 941–51.

31. Geraci G, Pisello F, Modica G, et al. Complications of elective esophago-gastro-duodenoscopy (EGDS). Personal experience and literature review. G Chir 2009; 30:502–6 [in Italian].

32. Sakran N, Goitein D, Raziel A, et al. Gastric leaks after sleeve gastrectomy: a multicenter experience with 2,834 patients. Surg Endosc 2013;27:240–5.

33. Morales MP, Miedema BW, Scott JS, et al. Management of postsurgical leaks in the bariatric patient. Gastrointest Endosc Clin N Am 2011;21:295–304.

34. Juza RM, Haluck RS, Pauli EM, et al. Gastric sleeve leak: a single institution's experience with early combined laparoendoscopic management. Surg Obes Relat Dis 2015;11:60–4.

35. Haito-Chavez Y, Law JK, Kratt T, et al. International multicenter experience with an over-the-scope clipping device for endoscopic management of GI defects (with video). Gastrointest Endosc 2014;80:610–22.

36. Juza RM, Pauli EM. Common post-operative anatomy that requires special endoscopic consideration. Tech Gastrointest Endosc 2018;20(4):201–10.

37. Yoshikane H, Hidano H, Sakakibara A, et al. Endoscopic repair by clipping of iatrogenic colonic perforation. Gastrointest Endosc 1997;46:464–6.

38. Binmoeller KF, Grimm H, Soehendra N. Endoscopic closure of a perforation using metallic clips after snare excision of a gastric leiomyoma. Gastrointest Endosc 1993;39:172–4.

39. Al Ghossaini N, Lucidarme D, Bulois P. Endoscopic treatment of iatrogenic gastrointestinal perforations: an overview. Dig Liver Dis 2014;46:195–203.

40. Morrell DJ, Winder JS, Johri A, et al. Over-the-scope clip management of non-acute, full-thickness gastrointestinal defects. Surg Endosc 2020;34:2690–702.

41. Alli VV, Strong AT, Allemang MT, et al. Results of the Ovesco-Over-Overstitch Technique for Managing Bariatric Surgical Complications. 16th World Congress of Endoscopic Surgery, Seattle, WA, April 11-14, 2018.
42. van den Berg MW, Kerbert AC, van Soest EJ, et al. Safety and efficacy of a fully covered large-diameter self-expanding metal stent for the treatment of upper gastrointestinal perforations, anastomotic leaks, and fistula. Dis Esophagus 2016;29:572–9.
43. Simon F, Siciliano I, Gillet A, et al. Gastric leak after laparoscopic sleeve gastrectomy: early covered self-expandable stent reduces healing time. Obes Surg 2013;23:687–92.
44. Southwell T, Lim TH, Ogra R. Endoscopic therapy for treatment of staple line leaks post-laparoscopic sleeve gastrectomy (LSG): experience from a large bariatric surgery centre in New Zealand. Obes Surg 2016;26:1155–62.
45. Donatelli G, Dumont JL, Cereatti F, et al. Treatment of Leaks Following Sleeve Gastrectomy by Endoscopic Internal Drainage (EID). Obes Surg 2015;25: 1293–301.
46. Maluf-Filho F, Hondo F, Halwan B, et al. Endoscopic treatment of Roux-en-Y gastric bypass-related gastrocutaneous fistulas using a novel biomaterial. Surg Endosc 2009;23:1541–5.
47. Papavramidis TS, Kotzampassi K, Kotidis E, et al. Endoscopic fibrin sealing of gastrocutaneous fistulas after sleeve gastrectomy and biliopancreatic diversion with duodenal switch. J Gastroenterol Hepatol 2008;23:1802–5.
48. Kowalski C, Kastuar S, Mehta V, et al. Endoscopic injection of fibrin sealant in repair of gastrojejunostomy leak after laparoscopic Roux-en-Y gastric bypass. Surg Obes Relat Dis 2007;3:438–42.
49. Casella G, Soricelli E, Rizzello M, et al. Nonsurgical treatment of staple line leaks after laparoscopic sleeve gastrectomy. Obes Surg 2009;19:821–6.
50. Schweitzer M, Steele K, Mitchell M, et al. Transoral endoscopic closure of gastric fistula. Surg Obes Relat Dis 2009;5:283–4.
51. Bege T, Emungania O, Vitton V, et al. An endoscopic strategy for management of anastomotic complications from bariatric surgery: a prospective study. Gastrointest Endosc 2011;73:238–44.
52. Spyropoulos C, Argentou MI, Petsas T, et al. Management of gastrointestinal leaks after surgery for clinically severe obesity. Surg Obes Relat Dis 2012;8: 609–15.
53. Weidenhagen R, Gruetzner KU, Wiecken T, et al. Endoscopic vacuum-assisted closure of anastomotic leakage following anterior resection of the rectum: a new method. Surg Endosc 2008;22:1818–25.
54. Leeds SG, Mencio M, Ontiveros E, et al. Endoluminal vacuum therapy: how I do it. J Gastrointest Surg 2019;23:1037–43.

Endoscopic Ultrasound

Shelini Sooklal, MD[a], Prabhleen Chahal, MD[b],*

KEYWORDS

- Endoscopic ultrasound • Fine-needle aspiration • Fine-needle biopsy • Biliary
- Pancreatitis • Adenocarcinoma

KEY POINTS

- The role of endoscopic ultrasound in the diagnosis and management of gastrointestinal malignancy, benign gastrointestinal, pancreatic, and biliary diseases continues to evolve.
- Therapeutic endoscopic ultrasound procedure for a variety of pancreatic and biliary indications shows a high technical and clinical success rate, with a low rate of adverse events.
- Endoscopic ultrasound plays a key role in the multidisciplinary management of complex surgical, oncologic patients and those with pancreaticobiliary disorders.

INTRODUCTION, HISTORY, AND BACKGROUND

Endoscopic ultrasound (EUS) provides high-resolution, real-time imaging of the gastrointestinal tract and surrounding extramural structures. It is a highly effective, efficient, and cost-effective method to assess a wide spectrum of benign and malignant gastrointestinal diseases.

Additionally, within the past several years, EUS has played an increasing role as an adjunct or alternative method to conventional surgical therapies. In the 1980s, EUS was used primarily as a diagnostic tool but has increasingly transitioned to a therapeutic modality.[1,2] The evolution of therapeutic EUS-guided procedures have steadily progressed because of its reported high technical and clinical success rates. The advent of novel procedures, such as gastrojejunostomy creation, gallbladder drainage (GBD), angiotherapy, drainage of postsurgical fluid collection, portal vein (PV) sampling, liver biopsy, contrast-enhanced harmonic EUS, and EUS-guided transluminal endoscopic retrograde cholangiopancreatography (ERCP) in patients with surgically altered anatomy[3] make EUS an exciting and ever-changing technology ripe with innovative advances.

[a] Department of Gastroenterology, Hepatology and Nutrition, Cleveland Clinic Foundation, 9500 Euclid Avenue, Cleveland, OH 44195, USA; [b] Advanced Endoscopy Fellowship, Department of Gastroenterology, Hepatology and Nutrition, Cleveland Clinic Foundation, 9500 Euclid Avenue, Cleveland, OH 44195, USA
* Corresponding author.
E-mail address: chahalp@ccf.org
Twitter: @SSooklalMD (S.S.); @ChahalPrabhleen (P.C.)

Surg Clin N Am 100 (2020) 1133–1150
https://doi.org/10.1016/j.suc.2020.07.003
0039-6109/20/© 2020 Elsevier Inc. All rights reserved.

DEFINITIONS AND ABBREVIATIONS
Equipment, Devices, and Techniques

- EUS
- Linear echoendoscope: EUS examinations are performed using a curvilinear echoendoscope or a radial echoendoscope. The curvilinear echoendoscope has an ultrasound transducer, which is located at the tip of the endoscope. The echoendoscope is attached to an ultrasound processor device throughout the procedure. It is an oblique viewing echoendoscope with a limited endoscopic field of view. Linear echoendoscopes produce ultrasound images in a sagittal plane (plane parallel to the long axis of the endoscope). Linear echoendoscopes have an instrument channel with a diameter ranging from 2.8 to 3.8 mm, and a lever (elevator) similar to a duodenoscope, allowing passage of different devices for therapeutic procedures.
- Radial echoendoscope: A radial echoendoscope is used to perform a diagnostic and staging examination. It provides a 360-degree field of view (axial view) of the wall layers of the esophagus, stomach, duodenum, rectum, and structures surrounding the gastrointestinal tract. The common applications include staging of esophageal, gastric, and rectal malignancy; assessment of gastrointestinal tract submucosal lesions; and diagnostic evaluation of the liver and pancreas (**Figs. 1** and **2**).
- Fine-needle aspiration (FNA): EUS-guided FNA (EUS-FNA) is a procedure by which EUS is used to identify and sample fluid collections or solid lesions in close proximity to the gastrointestinal tract. This is performed by the use of a hollow needle device passed through the echoendoscope channel and is used to puncture the gastrointestinal wall and adjacent wall of a fluid-filled structure or solid intramural and transmural lesions in real-time EUS examination. This needle is attached to a suction syringe providing negative pressure for aspiration of cytologic material and fluid contents for diagnostic purposes. There are several commercially available FNA devices, and 19-, 22-, and 25-gauge sizes are most commonly used. Fluid and cytologic material obtained is placed in a preservative medium and sent to the laboratory for analysis.
- Fine-needle biopsy (FNB): EUS-guided FNB (EUS-FNB) is a procedure by which EUS is used to identify and sample solid lesions in close proximity to the gastrointestinal tract. This is performed by the use of a hollow needle device passed through the echoendoscope channel and is used to puncture the gastrointestinal wall and adjacent solid lesion. Tissue cores or cells are obtained by use of the "slow-pull" technique or suction technique. The suction technique is the same as described for FNA, where the needle device is attached to a suction syringe

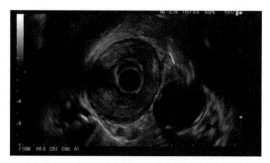

Fig. 1. Radial EUS image of a T2 distal esophageal adenocarcinoma.

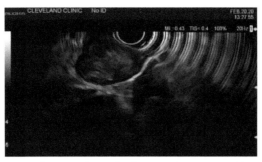

Fig. 2. Radial EUS image of an esophageal submucosal granular cell tumor.

providing 5 to 20 mL of negative pressure for aspiration of fluid contents for diagnostic purposes. The slow-pull technique describes the technique by which the stylet of the FNB needle device is slowly withdrawn while the needle is simultaneously and repeatedly advanced and withdrawn several times within the solid lesion to obtain a core of tissue within the needle. Several commercially available FNA/FNB devices are available, and 19-, 22-, and 25-gauge sizes are most commonly used. The tissue obtained is then placed in a preservative medium and submitted for analysis by a pathologist, or interpreted in real-time in the endoscopy unit where rapid on-site evaluation by a cytopathologist is available (**Table 1**).

PROCEDURAL APPROACH

EUS has a wide spectrum of uses for diagnostic and therapeutic modalities, in benign and malignant conditions.

Endoscopic Ultrasound in Benign Conditions

Gastrointestinal tract subepithelial lesions

EUS is used to evaluate and perform FNA or FNB of subepithelial lesions in the esophagus, stomach, duodenum, rectum, and sigmoid colon. A radial echoendoscope is often chosen to evaluate gastrointestinal tract subepithelial lesions. Because of its 360-degree field of view, each of the wall layers is clearly visualized in concentric circles, and the lesion is clearly seen originating from a particular wall layer.

Table 1
FNA and FNB reported sensitivity and specificity from randomized trials from recently published meta-analysis

Needle Type	Sensitivity (%)	Specificity (%)
22-gauge FNA	90.8	100
25-gauge FNA	89.9	100
22-gauge FNB	94.7	100
25-gauge FNB	87.9	100

Data from Facciorusso A, Wani S, Triantafyllou K, et al. Comparative accuracy of needle sizes and designs for EUS tissue sampling of solid pancreatic masses: a network meta-analysis. Gastrointest Endosc. 2019;90(6):893-903 and Guedes HG, Moura DTH, Duarte RB, et al. A comparison of the efficiency of 22G versus 25G needles in EUS-FNA for solid pancreatic mass assessment: A systematic review and meta- analysis. Clinics (Sao Paulo). 2018;73:e261.

Further diagnosis is ascertained by performing FNA or FNB, using a linear echoendoscope. When comparing FNA with FNB, traditional FNA only provides a cytologic specimen with scant cellularity and lacks architectural stroma sampling. However, FNB provides stromal architecture information because core tissue samples are obtained. This fact had made FNB a more attractive option for sampling solid lesions in recent times. A recent international multicenter randomized control trial by Bruno and colleagues[4] investigated FNA versus FNB techniques and found that a 20-gauge FNB needle outperformed the 25-gauge FNA needle in terms of histologic yield and diagnostic accuracy. This benefit was consistently seen in all the participating centers, and was irrespective of the indication for FNA or FNB.

Celiac plexus block and celiac plexus neurolysis

EUS-guided celiac plexus block (CPB) and celiac plexus neurolysis (CPN) are therapeutic options for pain control for patients with chronic pain caused by chronic pancreatitis (**Fig. 3**) or pancreatic malignancy. These options are often explored as an alternative to chronic opioid therapy, or when other analgesic modalities are ineffective despite maximal dose or are poorly tolerated because of the side effects leading to suboptimal pain control. CPB and CPN are performed using a linear echoendoscope through which a 19- or 22-gauge needle is passed and used for drug delivery (**Fig. 4**). CPB can block temporary transmission of pain signals from the celiac plexus resulting in temporary pain relief that can last from weeks to months. The medications injected during a CPB are a local anesthetic agent, such as bupivacaine or ropivacaine, sometimes used along with a corticosteroid medication, such as triamcinolone.

A single-center randomized control trial comparing the duration of pain relief with or without the addition of triamcinolone to an injected local anesthetic agent found that there was no increase in pain relief or lengthening the effects of CPB with addition of triamcinolone.[5] For CPN, concentrated alcohol (eg, 98% alcohol) is used. For CPB and CPN, EUS is used to identify the celiac artery origin from the abdominal aorta, then the celiac ganglia are identified adjacent to the celiac artery. Doppler flow is used to identify any interposing vessels that should be avoided; then under EUS guidance, the celiac ganglion is punctured, or alternatively the area adjacent to the ganglia are punctured, medication injected, and the needle withdrawn.[6]

Endoscopic ultrasound–guided angiotherapy

EUS is used in the treatment of gastric varices in patients with refractory or recurrent episodes of gastrointestinal bleeding caused by gastric varices. They are present in

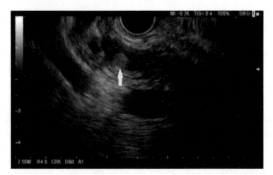

Fig. 3. Linear EUS image of a pancreatic duct stone in chronic pancreatitis.

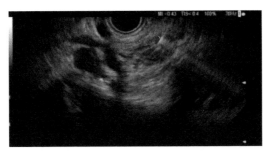

Fig. 4. Linear EUS image of EUS-guided celiac plexus neurolysis.

approximately 20% of patients with portal hypertension. EUS-guided angiotherapy refers to the ability of injecting a variety of agents (cyanoacrylate glue, microembolization coils, hyaluronate, sclerosants, and fibrin products) into gastric varices under EUS guidance.

Isolated gastric varices or gastroesophageal varices in the fundus are identified using Doppler flow. The main feeding varix is identified and punctured using a 19-gauge needle. Through the needle, cyanoacrylate glue is injected and/or microembolization coils are deployed until a cessation of Doppler flow in the varix is confirmed. A recent systematic review and meta-analysis evaluated the comparative effectiveness of EUS-guided interventions for the treatment of gastric varices (**Fig. 5**) and found that EUS combination therapy with coil embolization plus cyanoacrylate glue injection seems to be a preferred strategy for the treatment of gastric varices over EUS-based monotherapy of these interventions. Additionally, they found that the overall technical success, clinical success, and adverse events for EUS angiotherapy treatments was 100%, 97%, and 14%, respectively.[7]

Drainage of pancreatic fluid collections
Symptomatic, mature pancreatic fluid collections are endoscopically drained. Appropriate indications for intervention includes patients with persistent abdominal pain, fever, signs of infection, gastric outlet obstruction, failure to thrive, biliary obstruction caused by extrinsic compression by a large pancreatic collection, or nonresolving collections. Mature pancreatic fluid collections include pseudocysts and walled-off necrosis, the latter containing liquid plus solid components and may require subsequent endoscopic direct debridement or necrosectomy (**Fig. 6**).

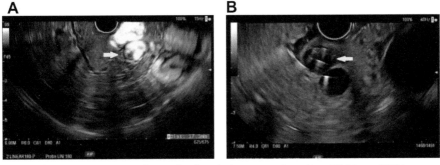

Fig. 5. (A) Linear EUS image of Doppler flow in large gastric varices. (B) Linear EUS image of EUS-guided coil embolization of gastric varices with cessation of Doppler flow.

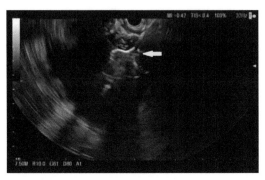

Fig. 6. Linear EUS image of EUS-guided cystogastrostomy of pancreatic walled-off necrosis using a 15 × 10 mm lumen-apposing metal stent.

EUS-guided transmural drainage of pancreatic collections has become the standard of care.[8]

Traditionally EUS-guided cystgastrostomy using double pigtail plastic stents was commonly performed but in recent times, the use of lumen-apposing metal stents (LAMS) has been more common because of their ease of use; high clinical success; and also provides access to the cyst cavity if subsequent debridement of necrotic contents is required, also known as step-up approach for management of symptomatic walled-off necrosis. A recent March 2020 study comparing an endoscopic approach with a minimally invasive surgical approach to the management of necrotizing pancreatitis again demonstrated that the endoscopic approach reduced the rate of major complications including death, new-onset multiorgan failure and multisystem dysfunction, enteropancreatic fistula formation, and visceral perforation. This study also demonstrated that the endoscopic approach reduced the rate of necrotizing pancreatitis-associated adverse events and costs.[9]

A recent systematic review and meta-analysis of metal versus plastic stents for drainage of pancreatic fluid collections published in the surgical literature found that use of metal stents for drainage of pancreatic fluid collections versus plastic stents was associated with improved clinical success (93.8% vs 86.2%), fewer adverse events (10.2% vs 25.0%), and reduced bleeding (2.8% vs 7.9%) compared with plastic stents.[10] Despite the previously mentioned data, one should be mindful of potential adverse events of bleeding, perforation, maldeployment, dislodgement, and buried stent syndrome associated with metal stents including LAMS. It is recommended that once deployed LAMS should be removed within 4 weeks to reduce the risk of complications.[11]

Drainage of postsurgical abdominal collections

Postsurgical fluid collections can occur because of anastomotic leak and sometimes require drainage if they become symptomatic. They have traditionally been drained percutaneously or surgically. EUS is safe and effective in accessing and draining intra-abdominal collections by the use of plastic pigtail stents or LAMS (**Fig. 7**). This method of internal drainage allows patients to be free of external drainage catheters, which require special care and may require interval exchange.[12–14]

Mediastinal adenopathy, intra-abdominal adenopathy, and masses

Mediastinal cystic lesions account for approximately 15% to 20% of all mediastinal masses and are difficult to differentiate because of similar imaging characteristics.

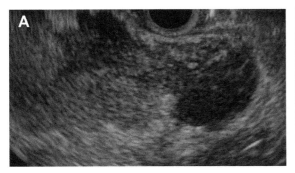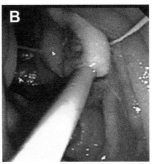

Fig. 7. (*A*) Linear EUS image of a mesenteric abscess. (*B*) Endoscopic image of EUS-guided drainage with placement of plastic pigtail stents within mesenteric abscess from third portion duodenum.

EUS-FNA offers a minimally invasive pathway to acquire tissue and to identify the pathologic type before surgery. Furthermore, EUS-FNA offers the advantages of reaching the lower mediastinum and aortopulmonary windows that endobronchial ultrasound–guided transbronchial aspiration cannot access.[15,16] Additionally, posterior and inferior mediastinal masses and adenopathy are accessible via EUS-FNA.

Similarly, EUS-FNA/FNB is used to obtain cellular material to diagnose abdominal and pelvic masses (**Figs. 8** and **9**). It is used in lieu of exploratory laparotomy and guide further management.

Apart from providing adequate diagnostic tissue in lymphoproliferative disorders, EUS is highly useful for pancreatic condition, such as autoimmune pancreatitis, and nonpancreatic conditions, such as retroperitoneal masses including adrenal metastasis, leiomyosarcoma, and paragangliomas.

Endoscopic ultrasound–guided pancreatic duct drainage

One of the evolving, but still a rare therapeutic indications of EUS is pancreatic ductal access and drainage. This technique is used in patients with prior failed ERCP, and in patients with sequelae of chronic pancreatitis including pancreatic duct strictures, stones, disruptions, or leaks. A variety of stents including plastic, self-expanding metal stents, or LAMS are used for pancreatic duct drainage. Immediate and delayed complications can occur in up to 20% and 11%, respectively, and include pancreatitis,

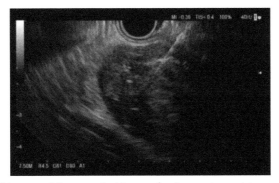

Fig. 8. Linear EUS image of fine-needle biopsy of a 4-cm retrogastric ganglioneuroma.

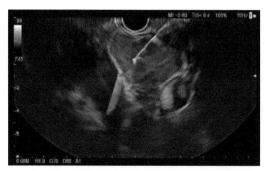

Fig. 9. Linear EUS image of fine-needle biopsy of porta hepatis lymphadenopathy.

pancreatic duct leak, pancreatic fluid collection formation, infection, bleeding, and perforation.[17]

In 2015, Fujii-Lau and Levy summarized the current literature on EUS-guided pancreatic duct drainage, reviewing the published experience of 222 patients. Including antegrade and rendezvous techniques, technical success was achieved in 170/222 patients (76.6%).[18–20]

Endoscopic ultrasound–guided transluminal endoscopic retrograde cholangiopancreatography in surgically altered anatomy

EUS-directed transgastric ERCP (EDGE) consists of accessing the excluded stomach from the gastric pouch or roux limb and then restoring continuity between the remnant stomach and the gastric pouch with a removable LAMS. Subsequently, conventional ERCP is performed through the LAMS. Traditionally, ERCP in surgically altered anatomy was attempted either by using balloon enteroscopy or in the operating room tag-teaming with a surgeon for a laparoscopic-assisted ERCP (LA-ERCP). Balloon enteroscopy is technically challenging and lengthy, with a reported dismal technical success rate of 50% to 63%. LA-ERCP has a high success rate, but is invasive, costly, and can result in longer length of inpatient hospitalization.[21]

A retrospective study of patients at four tertiary centers with Roux-en-Y anatomy who had undergone EDGE or LA-ERCP for a biliary indication found that there was no significant difference in the technical outcomes of either procedure, where the technical success of EDGE was 96.5% and LA-ERCP was 100%. The overall adverse event rate was also similar, 24% for EDGE and 19% for LA-ERCP. The EDGE procedure may offer a significant overall clinical and cost benefit given its noninferiority to LA-ERCP, while having a shorter procedure duration, length of hospitalization, and lack of skin incisions.[22]

Endoscopic ultrasound–guided liver interventions

EUS allows identification and assessment of small, less than 1 cm liver lesions with simultaneous performance of FNB for histologic diagnosis. Multiple studies have shown that the sensitivity of cross-sectional imaging for small liver lesions (<1 cm) ranges from 55% to 80%. EUS has shown to increase detection of up to 28% additional lesions that were initially missed with cross-sectional imaging. Multiple studies have demonstrated excellent diagnostic yield (90%–100%) and low rates of adverse events. The reported performance of EUS-guided liver biopsy meets current recommendations by the American Association for the Study of Liver Disease that recommends a total specimen length of 30 mm and number of complete portal triad greater than 11.[23,24]

The Doppler capability of EUS facilitates assessment and access to vascular structures, such as the PV. The evolving field of "endohepatology" also includes EUS-guided PV access for PV sampling for measurement of circulating tumor cells, EUS-guided PV pressure gradient measurement,[25–27] EUS-guided fiducial placement for tumor marking, and EUS-guided radiofrequency ablation (RFA) of hepatic lesions.[28]

Endoscopic ultrasound–guided gallbladder drainage

Cholecystectomy is the standard of care for acute calculous cholecystitis; however, poor surgical candidates may require alternative interventions. Traditionally, percutaneous cholecystostomy (PT) has been used to decompress the gallbladder in such patients. EUS allows good visualization of the gallbladder and facilitates internal drainage without the need for external tubes (**Fig. 10**). EUS-guided GBD (EUS-GBD) was first described a decade ago using double pigtail plastic stents, but lately, this has been performed using EUS deployment of a cautery-enhanced LAMS between the gallbladder lumen and the gastric or duodenal lumen.

In a landmark 2020 multicenter randomized controlled study including five centers and consisting of 80 patients, patients with acute calculous cholecystitis who were too high risk for surgery were randomized to EUS-GBD or PT-GBD. There was no difference in technical success, 97% for EUS-GBD and 100% for PT-GBD. Clinical success was 92% in both groups. However, EUS-GBD significantly reduced 1-year adverse events, 30-day adverse events, reinterventions after 30 days, number of unplanned readmissions, and recurrent cholecystitis.[29] A recent 2020 metanalysis of more than 1200 patients comparing the same group of patients as described previously found that the clinical success of EUS-GBD was significantly superior to PT-GBD and endoscopic transpapillary GBD (96% vs 89% vs 88%, respectively). The complication rate was similar among all three groups.[30]

Endoscopic Ultrasound in Malignant Conditions

Pancreatic and biliary masses, pancreatic cystic neoplasms

EUS-FNB/FNA has a reported diagnostic sensitivity of 82% and 71%, respectively, for detecting malignancy in solid pancreatic tumors (**Fig. 11**).[31] Immediate cytologic evaluation by an on-site cytopathologist can help to improve diagnostic yield. Differentiation of premalignant mucinous from benign nonmucinous cysts by EUS with FNA for fluid analysis provides high-quality imaging of the cyst and fluid sampling leads to high diagnostic accuracy. Cyst fluid analysis is performed to quantify carcinoembryonic, glucose, amylase, cytology, and mucin stain evaluation, which assists in differentiation between various cyst types.

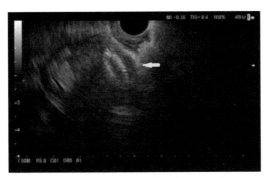

Fig. 10. Linear EUS image of EUS-guided gallbladder drainage for acute calculous cholecystitis using a lumen-apposing metal stent.

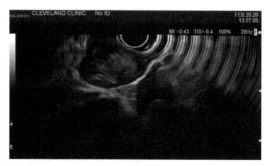

Fig. 11. Linear EUS image of fine-needle aspiration of a pancreatic head cyst.

Endoscopic ultrasound–guided gastroenterostomy

Gastric outlet obstruction by mechanical obstruction of the distal stomach or proximal duodenum can occur because of extrinsic compression from tumor or intra-abdominal collection. Enteral stent placement with the use of fluoroscopy has been the standard of care. When enteral stents become occluded because of tumor ingrowth, or become ineffective to relieve gastric outlet obstruction caused by continued tumor growth, EUS-guided gastroenterostomy using a LAMS may offer an alternative option to provide symptomatic relief. The obstructed proximal duodenum is bypassed with LAMS placement from the stomach to the duodenum (gastro-duodenostomy) or to the jejunum (gastrojejunostomy) (**Fig. 12**). EUS-guided gastroenterostomy performed for benign or malignant gastric outlet obstruction had high technical success (90%–92%) and a complication rate of 11.5%, comparable with a surgical or laparoscopic approach.[32,33]

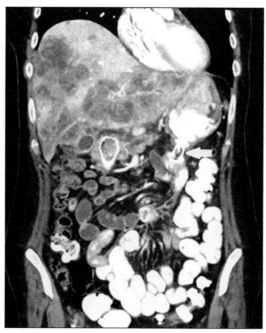

Fig. 12. Coronal computed tomography image EUS-guided gastrojejunostomy with LAMS in patient with metastatic cholangiocarcinoma.

Endoscopic ultrasound–guided ablative interventions
The utility of EUS to guide locoregional therapies for pancreatic lesions is a minimally invasive option that may be a viable, pancreas-saving alternative to surgery or surveillance in select patients. Alcohol ablation, paclitaxel ablation, and RFA of pancreatic cystic lesions has been described. Additionally, EUS-guided RFA has been described as a treatment modality for pancreatic insulinomas (**Fig. 13**). EUS-guided RFA allows precise delivery of antitumor treatment combining tumor necrosis and enhancement of the immune response. In a prospective, multicenter French study 14 pancreatic neuroendocrine tumors were treated with RFA. Twelve lesions completely disappeared (86% efficacy) when assessed at 1 year after the procedure. Most complications are related to thermal injury to the pancreatic parenchyma and surrounding structures.[34–36]

Anatomy

Native anatomy
EUS is performed for diagnostic and therapeutic purposes of structures that are viewed and accessed by the echoendoscope. The oblique-viewing echoendoscope is safely advanced up to the third portion of the duodenum in a native anatomy. Per rectum, the echoendoscope is safely advanced up to the distal sigmoid colon and descending colon. The structures surrounding these luminal sites can then be assessed for diagnostic and therapeutic interventions.

With the echoendoscope positioned in the esophagus, the following is performed:

- Assessment and FNA/FNB of esophageal subepithelial lesions
- Staging of esophageal malignancy
- FNA/FNA of paraesophageal lymph nodes
- FNA/FNB of paraesophageal and mediastinal masses
- Assessment of esophageal varices and gastroesophageal varices

With the echoendoscope positioned in the stomach, the following is performed:

- Assessment and FNA/FNB of gastric subepithelial lesions
- Staging of gastric malignancy
- CPB and CPN
- EUS-guided angiotherapy of gastric varices
- Assessment of the pancreas, FNA/FNB of pancreatic cystic and solid lesions
- EUS-guided drainage of pancreatic fluid collections
- EUS-guided drainage of postsurgical abdominal collections

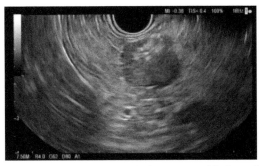

Fig. 13. Linear EUS image of EUS-guided radiofrequency ablation of a pancreatic body insulinoma.

- Assessment of the left lobe of the liver and FNB of lesions of the left lobe of the liver
- EUS-GBD
- EDGE to access the remnant stomach after gastric bypass surgery
- EUS-guided gastrojejunostomy
- EUS-guided pancreaticogastrostomy for pancreatic duct obstruction caused by pancreatic duct stones
- EUS-guided hepaticogastrostomy for biliary obstruction caused by tumor (**Fig. 14**)
- FNA/FNB of intra-abdominal lymphadenopathy, metastatic lesions

With the echoendoscope positioned in the duodenum, the following is performed:

- Assessment of the pancreatic head and uncinate of the pancreas, FNA/FNB of pancreatic cystic and solid lesions
- Assessment and FNA/FNB of duodenal subepithelial lesions
- EUS-GBD
- EUS-guided drainage of postsurgical abdominal collections
- EUS-guided biliary drainage
- FNA/FNB of intra-abdominal lymphadenopathy, metastatic lesions
- Assessment, staging, sampling of ampullary lesions, and evaluation of intraductal extension
- Assessment and FNA/FNB of pericaval, periaortic, portahepatic, and gastrohepatic masses and adenopathy

With the echoendoscope positioned in the rectum, the following is performed:

- Staging of rectal cancer
- Assessment and FNA/FNB of pelvic lesions and pelvic lymphadenopathy
- Assessment and FNA/FNB of rectal subepithelial lesions
- Assessment of anal sphincter, Crohn disease fistulae
- EUS-guided drainage of pelvic collections

Surgically altered anatomy

Performing EUS in surgically altered upper gastrointestinal tract anatomy is challenging. Patients who have had Roux-en-Y gastrojejunostomy, Billroth I and Billroth II surgery, post Whipple anatomy, and so forth present unique challenges to performing EUS in terms of technical difficulty navigating the oblique-viewing echoendoscope

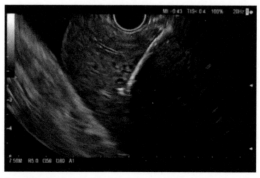

Fig. 14. Linear EUS image of EUS-guided left hepaticogastrostomy for biliary obstruction caused by metastatic ovarian carcinoma.

safely, and the echoendoscopic views obtained from the surgically altered gastrointestinal tract lumen. For example, in patients with Roux-en-Y gastrojejunostomy, the pancreatic body and tail may be visualized from the gastric pouch, but views of the pancreatic head are limited, because the pancreatic head is best evaluated with the echoendoscope in the duodenal bulb. Adequate examination of the head of the pancreas may require additional techniques and devices, such as changing to a forward-viewing echoendoscope for easier navigation through the jejunal limb, or balloon-assisted enteroscopy for placement of a catheter or guidewire to aid echoendoscope advancement.[37]

Preoperative/Preprocedure Planning

Anesthesia preprocedure assessment
In most endoscopy units in the United States, EUS procedures are performed with monitored anesthesia care anesthesia, or general anesthesia with endotracheal intubation. The choice of anesthesia is made by the anesthesiologist after input from the endoscopist on the day of the procedure based on a combination of factors including airway assessment, medical comorbidities, and duration and complexity of the planned procedure.

Additionally, 1 to 2 weeks before the procedure date, outpatients identified with a history of multiple medical comorbidities, such as significant cardiac or respiratory diseases, may be referred for preprocedure anesthesia assessment by a physician for optimization of patient before the endoscopy.

Anticoagulation
The American Society for Gastrointestinal Endoscopy published guidelines in 2016 outlining the management of antithrombotic agents for patients undergoing gastrointestinal endoscopy procedures. These guidelines categorize a diagnostic EUS procedure as low risk for bleeding, and EUS with FNA/FNB or any therapeutic EUS procedure as high risk for bleeding.

If a diagnostic EUS is planned, patients may remain on therapeutic doses of anticoagulation. In the event of possible intervention, or a planned therapeutic EUS procedure, anticoagulation medications need to be stopped before the procedure. As a general rule of thumb, aspirin, 81 mg daily, is continued for all EUS procedures; antiplatelet agents and warfarin should be stopped 5 days before the procedure; and the newer direct oral anticoagulant medications should be stopped 2 days before the procedure. The American Society for Gastrointestinal Endoscopy guideline mentioned previously details many antiplatelet and anticoagulant agents, their duration of action, and the approach to reversal based on procedural urgency (ie, elective vs urgent).[38]

Restarting antiplatelet or anticoagulation medications usually is recommended 24 to 48 hours post-procedure, but is dependent on several factors including endoscopist discretion, bleeding risk of therapeutic intervention performed, and patients' underlying comorbidities necessitating need for anticoagulation.

Laboratory tests and imaging
Laboratory analysis within normal limits or at acceptable levels for endoscopic procedures (international normalized ratio <1.5, platelets >50,000, hemoglobin >7) and cross-sectional imaging are required for proper procedure planning and safe outcomes.

Preparation and Patient Positioning

Patient preparation
Before EUS, patients are given standard pre-endoscopy instructions including:

- Remain nil per oral from midnight before the procedure
- Stop anticoagulant and antiplatelet medications if therapeutic EUS is planned
- Patients with diabetes mellitus on oral hypoglycemics or insulin should contact their prescribing physician for dose adjustment
- Patients should be accompanied by a responsible adult who will accompany them home after the procedure
- Patients taking aspirin, 81 mg once daily, or nonsteroidal anti-inflammatory medications can continue these medications without interruption

Patient positioning

By convention, as for all upper endoscopy procedures, EUS procedures are generally performed in the left lateral decubitus position, with the knees flexed. In special circumstances, EUS may be performed in the prone position (eg, if EUS is being performed before ERCP and the patient has already been positioned for ERCP). EUS can also be performed in the supine position if there are anesthesia concerns requiring close airway management during the duration of sedation or the patient is unable to be positioned in the left lateral decubitus position because of joint concerns or reduced mobility.

Recovery and Rehabilitation (Including Post-Procedure Care)

Recovery

Most EUS procedures are performed with monitored anesthesia care anesthesia, and propofol boluses and infusions are generally the drug of choice. Propofol is metabolized rapidly in the liver via hydroxylation and conjugation with glucuronide and sulfate, and its metabolites are excreted by the kidneys. The onset of effect for propofol is 0.5 to 1 minute, and the duration of effect is 4 to 8 minutes.[39–42] Therefore, patients are awake within minutes after the conclusion of the procedure and are transported to the post-procedure recovery unit.

After most endoscopy procedures, patients are observed for approximately 30 minutes in the post-procedure recovery unit, and if hemodynamically stable and pain free, are discharged home in the company of a responsible adult. Certain EUS procedures, such as CPB or CPN, may require longer periods of post-procedure observation. Loss of sympathetic tone to the vessels innervated by the celiac plexus may result in post-procedural hypotension. Therefore, these patients are observed for approximately 90 minutes, and are discharged home if no hypotension is noted. They may also receive intravenous fluid bolus preprocedural if deemed to be at higher risk for hypotension.

Patients are also given standard postendoscopy instructions including avoiding driving or decision-making until the next day, and consuming small, nonfatty meals for the remainder of the day to prevent nausea. They can resume normal activities and return to work the next day.

Resuming anticoagulation and antiplatelet medications

Patients can usually resume antiplatelet and anticoagulation medications the same day if a diagnostic EUS was performed, that is, without FNA/FNB or any therapeutic interventions (low bleeding risk). For therapeutic EUS procedures, including FNA/FNB, recommended resumption of antiplatelets or anticoagulation is at the discretion of the performing endoscopist who assesses the risk of post-procedure bleeding based on the type of intervention, intraprocedural bleeding, and so forth. Generally, antiplatelet and anticoagulation medications are resumed 48 to 72 hours after a therapeutic EUS procedure. Some patients may require prophylactic antibiotics for few days after therapeutic interventions, such as FNA of pancreatic cyst or ductal drainage procedures.

Rehabilitation

Rehabilitation is generally not necessary after uncomplicated EUS procedures. Patients return to normal daily activities the day after their procedure.

MANAGEMENT

The management of patients requiring EUS procedures is often a multidisciplinary effort, and is often done in conjunction with hepatobiliary surgeons, colorectal surgeons, intervention radiologists, pathologists, and oncologists. In large academic institutions, the decision to proceed with various therapeutic EUS procedures is often made after multidisciplinary conferences and tumor board discussions. After EUS procedures, patients may be referred to interventional radiologists for management or placement of biliary or percutaneous drainage catheters. After FNA/FNB is performed and pathology results are confirmed, patients may be referred to surgeons or oncologists as needed. If stents are placed during EUS procedures (eg, LAMS or self-expanding metal stents), patients are followed in the outpatient gastroenterology setting to monitor symptoms, review of follow-up imaging, and also plan for repeat procedures for stent removal or replacement.

SUMMARY

The role of EUS in the diagnosis and management of gastrointestinal malignancy, pancreatic diseases, and biliary diseases continues to evolve. Therapeutic EUS procedures for a variety of pancreatic and biliary indications shows a high technical and clinical success rate, with a low rate of adverse events. EUS plays a key role in the multidisciplinary management of complex surgical and oncology patients and those with pancreaticobiliary disorders.

CLINICS CARE POINTS

- EUS is a valuable diagnostic and therapeutic tool, and its applications in the management of complex patients continues to evolve.
- EUS-FNA/FNB of intra-abdominal solid and cystic lesions has overall greater than 90% diagnostic yield.
- EUS therapeutic interventions in the management of oncology patients and complex pancreatobiliary patients has a high technical and clinical success rate with a low rate of complications, and may be a viable alternative to surgical and percutaneous approaches in select patients.

DISCLOSURE

S. Sooklal and P. Chahal have nothing to disclose.

REFERENCES

1. DiMagno EP, Buxton JL, Regan PT, et al. Ultrasonic endoscope. Lancet 1980; 1(8169):629–31.
2. Wiersema MJ, Kochman ML, Cramer HM, et al. Endosonography-guided real-time fine-needle aspiration biopsy. Gastrointest Endosc 1994;40(6):700–7.
3. Siddiqui UD, Levy MJ. EUS-guided transluminal interventions. Gastroenterology 2018;154(7):1911–24.

4. Bruno MJ, Cahen DL, Poley JW, et al. A multicenter randomized trial comparing a 25-gauge EUS fine-needle aspiration device with a 20-gauge EUS fine-needle biopsy device. Gastrointest Endosc 2019;89(2):329–39.
5. Stevens T, et al. Adding triamcinolone to endoscopic ultrasound–guided celiac plexus blockade does not reduce pain in patients with chronic pancreatitis. Clin Gastroenterol Hepatol 2012;10:186–91.
6. Simons-Linares CR, Wander P, Vargo J, et al. Endoscopic ultrasonography: an inside view. Cleve Clin J Med 2020;87(3):175–83.
7. McCarty TR, Bazarbashi AN, Hathorn KE, et al. Combination therapy versus monotherapy for EUS-guided management of gastric varices: a systematic review and meta-analysis. Endosc Ultrasound 2019;9(1):6–15.
8. Parsa N, Nieto JM, Powers P, et al. Endoscopic ultrasound-guided drainage of pancreatic walled-off necrosis using 20-mm versus 15-mm lumen-apposing metal stents: an international, multicenter, case-matched study. Endoscopy 2020;52(3):211–9.
9. Bang JY, Arnoletti JP, Holt BA, et al. An endoscopic transluminal approach, compared with minimally invasive surgery, reduces complications and costs for patients with necrotizing pancreatitis. Gastroenterology 2019;156(4):1027–40.
10. Halloran C, Ramesh J, Cicconi S, et al. A systematic review and meta-analysis of metal versus plastic stents for drainage of pancreatic fluid collections: metal stents are advantageous. Surg Endosc 2019;33(5):1412–25.
11. Baron TH, DiMaio CJ, Wang AY, et al. American Gastroenterological Association clinical practice update: management of pancreatic necrosis. Gastroenterology 2020;158(1):67–75.
12. Donatelli G, Fuks D, Cereatti F, et al. Endoscopic transmural management of abdominal fluid collection following gastrointestinal, bariatric, and hepato-biliopancreatic surgery. Surg Endosc 2018;32(5):2281–7.
13. Simons-Linares CR, Rodriguez J, Chahal P. EUS-guided drainage of postoperative subphrenic fluid collection through gastric pouch with a lumen-apposing metal stent in a patient with Roux-en-Y gastric bypass. Obes Surg 2018;28(10):3301–3.
14. Simons-Linares CR, Chahal P. Successful EUS-guided drainage of a persistent subdiaphragmatic fluid collection in a patient with Crohn's disease. Inflamm Bowel Dis 2019;25(7):e85–6.
15. Zhao Y, Wang R, Wang Y, et al. Application of endoscopic ultrasound- guided-fine needle aspiration combined with cyst fluid analysis for the diagnosis of mediastinal cystic lesions. Thorac Cancer 2019;10(2):156–62.
16. Herth FJF, Rabe KF, Gasparini S, et al. Transbronchial and transoesophageal (ultrasound- guided) needle aspirations for the analysis of mediastinal lesions. Eur Respir J 2006;28:1264–75.
17. Tyberg A, Sharaiha RZ, Kedia P, et al. EUS-guided pancreatic drainage for pancreatic strictures after failed ERCP: a multicenter international collaborative study. Gastrointest Endosc 2017;85(1):164–9.
18. Chapman C, Waxman I, Siddiqui U. Endoscopic ultrasound (EUS)-guided pancreatic duct drainage: the basics of when and how to perform EUS-guided pancreatic duct interventions. Clin Endosc 2016;49(2):161–7.
19. Fujii-Lau LL, Levy MJ. Endoscopic ultrasound-guided pancreatic duct drainage. J Hepatobiliary Pancreat Sci 2015;22:51–7.
20. Tyberg A, Nieto J, Salgado S, et al. Endoscopic ultrasound (EUS)-directed transgastric endoscopic retrograde cholangiopancreatography or EUS: mid-term analysis of an emerging procedure. Clin Endosc 2017;50(2):185–90.

21. Abbas AM, Strong AT, Diehl DL, et al, LA- ERCP Research Group. Multicenter evaluation of the clinical utility of laparoscopy-assisted ERCP in patients with Roux-en-Y gastric bypass. Gastrointest Endosc 2018;87(4):1031–9.
22. Kedia P, Tarnasky PR, Nieto J, et al. EUS-directed transgastric ERCP (EDGE) versus laparoscopy-assisted ERCP (LA- ERCP) for Roux-en-Y gastric bypass (RYGB) anatomy: a multicenter early comparative experience of clinical outcomes. J Clin Gastroenterol 2019;53(4):304–8.
23. Nieto J, Khaleel H, Challita Y, et al. EUS-guided fine-needle core liver biopsy sampling using a novel 19-gauge needle with modified 1-pass, 1 actuation wet suction technique. Gastrointest Endosc 2018;87(2):469–75, 74.
24. Parekh PJ, Majithia R, Diehl DL, et al. Endoscopic ultrasound-guided liver biopsy. Endosc Ultrasound 2015;4(2):85–91.
25. Catenacci DV, Chapman CG, Xu P, et al. Acquisition of portal venous circulating tumor cells from patients with pancreaticobiliary cancers by endoscopic ultrasound. Gastroenterology 2015;149(7):1794–803.
26. Samarasena JB, Yu AR, Chang KJ. EUS-guided portal pressure measurement (with videos). Endosc Ultrasound 2018;7(4):257–62.
27. Kalva NR, Vanar V, Forcione D, et al. Efficacy and safety of lumen apposing self-expandable metal stents for EUS guided cholecystostomy: a meta-analysis and systematic review. Can J Gastroenterol Hepatol 2018;2018:7070961.
28. Chua T, Faigel DO. Endoscopic ultrasound-guided ablation of liver tumors. Gastrointest Endosc Clin N Am 2019;29(2):369–79.
29. Teoh AYB, Kitano M, Itoi T, et al. Endosonography-guided gallbladder drainage versus percutaneous cholecystostomy in very high-risk surgical patients with acute cholecystitis: an international randomised multicentre controlled superiority trial (DRAC 1). Gut 2020;69(6):1085–91.
30. Mohan BP, Khan SR, Trakroo S, et al. Endoscopic ultrasound-guided gallbladder drainage, transpapillary drainage, or percutaneous drainage in high risk acute cholecystitis patients: a systematic review and comparative meta- analysis. Endoscopy 2020;52(2):96–106.
31. Oppong KW, Bekkali NLH, Leeds JS, et al. Fork-tip needle biopsy versus fine-needle aspiration in endoscopic ultrasound-guided sampling of solid pancreatic masses: a randomized crossover study. Endoscopy 2020. https://doi.org/10.1055/a-1114-5903.
32. Khashab MA, Bukhari M, Baron TH, et al. International multicenter comparative trial of endoscopic ultrasonography-guided gastroenterostomy versus surgical gastrojejunostomy for the treatment of malignant gastric outlet obstruction. Endosc Int Open 2017;5(4):E275–81.
33. Canakis A, Law R, Baron T. An updated review on ablative treatment of pancreatic cystic lesions. Gastrointest Endosc 2019;91(3):520–6.
34. Barthet M, Giovannini M, Lesavre N, et al. Endoscopic ultrasound-guided radiofrequency ablation for pancreatic neuroendocrine tumors and pancreatic cystic neoplasm: a prospective multicenter study. Endoscopy 2019;51:836–42.
35. Gaidhane M, Smith I, Ellen K, et al. Endoscopic ultrasound-guided radiofrequency ablation of the pancreas on a porcine model. Gastroenterol Res Pract 2012;431–51.
36. Kluz M, Staroń R, Krupa L, et al. Successful endosonography-guided radiofrequency ablation of pancreatic insulinoma. Pol Arch Intern Med 2019. https://doi.org/10.20452/pamw.15100.
37. Tanaka K, Hayashi T, Utsunomiya R, et al. Endoscopic ultrasound-guided fine needle aspiration for diagnosing pancreatic mass in patients with surgically

altered upper gastrointestinal anatomy. Dig Endosc 2020. https://doi.org/10. 1111/den.13625.

38. ASGE Standards of Practice Committee, Acosta R, Abraham NS, Chandrasekhara V, et al. The management of antithrombotic agents for patients undergoing GI endoscopy. Gastrointest Endosc 2016;83(1):3–16.

39. Moon SH. Sedation regimens for gastrointestinal endoscopy. Clin Endosc 2014; 47(2):135–40.

40. Jacobson BC, Chak A, Hoffman B, et al. Quality indicators for endoscopic ultra-sonography. Gastrointest Endosc 2006;63(4 Suppl):S35–8.

41. Paik WH, Lee TH, Park DH, et al. EUS-guided biliary drainage versus ERCP for the primary palliation of malignant biliary obstruction: a multicenter randomized clinical trial. Am J Gastroenterol 2018;113(7):987–99.

42. Khan MA, Atiq O, Kubiliun N, et al. Efficacy and safety of endoscopic gallbladder drainage in acute cholecystitis: Is it better than percutaneous gallbladder drainage? Gastrointest Endosc 2017;85(1):76–87.

Endoscopic Management of Pancreaticobiliary Disease

Catherine F. Vozzo, DO[a], Madhusudhan R. Sanaka, MD[b],*

KEYWORDS

- Pancreaticobiliary disease • ERCP • EUS • Therapeutic endoscopy • Pancreas
- Biliary

KEY POINTS

- Endoscopic retrograde cholangiopancreatography (ERCP) and endoscopic ultrasound comprise the endoscopic armamentarium to manage pancreaticobiliary diseases.
- Diagnostic ERCP is mostly replaced by computed tomography, magnetic resonance cholangiopancreatography, and EUS due to a lower risk of complications.
- Endoscopic therapy of biliary disease is performed primarily with ERCP, in particular choledocholithiasis, obstructive jaundice, and biliary strictures.
- EUS is rapidly emerging as a therapeutic interventional tool in the recent years.
- Multidisciplinary team approach to management of pancreaticobiliary disease is important for optimal outcomes.

INTRODUCTION

Diagnostic and therapeutic modalities of pancreatic and biliary disease have changed significantly over the past 50 years with the advancement of endoscopic retrograde cholangiopancreatography (ERCP) and endoscopic ultrasound (EUS).[1] Pancreaticobiliary endoscopy differentiates itself from luminal endoscopy with the use of fluoroscopy, side-viewing duodenoscopes, and echoendosonography. ERCP and EUS initially were used as diagnostic procedures. At present, these techniques are used for management of a plethora of benign and malignant diseases of the pancreatic and biliary system.

ERCP is performed with a side-viewing duodenoscope that allows for the identification and proper orientation of the major papilla for cannulation. The bile duct or pancreatic duct then is cannulated with endoscopic and fluoroscopic guidance. ERCP enables various interventions with the use of several devices, including stents, guide wires, and catheters. This review provides a brief background on each disease

[a] Department of Gastroenterology, Cleveland Clinic, 9500 Euclid Avenue / A30, Cleveland, OH 44195, USA; [b] Department of Gastroenterology, Cleveland Clinic, 9500 Euclid Avenue / Q30, Cleveland, OH 44195, USA
* Corresponding author.
E-mail address: sanakam@ccf.org

Surg Clin N Am 100 (2020) 1151–1168
https://doi.org/10.1016/j.suc.2020.08.006
0039-6109/20/© 2020 Elsevier Inc. All rights reserved.

entity and how it can be managed with therapeutic endoscopy. It concludes by reviewing the outcomes and general complications of ERCP and EUS.

THE PANCREAS
Pancreatitis

Identifying the etiology

Pancreatitis most commonly is due to alcohol abuse and gallstones. The cause of acute pancreatitis (AP) can be established with a thorough history, physical examination, blood tests, and imaging studies in approximately 80% of patients.[2] In those remaining patients without a clear etiology, computerized tomography (CT), EUS, and/or magnetic resonance cholangiopancreatography (MRCP) should be performed after resolution of the acute phase of pancreatitis.[3] Diagnostic ERCP is not recommended because of the low yield and its associated risk of complications, including iatrogenic pancreatitis. EUS can assist in identifying the cause of idiopathic AP by providing better detection of biliary sludge and stones. It also allows for tissue and fluid acquisition to help with the diagnosis. In idiopathic pancreatitis, EUS was shown to have a higher diagnostic yield than MRCP (29% vs 10.5%, respectively).[4] Once a clear etiology of pancreatitis has been identified, such as gallstone pancreatitis or pancreas divisum (PD), therapeutic ERCP can provide definitive management.

Managing complications of pancreatitis

Pancreatic fluid collections Local complications of AP include acute fluid collections (<4 weeks after onset), pseudocysts (>4 weeks after onset), acute necrotic collections (<4 weeks), and walled-off necrosis (WON) (>4 weeks). In the acute phase (<4 weeks) there is no indication for intervention because collections typically are reabsorbed. If intervention is performed too early, there is a risk of infection and other complications. Mature fluid collections that are symptomatic may require endoscopic, percutaneous, or surgical drainage. Endoscopic approaches to the drainage of pancreatic fluid collections are discussed later.

EUS-guided transgastric drainage of pseudocysts aims to create a fistulous connection between the gastrointestinal lumen and the cyst cavity. See **Fig. 1** for a EUS image of a large pseudocyst. The target lesion is visualized and the puncture route is determined by excluding intervening vessels.[5] As a general rule, the distance between the pancreatic fluid collections and gastrointestinal tract wall should not exceed 10 mm. The cyst is punctured with a 19-gauge fine-needle aspiration (FNA) needle. A guide wire then is inserted into the cystic cavity by removing the stylet.

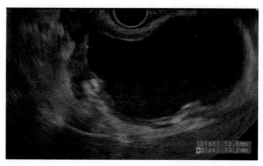

Fig. 1. Endosonographic image of a large (5.3-cm × 3.3-cm) mature pseudocyst.

The fistulous tract then is dilated to facilitate stent placement. Plastic or metal stents may be placed across the tract for pseudocyst drainage.[6]

Endoscopic necrosectomy involves creating a large fistulous cavity into the WON, allowing for spontaneous drainage via lumen-apposing metal stents (LAMSs). Débridement of the necrotic tissue can be through nasocystic tubes or percutaneous drains. An alternative technique, direct endoscopic necrosectomy (DEN), requires advancing the endoscope directly into the necrotic cavity to remove necrotic debris and control infection (**Fig. 2**). DEN has better outcomes in patients with WON compared with irrigation with plastic stents but may be associated with complications including air embolism, bleeding, and perforation. Therefore, patients should be selected carefully based on the amount of solid debris within the WON.[7] The procedure can be repeated every few days until all the necrotic tissue is cleared.

Chronic pancreatitis Chronic pancreatitis (CP) is a disorder that results in destruction of the pancreatic tissue and ducts, leading to exocrine and endocrine pancreatic insufficiency. Moderate to severe CP is easily diagnosed with a CT scan or magnetic resonance imaging. A diagnosis of early or mild CP is less obvious and may require MRCP or EUS. EUS is a safe and minimally invasive way to obtain structural information of the pancreas. Criteria for diagnosis of CP with EUS are outlined in **Box 1**. The predictive value for diagnosis of CP is approximately 85% when 5 or more EUS criteria are present.[8]

Endoscopic management of CP may include pain relief via EUS-guided celiac plexus block and treating the associated sequela, including pseudocysts, pancreatic strictures or stones, and pancreatic duct leaks. Pseudocyst management in CP is similar to that outlined in AP. Management of CP pain, pancreatic strictures, and stones is discussed later.

The celiac plexus transmits pain from the pancreas and is located easily with EUS as it surrounds the celiac trunk at its origin from the aorta. The linear echoendoscope is advanced to the posterior lesser curve of the proximal stomach and the injection target is the region directly adjacent and anterior to the celiac takeoff. The endoscopist can perform either celiac plexus neurolysis (injection of absolute ethanol that permanently destroys the plexus) or celiac plexus block (injection of local anesthetic and corticosteroids that temporarily block the plexus and reduce inflammation). Expert

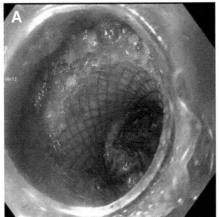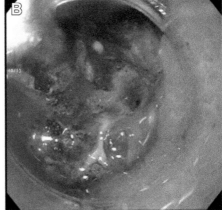

Fig. 2. (*A*) and (*B*), images of DEN.

Box 1
Endoscopic ultrasound criteria for chronic pancreatitis

Parenchymal changes
- Inhomogeneity
- Hyperechoic foci
- Hyperechoic strands
- Lobularity
- Pseudocysts

Ductal changes
- Ductal dilation
- Hyperechoic main duct margins
- Irregular main duct margins
- Visible side branches

---

guidelines advise against celiac plexus neurolysis for CP-related pain because neurolysis can induce fibrosis and limit future surgical options.[9] Celiac plexus neurolysis generally is reserved for patients with pancreatic cancer-related pain. Celiac plexus block is successful in controlling CP pain in approximately half of the patients.[10] Notable complications of EUS-guided celiac plexus block include transient sympathetic tone blockade (diarrhea, hypotension, and abdominal pain).

Pancreatic ductal endotherapy for strictures or stones is performed to relieve obstruction of the main pancreatic duct, which may be causing abdominal pain and recurrent pancreatitis. Catheter or balloon dilation with placement of plastic stents is the mainstay in management of pancreatic duct strictures. Hard or calcified pancreatic stones may not be removed successfully with standard endotherapy. Extracorporeal shock wave lithotripsy (ESWL) sometimes is needed to fragment stones to assist with their removal (either endoscopically or pass naturally).[11]

Pancreatic ductal leaks and disruptions can occur as a result of AP, CP, pancreatic surgery, or trauma. Leaks may arise from the head, body, or tail of the pancreas and fluid may track into the mediastinum or abdomen with resultant pleural effusions or ascites. In the setting of a large pancreatic fluid collection, transmural drainage may be used (as discussed previously). Drainage with transpapillary stenting can be performed with the intent of crossing the site of the leak and is associated with resolution of pancreatic ductal disruption.[12]

Pancreas Divisum

PD occurs when the dorsal and ventral pancreatic buds fail to fuse during fetal development. PD is a common genetic abnormality, with an estimated prevalence of 5% to 10% of the population.[13] In patients with PD, pancreatic juices drain primarily through the minor papilla. It is hypothesized that PD causes pancreatitis by impaired drainage through a narrow minor papilla. Prior to 2012, there was debate on whether PD alone could cause acute recurrent or CP. New research has shown that PD alone should no longer be considered a cause of pancreatitis, but that certain genetic mutations (CFTR, SPINK1, and PRSS1) may predispose patients with PD to recurrent AP and CP.[14]

PD typically is diagnosed incidentally on CT scan or an MRCP. Secretin-enhanced MRCP is the imaging modality of choice for diagnosis of PD.[15] No treatment is recommended for asymptomatic patients. Identifying which patients with pancreatitis and PD might benefit from intervention remains a clinical challenge.[16] Patients with evidence of minor papilla stenosis, dorsal body pancreatitis, and/or dorsal duct dilation may benefit from therapeutic intervention.

Endoscopic intervention aims at enhancing the dorsal duct drainage. Multiple techniques have been used, including minor papilla sphincterotomy, stenting, balloon dilation, and surgical sphincteroplasty. Endoscopic minor papilla sphincterotomy currently is preferred over surgery. The SpHincterotomy for Acute Recurrent Pancreatitis (SHARP) trial is under way to answer whether or not minor papilla endoscopic sphincterotomy an reduce the risk of AP caused by PD.[17]

The first step in endoscopic minor papilla sphincterotomy is identifying the minor papilla, which may be small or stenotic. It typically is located anteriorly and proximally to the major papilla. Localization can be aided by intravenous secretin injection, which may cause the orifice to open. Wire-guided cannulation is recommended. Once the guide wire is positioned deeply within the dorsal duct, a minor papillotomy can be performed with a pull-type sphincterotome. If the catheter cannot be advanced over the wire due to stenosis, a needle-knife sphincterotomy can be made over the wire. After sphincterotomy, a 4F to 7F stent should be inserted into the dorsal duct and left in place for 2 weeks to 4 weeks.[18]

Pancreatic Cystic Neoplasms

Pancreatic cystic neoplasms encompass a diverse group of cystic lesions affecting the pancreas. These include intraductal papillary mucinous cystic neoplasms, mucinous cystic neoplasms, serous cystic neoplasms, solid pseudopapillary neoplasms, and cystic neuroendocrine tumors. Accurate diagnosis is key because the management of different types of cystic neoplasms varies dramatically. Diagnostic imaging modalities include dedicated pancreatic CT or MRCP. If there are concerning features on initial imaging, then EUS may be indicated. Concerning features include mural nodules or associated mass, dilatation of the main pancreatic duct, thickened wall, or a cyst size greater than 3 cm.[19] EUS should not be used as a first-line examination for cysts with a clear diagnosis and/or without concerning features because it is unlikely to alter the management plan. In addition, patients who are nonoperative candidates should not undergo further evaluation of incidental pancreatic cysts, irrespective of their size.[19]

EUS also can be used to obtain cyst fluid for analysis. EUS-FNA for pancreatic cysts is very safe with low risk of complications (approximately 1%), including infection, bleeding, and AP.[20] Antibiotic prophylaxis is used commonly but not evidence based. EUS-FNA typically is performed with either a 19-gauge, 22-gauge, or a 25-gauge FNA needle. The area of interest is visualized by EUS and placed within the center of the imaging field. Doppler imaging is used to locate vascular structures within or around the lesion. The aspirated fluid usually is sent for CEA, amylase, and cytology to assist with diagnosis (**Fig. 3**). Needle confocal microscopy and microforceps biopsy are recently emerging diagnostic tools for pancreatic cystic neoplasms and may lead to improved tissue acquisition and diagnostic yield.[21,22]

Pancreatic Cancer

There has been no improvement in survival of pancreatic cancer patients over the past 3 decades. The main reason for this is failure to detect pancreatic cancer in the early stages. When a CT is indeterminate, EUS is highly sensitive and accurate in detecting pancreatic neoplasms, in particular those less than 2 cm in size.[23] Diagnosis with ERCP can be performed with brushing or biopsies of biliary strictures, although a recent meta-analysis revealed poor sensitivity (45% and 48% for brushings and

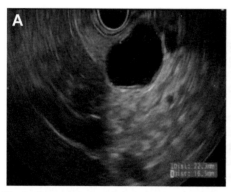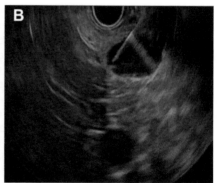

Fig. 3. Pancreatic cyst. (*A*) Endosonographic image of a pancreatic cyst with some debris. (*B*) FNA needle advanced into cyst for fluid analysis.

biopsies, respectively).[24] Other ERCP techniques, including cholangioscopy and probe-based confocal laser endomicroscopy, might improve diagnostic accuracy.

Common complications of pancreatic cancer include biliary obstruction, duodenal obstruction, and pancreatic ductal obstruction that may lead to jaundice, pain, pseudocysts, or leaks. Biliary obstruction occurs as a result of the pancreatic cancer's proximity to the common bile duct and its management are discussed later. Pain may be alleviated through EUS-guided celiac plexus block or neurolysis.

Duodenal obstruction can occur if a pancreatic head cancer invades through duodenal wall. This can be managed endoscopically via placement of duodenal self-expandable metal stent (SEMS) or EUS-guided gastrojejunostomy (GJY) using LAMS. The technical and clinical success rates of SEMSs were reported to be 97% and 89%, respectively.[25] Patients planned for SEMS should have a life expectancy less than 6 months. Alternatively, the technical and clinic success rates of GJY were reported to be 90% to 92% and 85% to 92%, respectively.[26,27] Recent studies have shown that GJY provided longer patency and survival time but more studies are needed before definitive conclusions can be drawn.[28]

THE BILIARY SYSTEM
Cholecystitis

A vast majority of patients with cholecystitis are treated with laparoscopic cholecystectomy. In a small portion of patients who cannot undergo surgery, percutaneous drainage of the gallbladder (PCGBD) is performed. This may be undesirable given the adverse events, including dislodgement of the drainage catheter, peritonitis, bleeding, and poor quality of life due to percutaneous drain. Endoscopic alternatives to a percutaneous drain include endoscopic transpapillary drainage of the gallbladder (ETGBD) and EUS-guided transmural drainage of the gallbladder (EUSGBD) usually with LAMS placement. Both are emerging techniques and currently are being studied but not widely used in practice. A recent meta-analysis revealed that clinical success of EUSGBD was superior to the other approaches (ETGBD and PCGBD). Complication rates were comparable between the groups. Pooled technical and clinical success rates were, respectively, ETGBD 83% and 88%, EUSGBD 95% and 96%, and PCGBD 98.7% and 89.3%.[29] Based on these findings, endoscopic alternatives should be considered in patients who are nonoperative candidates.

Choledocholithiasis

Choledocholithiasis (bile duct stones) can be seen in approximately 10% to 15% of patients with cholelithiasis (gallbladder stones). Choledocholithiasis also may be seen in patients who have undergone cholecystectomy in the past.[30] The American Society for Gastrointestinal Endoscopy proposed a strategy to assign risk of choledocholithiasis in patients with symptomatic cholelithiasis outlined in **Box 2**.[31]

Patients at high risk for choledocholithiasis should undergo ERCP. The standard technique for stone removal includes endoscopic biliary sphincterotomy to widen the papillary orifice and extraction using a balloon or a basket. The steps involved in ERCP with stone extraction include selective biliary cannulation, biliary sphincterotomy, and stone extraction (**Fig. 4**). Stones measuring less than 10 mm usually are removed intact by using an extraction balloon or retrieval basket. Biliary stones greater than 20 mm usually require fragmentation prior to removal.[32] Fragmentation can be performed with either mechanical lithotripsy, ESWL, electrohydraulic lithotripsy, or laser lithotripsy.

Mirizzi syndrome is uncommon and occurs when there is extrinsic compression of the common hepatic duct by a biliary stone in the cystic duct or gallbladder. In most cases, the stone cannot be removed endoscopically and surgical intervention is required.

Altered anatomy due to prior Billroth II and Roux-en-Y surgeries pose a challenge in the management of choledocholithiasis because a longer segment of small bowel needs to be navigated to reach the major papilla. The length of the Roux limb varies in each patient. Biliary access can be achieved with a device-assisted forward-viewing enteroscopy, laparoscopy-assisted ERCP, transgastric ERCP though a percutaneous gastrostomy tube, or EUS-directed transgastric ERCP (EDGE) using LAMS. A 2018 study compared EDGE versus enteroscopy-assisted ERCP, and the technical success was higher in the EDGE group (100% vs 60%, respectively).[33]

In the EDGE procedure, a connection between the gastric pouch or proximal jejunum and the excluded stomach is created by placing a LAMS between the 2 entities. A traditional ERCP then can be performed by advancing the duodenoscope through the LAMS into excluded stomach and into the duodenum. It is advisable to wait and perform ERCP at least 1 week to 2 weeks after creation of the gastrogastrostomy to avoid the risk of dislodging the LAMS and resultant perforation between the 2 stomachs. A study comparing laparoscopy-assisted ERCP to that of EGDE showed a technical success of 96.5% and clinical success of 96.5% with EDGE, similar to that of laparoscopy-assisted ERCP. Adverse events also were similar; however, EDGE procedure was faster and patients had a shorter length of hospital stay.[34]

Box 2
Likelihood of common bile duct stone

The probability of a common bile duct stone is high (>50%) if at least one very strong predictor is present:
- Total bilirubin of >4 mg/dL
- Common bile duct stone on ultrasound
- Clinical ascending cholangitis

The probability of a common bile duct stone is high (>50%) if 2 strong predictors are present:
- Total bilirubin between 1.8 mg/dL and 4 mg/dL
- Dilated common bile duct on ultrasound

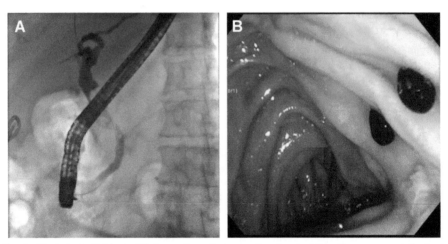

Fig. 4. Choledocholithiasis. (*A*) Several small stones visualized within the common bile duct. (*B*) Removed bile duct stones within the duodenal lumen.

Biliary Strictures

Benign and indeterminate strictures

There are several causes of benign biliary strictures, including postsurgical (cholecystectomy and liver transplantation), CP, primary sclerosing cholangitis (PSC), acquired immunodeficiency syndrome cholangiopathy, ischemia, trauma, infection (clonorchiasis), and radiation.[35] MRCP and/or CT are essential in the initial evaluation of strictures to exclude a malignant etiology.[36] Various classification systems are used to describe bile duct strictures. Most commonly used is the Bismuth classification, which is organized into types I to V based on the location of the stricture.[37] See **Fig. 5** for an anatomic representation of the Bismuth classification of strictures.[38]

Indeterminate biliary strictures are those that cannot be readily identified as either benign or malignant based on imaging and tissue sampling. ERCP with brush cytology or intraductal biopsy is performed to obtain a diagnosis.[35] In addition, EUS with FNA can be performed to improve the diagnostic accuracy.[39] Peroral cholangioscopy can be used as an adjunct to ERCP to allow for direct visualization of the stricture and targeted biopsies utilizing an ultraslim endoscope. SpyGlass DS (Boston Scientific, Marlborough, MA) is a new digital version of the single operator cholangiopancreatoscope and consists of a sterile, single-use catheter, a digital controller, and biliary biopsy forceps.[40] The strongest feature suggestive of malignancy on cholangioscopy is the presence of dilated tortuous vessels, with a reported positive predictive value of 100%.[41]

Benign biliary strictures are managed with standard biliary cannulation techniques.[42] First, a cholangiogram is obtained to estimate the diameter and length of the stricture. Stricture dilation or stricturoplasty then is performed using a balloon dilator, typically 4 mm to 12 mm in diameter. Balloon dilation alone is not advisable because the recurrence rate can be as high as 47%.[35] After dilation, current data support the use of either multiple plastic stents or fully covered SEMSs (FCSEMSs).[43] Based on a meta-analysis, they appear to be similar in efficacy, but FCSEMSs require fewer ERCPs to achieve clinical success.[44] Temporary single plastic stent placement is not advisable because it is associated with poor patency rates. Complications

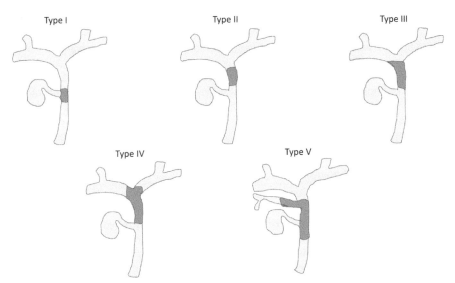

Fig. 5. Bismuth classification for biliary strictures. Type I strictures are located greater than 2 cm from the confluence. Type II strictures are located less than 2 cm from the confluence. Type III strictures leave the confluence ceiling intact. Type IV strictures interrupt the confluence. Type V strictures involve an aberrant right intrahepatic duct in addition to the stricturing pattern found in types I, II, and III. (*Data from* Zepeda-Gómez S, Baron T. Benign biliary strictures: current endoscopic management. Nat Rev Gastroenterol Hepatol. 2011;8(10):573-581).

associated with plastic stents include stent dysfunction, including clogging or migration, and a very low risk of cholecystitis.[42] The most common complication associated with FCSEMSs is stent migration.[42]

Malignant strictures
Malignant obstructive jaundice is a common complication of advanced pancreaticobiliary tumors. Types of pancreaticobiliary malignancies include ampullary adenocarcinoma, pancreatic adenocarcinoma, cholangiocarcinoma, and metastatic disease.[45] Management of malignant biliary strictures can be divided into distal bile duct strictures and perihilar/proximal bile duct strictures. In either instance (hilar or distal), if the lesion is surgically resectable and if surgery is planned in the next 1 week to 2 weeks, routine preoperative biliary drainage is not advised except in situations of cholangitis, intense pruritis, or preoperative neoadjuvant chemoradiation.[42,45]

Palliative stenting of distal bile duct strictures relieves symptoms of biliary obstruction and improves quality of life.[46] The endoscopist must decide which type of stent (plastic stent vs SEMSs) to utilize based on several factors. Compared with plastic stents, SEMSs are associated with longer patient survival, fewer interventions, and lower risk of stent dysfunction.[47] The mean patency of plastic stents is 3 months to 4 months in contrast to SEMSs, which have a mean patency of 9 months to 12 months. SEMSs initially were thought to be more costly; however, a meta-analysis found no difference in cost.[48] The 2017 European Society of Gastrointestinal Endoscopy (ESGE) guidelines support the use of SEMSs over plastic stents in all cases of malignant extrahepatic biliary obstruction.[42] No specific designs of SEMSs (covered vs uncovered) have shown a clear benefit in clinical outcomes.[49]

Palliative stenting of hilar bile duct strictures technically is more challenging and less likely to be clinically successful.[50] Therefore, these patients should be referred to high-volume centers with a multidisciplinary hepatobiliary team. Bismuth type III and IV may benefit from a combination of percutaneous biliary drainage and ERCP drainage. Evidence suggests that drainage of greater than 50% of the liver volume leads to a lower incidence of cholangitis and longer patient survival.[51] During ERCP, it is important to avoid opacification of biliary ducts that will not be drained due to an increased risk of cholangitis. Finally, uncovered stents are preferred for drainage of malignant hilar obstruction owing to limited data with the use of covered stents and concern for occlusion of smaller biliary branches joining at the hilum.[52]

Primary Sclerosing Cholangitis

PSC is a chronic inflammatory hepatobiliary tract disease of unknown etiology. Complications of PSC include fibrosis and bile duct strictures. MRCP is preferred over ERCP to establish a diagnosis of PSC.[53] The cholangiographic features of PSC include multifocal intrahepatic and extrahepatic bile duct strictures (beaded appearance) and slight biliary dilatation. Patients with PSC may benefit from endoscopic therapy for dominant strictures or biliary stones.[54] Dominant strictures are defined as strictures less than 1.5 mm in diameter in extrahepatic ducts and less than 1 mm in diameter in intrahepatic ducts. Most dominant strictures are benign; however, malignancy should be ruled out with brush cytology, intraductal biopsy, or direct cholangioscopy. Routine cytology brushing and biopsy have low sensitivity. Fluorescence in situ hybridization increases the sensitivity modestly for detection of cholangiocarcinoma.[55]

Endoscopic treatment of dominant strictures in PSC is different compared with other strictures described in previous sections. Antibiotic prophylaxis is recommended to reduce cholangitis in all PSC patients undergoing ERCP. Often balloon or catheter dilation (using 4–6 mm balloons) is sufficient to relieve biliary obstruction and reduce the risk of cholangitis. Placement of biliary stents, while effective in treating the stricture, could increase the risk of postprocedural complications (cholangitis), with a relative risk of 6.8.[56] If a stent is used to treat a stricture that is, refractory to balloon dilation, it is recommended that the stent be removed as early as possible, typically 1 week to 2 weeks after insertion.[57]

Cholangitis

Fever, right upper quadrant pain, jaundice, hypotension, and altered mental status encompass Reynolds pentad, a classic description for acute cholangitis. The Tokyo guidelines were created in 2006 to add objective measures to increase the diagnosis of cholangitis. They define severe disease (grade III) as the presence of organ dysfunction whereas moderate disease (grade II) can be seen with 2 of the following 5 criteria: white blood cells greater than 12,000 μL or less than 4000 μL; fever greater than 39°C; age greater than 75 years; bilirubin greater than 5mg/dL; and albumin less than 0.7 × lower limit of normal. Acute cholangitis occurs most commonly in the setting of bile duct stones and bile duct stents.[58] Alternative etiologies include biliary strictures, malignant obstruction, post-ERCP, Mirizzi syndrome, and parasitic infections.[59]

Treatment of acute cholangitis includes supportive care, antibiotics, and biliary drainage. Biliary drainage should be performed within 24 hours to 48 hours in mild to moderate disease or within 24 hours in severe cholangitis or those with mild/moderate disease who did not respond to conservative management.[60] Endoscopic sphincterotomy with stone extraction and/or stent insertion is the treatment of choice but may vary depending on the initial etiology of cholangitis (**Fig. 6**). An alternative for

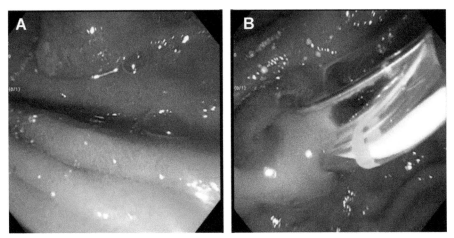

Fig. 6. Cholangitis. (*A*) Protuberant duodenal papilla. (*B*) Sphincterotomy and subsequent pustular drainage.

patients in whom ERCP is unsuccessful or in those with surgically altered anatomy is percutaneous transhepatic biliary drainage (PTBD) or recently emerging EUS-guided transluminal biliary drainage (or EUS-guided hepaticoenterostomy).[61]

EUS-guided transluminal biliary drainage is performed by passing a 19-gauge needle through the intestinal lumen (stomach or duodenum) into the biliary tract and contrast is injected to confirm proper location by fluoroscopy. A guide wire then is inserted into the biliary tract. The tract between bile duct and intestinal wall is dilated using a biliary dilation catheter or a balloon. Then a biliary stent is deployed into the bile duct.[62] Although there are few data for this procedure in the setting of acute cholangitis, this appears to be a promising technique in the urgent setting because of the ability to obtain quick source control over an alternative like EDGE in surgically altered anatomy.[63,64]

Sphincter of Oddi Dysfunction

Biliary sphincter of Oddi dysfunction (SOD) may present with signs and symptoms of biliary or pancreatic disease. It traditionally was categorized into types I, II, and III. This has been abandoned for a new classification that is more clinically accurate. Patients labeled as SOD type I have biliary-like pain, abnormal liver function tests ($>2\times$ normal) on 2 occasions and a dilated bile duct (>8 mm on ultrasound). These patients now are recognized as having an organic problem (sphincter fibrosis or microlithiasis) that should be termed, *sphincter of Oddi stenosis*.[65] SOD type II patients present with biliary-like pain and either elevated liver function tests or biliary ductal dilation that now is called, *suspected functional biliary sphincter disorder*. SOD type III patients have only biliary-like pain, and generally this term has been discarded and ERCP approaches no longer are appropriate in these patients.[65]

ERCP with biliary sphincterotomy is the treatment of choice for those with definite evidence of biliary stenosis or microlithiasis (formerly SOD type I). ERCP for the diagnosis of suspected functional biliary sphincter disorders is now limited and largely has been replaced by CT, MRCP, and EUS. ERCP in these patients portends a high risk of post-ERCP pancreatitis (10%–15%) even in expert hands. In SOD type II, ERCP with sphincter manometry may assist with diagnosis, because elevated basal biliary pressures predicted the outcome of biliary sphincterotomy.[66,67] The acceptable upper limit of normal for basal biliary pressure is 35 mm Hg to 40 mm Hg.[68] Manometry is performed with a pull-back technique, using a water-perfused catheter system. Provider confidence in the accuracy of sphincter manometry has declined in recent years, however, due to the concerns over reproducibility.[69] Most centers now are performing empiric ERCP with biliary sphincterotomy without manometry in patients with a high probability of SOD type II.

Ampullary Adenomas

Ampullary adenomas are a special subset of duodenal lesions that can present sporadically or in patients with familial adenomatous polyposis. Sporadic ampullary adenomas are rare and often asymptomatic, but, when identified, should be resected because of potential for cancerous transformation.[70] Until 1982, ampullary adenomas were treated surgically with pancreaticoduodenectomy.[71] Now, endoscopic ampullectomy is considered first line because it is less invasive and has a lower morbidity.[72] Determining which lesions can be removed safely endoscopically remains unclear. Lesions with the following high-risk features should have EUS for staging purposes prior to considering endoscopic intervention: size greater than 1 cm, high-grade dysplasia, ulceration, irregular margins, spontaneous bleeding, or firmness.[73] It generally is agreed that lesions larger than 4 cm should be referred to surgery.[74] Surgical excision also is recommended for lesions with carcinoma, lymph node involvement, or when an experienced endoscopist is not available.[75]

En bloc resection is preferred and should be attempted in all cases. It generally is recommended to avoid the use of submucosal injection because it may alter the anatomy of the lesion and decrease the chance of complete resection.[73] Endoscopic ampullectomy is performed using a snare with electrocautery similar to polypectomy. Adjunctive tissue ablation of any residual adenomatous tissue can be carried out with argon plasma coagulation, monopolar, or bipolar coagulation. Current data support temporary prophylactic pancreatic duct stenting to prevent pancreatitis after ampullectomy.[76,77]

COMPLICATIONS ASSOCIATED WITH PANCREATICOBILIARY ENDOSCOPY
Complications of Endoscopic Retrograde Cholangiopancreatography

The declining use of diagnostic ERCP over the past 2 decades largely is related to the risk of adverse events and that less-invasive imaging modalities now are available. Post-ERCP complications occur in 5% to 10% of patients.[78–81] Complications include pancreatitis, bleeding, perforation, cholangitis, cholecystitis, stent-related adverse events, cardiopulmonary events, endoscopic-related infection, and death. The most common adverse event is pancreatitis in approximately 5% of patients.[80,81] Established risk factors for post-ERCP pancreatitis include patient-related factors (suspected SOD, female sex, history of previous pancreatitis, and post-ERCP pancreatitis) and procedure-related factors (difficult cannulation, pancreatic guidewire passage more than once, and contrast injection into the pancreatic duct).[82] Prevention of post-ERCP pancreatitis has been studied widely and society guidelines support the use of early precut sphincterotomy for challenging biliary cannulation, pancreatic duct stenting in high-risk patients, administration of rectal indomethacin, and periprocedural intravenous hydration with lactated Ringer solution.[82,83]

Bleeding after ERCP is related most commonly to biliary or pancreatic sphincterotomy. Risk factors include coagulopathy, active cholangitis, anticoagulation within 3 days of the procedure, low endoscopist case volume, and bleeding noted during the procedure. Papillary balloon dilation can be used as an alternative to sphincterotomy to decrease the risk of bleeding. This is associated, however, with increased risk of post-ERCP pancreatitis and should be used only in carefully selected patients.[52]

Infectious complications include acute cholangitis, sepsis, cholecystitis, and duodenoscope-related infections. Acute cholangitis occurs more often in patients with hilar cholangiocarcinoma, PSC, and history of liver transplantation. In such patients, it is important to provide periprocedural antibiotics and avoid contract injection into regions not intended to be drained through stenting.[84] Finally, sterilization of duodenoscope is difficult due to the elevator mechanism leading to transmission of multidrug-resistant organisms. There have been several cases of duodenoscope-related infections, including some deaths in the recent years. The Food and Drug Administration revised the reprocessing protocol to include 1 or more supplemental reprocessing measures beyond the standard, which included repeat high-level disinfection, microbiological culture, ethylene oxide gas sterilization, and liquid chemical sterilization.[85] Despite adding this extra step, outbreaks still have occurred. Future solutions include disposable endoscope parts or disposable endoscopes to prevent infection.[85]

Complications of Endoscopic Ultrasound

Diagnostic EUS is associated with very low complication rates, ranging from 0.03% to 0.15%, similar to that of upper endoscopy.[86] Risk of perforation with EUS is slightly higher compared with traditional upper endoscopy. Complications after EUS-guided fine-needle biopsy are similarly low, at 0.3% to 6.3%, and include postprocedural pain, AP, infection, and hemorrhage.[86,87] Interventional EUS procedures are associated with higher complication rates: 5% to 11% for EUS-guided drainage of pancreatic fluid collections,[88] up to 17% for EUS-guided biliary drainage,[89] 5% to 43% for EUS-guided pancreatic duct drainage, and approximately 10% for EUS-guided gallbladder drainage.[88]

SUMMARY

Endoscopic treatments are effective in the management of a wide spectrum of pancreaticobiliary diseases with a plethora of medical and endoscopic treatment options. Although the use of ERCP has decreased, it remains the primary modality for managing indeterminant biliary strictures, obstructive jaundice, and choledocholithiasis. EUS serves as a safe diagnostic tool and continues to grow as an interventional tool.

CLINICS CARE POINTS

- ERCP is not routinely recommended to identify the etiology of pancreatitis
- Endoscopic ultrasound is a safe and minimally invasive way to obtain structural information about the pancreas
- Pancreas divisum alone should no longer be consider a cause of pancreatitis, but certain genetic mutations may predispose patients with PD to recurrent acute pancreatitis
- Patients at high risk for choledocholithiasis should undergo ERCP for definitive management
- Dominant strictures in primary sclerosing cholangitis are treated differently compared with other biliary strictures

DISCLOSURE

The authors have no conflicts to disclose pertinent to this article.

REFERENCES

1. Kozarek RA. The Past, present, and future of endoscopic retrograde cholangio-pancreatography. Gastroenterol Hepatol (N Y). 2017;13(10):620–2. Available at: https://www.ncbi.nlm.nih.gov/pubmed/29230140.
2. Wang G-J, Gao C-F, Wei D, et al. Acute pancreatitis: etiology and common pathogenesis. World J Gastroenterol 2009;15(12):1427–30.
3. Vivian E, Cler L, Conwell D, et al. Acute pancreatitis task force on quality: development of quality indicators for acute pancreatitis management. Am J Gastroenterol 2019;114(8):1322–42. Available at: https://journals.lww.com/ajg/Fulltext/2019/08000/Acute_Pancreatitis_Task_Force_on_Quality_.24.aspx.
4. Thevenot A, Bournet B, Otal P, et al. Endoscopic ultrasound and magnetic resonance cholangiopancreatography in patients with idiopathic acute pancreatitis. Dig Dis Sci 2013;58(8):2361–8.
5. Elmunzer BJ. Endoscopic drainage of pancreatic fluid collections. Clin Gastroenterol Hepatol 2018;16(12):1851–63.e3.
6. Fukami N. EUS for pancreaticobiliary duct access and drainage. In: Adler DG, editor. Advanced pancreaticobiliary endoscopy. 1st edition. Switzerland: Spinger International Publishing; 2016. p. 193–204.
7. Baron TH, DiMaio CJ, Wang AY, et al. American gastroenterological association clinical practice update: management of pancreatic necrosis. Gastroenterology 2020;158(1):67–75.e1.
8. Sahai AV, Zimmerman M, Aabakken L, et al. Prospective assessment of the ability of endoscopic ultrasound to diagnose, exclude, or establish the severity of chronic pancreatitis found by endoscopic retrograde cholangiopancreatography. Gastrointest Endosc 1998;48(1):18–25.
9. Wallace MB, Hawes RH. Endoscopic ultrasound in the evaluation and treatment of chronic pancreatitis. Pancreas 2001;23(1):26–35.
10. Kaufman M, Singh G, Das S, et al. Efficacy of endoscopic ultrasound-guided celiac plexus block and celiac plexus neurolysis for managing abdominal pain associated with chronic pancreatitis and pancreatic cancer. J Clin Gastroenterol 2010;44(2):127–34. Available at: https://journals.lww.com/jcge/Fulltext/2010/02000/Efficacy_of_Endoscopic_Ultrasound_guided_Celiac.13.aspx.
11. Dumonceau J-M, Delhaye M, Tringali A, et al. Endoscopic treatment of chronic pancreatitis: European society of gastrointestinal endoscopy (ESGE) clinical guideline. Endoscopy 2012;44(8):784–800.
12. Telford JJ, Farrell JJ, Saltzman JR, et al. Pancreatic stent placement for duct disruption. Gastrointest Endosc 2002;56(1):18–24.
13. Barth BA, Husain SZ. No title. In: Feldman M, Friedman LS, Brandt LJ, editors. Sleisenger and Fordtran's gastrointestinal and liver disease. 10th edition. Philadelphia: Elsevier; 2016. p. 923–33.e4.
14. Bertin C, Pelletier A-L, Vullierme MP, et al. Pancreas divisum is not a cause of pancreatitis by itself but acts as a partner of genetic mutations. Am J Gastroenterol 2012;107(2):311–7. Available at: https://journals.lww.com/ajg/Fulltext/2012/02000/Pancreas_Divisum_Is_Not_a_Cause_of_Pancreatitis_by.26.aspx.
15. Sherman S, Freeman ML, Tarnasky PR, et al. Administration of secretin (RG1068) increases the sensitivity of detection of duct abnormalities by magnetic

resonance cholangiopancreatography in patients with pancreatitis. Gastroenterology 2014;147(3):646–54.e2.

16. Fogel EL, Toth TG, Lehman GA, et al. Does endoscopic therapy favorably affect the outcome of patients who have recurrent acute pancreatitis and pancreas divisum? Pancreas 2007;34(1):21–45.

17. Coté GA, Durkalski-Mauldin VL, Serrano J, et al. SpHincterotomy for acute recurrent pancreatitis randomized trial: rationale, methodology, and potential implications. Pancreas 2019;48(8):1061–7.

18. Vila JJ, Kutz M. Sphincterotomy of the minor papilla. Video J Encycl GI Endosc 2013;1(2):588–92.

19. Elta GH, Enestvedt BK, Sauer BG, et al. ACG clinical guideline: diagnosis and management of pancreatic cysts. Am J Gastroenterol 2018;113(4):464–79.

20. Polkowski M, Jenssen C, Kaye P, et al. Technical aspects of endoscopic ultrasound (EUS)-guided sampling in gastroenterology: European society of gastrointestinal endoscopy (ESGE) technical guideline - March 2017. Endoscopy 2017; 49(10):989–1006.

21. Cheesman AR, Zhu H, Liao X, et al. Impact of EUS-guided microforceps biopsy and needle-based confocal laser endomicroscopy on the diagnostic yield and clinical management of pancreatic cystic lesions. Gastrointest Endosc 2019. https://doi.org/10.1016/j.gie.2019.12.022.

22. Zhang M-M, Zhong N, Wang X, et al. Endoscopic ultrasound-guided needle-based confocal laser endomicroscopy for diagnosis of gastric subepithelial tumors: a pilot study. Endoscopy 2019;51(6):560–5.

23. Wang W, Shpaner A, Krishna SG, et al. Use of EUS-FNA in diagnosing pancreatic neoplasm without a definitive mass on CT. Gastrointest Endosc 2013;78(1): 73–80.

24. Navaneethan U, Njei B, Lourdusamy V, et al. Comparative effectiveness of biliary brush cytology and intraductal biopsy for detection of malignant biliary strictures: a systematic review and meta-analysis. Gastrointest Endosc 2015;81(1):168–76.

25. Dormann A, Meisner S, Verin N, et al. Self-expanding metal stents for gastroduodenal malignancies: systematic review of their clinical effectiveness. Endoscopy 2004;36(6):543–50.

26. Tyberg A, Perez-Miranda M, Sanchez-Ocana R, et al. Endoscopic ultrasound-guided gastrojejunostomy with a lumen-apposing metal stent: a multicenter, international experience. Endosc Int Open 2016;4(3):E276–81.

27. Khashab MA, Kumbhari V, Grimm IS, et al. EUS-guided gastroenterostomy: the first U.S. clinical experience (with video). Gastrointest Endosc 2015;82(5):932–8.

28. Jang S, Stevens T, Lopez R, et al. Superiority of gastrojejunostomy over endoscopic stenting for palliation of malignant gastric outlet obstruction. Clin Gastroenterol Hepatol 2019;17(7):1295–302.e1.

29. Mohan BP, Khan SR, Trakroo S, et al. Endoscopic ultrasound-guided gallbladder drainage, transpapillary drainage, or percutaneous drainage in high risk acute cholecystitis patients: a systematic review and comparative meta-analysis. Endoscopy 2019. https://doi.org/10.1055/a-1020-3932.

30. Ko CW, Lee SP. Epidemiology and natural history of common bile duct stones and prediction of disease. Gastrointest Endosc 2002;56(6 Suppl):S165–9.

31. Maple JT, Ben-Menachem T, Anderson MA, et al. The role of endoscopy in the evaluation of suspected choledocholithiasis. Gastrointest Endosc 2010; 71(1):1–9.

32. Yasuda I, Itoi T. Recent advances in endoscopic management of difficult bile duct stones. Dig Endosc 2013;25(4):376–85.

33. Bukhari M, Kowalski T, Nieto J, et al. An international, multicenter, comparative trial of EUS-guided gastrogastrostomy-assisted ERCP versus enteroscopy-assisted ERCP in patients with Roux-en-Y gastric bypass anatomy. Gastrointest Endosc 2018;88(3):486–94.
34. Kedia P, Sharaiha RZ, Kumta NA, et al. Internal EUS-directed transgastric ERCP (EDGE): game over. Gastroenterology 2014;147(3):566–8.
35. Visrodia KH, Tabibian JH, Baron TH. Endoscopic management of benign biliary strictures. World J Gastrointest Endosc 2015;7(11):1003–13.
36. Shanbhogue AKP, Tirumani SH, Prasad SR, et al. Benign biliary strictures: a current comprehensive clinical and imaging review. Am J Roentgenol 2011;197(2): W295–306.
37. Judah JR, Draganov PV. Endoscopic therapy of benign biliary strictures. World J Gastroenterol 2007;13(26):3531–9.
38. Bismuth H, Majno PE. Biliary strictures: classification based on the principles of surgical treatment. World J Surg 2001;25(10):1241–4.
39. Chiang A, Theriault M, Salim M, et al. The incremental benefit of EUS for the identification of malignancy in indeterminate extrahepatic biliary strictures: a systematic review and meta-analysis. Endosc Ultrasound 2019;8(5):310–7.
40. Parsa N, Khashab MA. The role of peroral cholangioscopy in evaluating indeterminate biliary strictures. Clin Endosc 2019;52(6):556–64.
41. Kim HJ, Kim MH, Lee SK, et al. Tumor vessel: a valuable cholangioscopic clue of malignant biliary stricture. Gastrointest Endosc 2000;52(5):635–8.
42. Dumonceau J-M, Tringali A, Papanikolaou IS, et al. Endoscopic biliary stenting: indications, choice of stents, and results: European Society of gastrointestinal endoscopy (ESGE) clinical guideline - updated October 2017. Endoscopy 2018;50(9):910–30.
43. Ma MX, Jayasekeran V, Chong AK. Benign biliary strictures: prevalence, impact, and management strategies. Clin Exp Gastroenterol 2019;12:83–92.
44. Khan MA, Baron TH, Kamal F, et al. Efficacy of self-expandable metal stents in management of benign biliary strictures and comparison with multiple plastic stents: a meta-analysis. Endoscopy 2017;49(7):682–94.
45. Anderson MA, Appalaneni V, Ben-Menachem T, et al. The role of endoscopy in the evaluation and treatment of patients with biliary neoplasia. Gastrointest Endosc 2013;77(2):167–74.
46. Abraham NS, Barkun JS, Barkun AN. Palliation of malignant biliary obstruction: a prospective trial examining impact on quality of life. Gastrointest Endosc 2002; 56(6):835–41.
47. Almadi MA, Barkun A, Martel M. Plastic vs. self-expandable metal stents for palliation in malignant biliary obstruction: a series of meta-analyses. Am J Gastroenterol 2017;112(2):260–73.
48. Zorrón Pu L, de Moura EGH, Bernardo WM, et al. Endoscopic stenting for inoperable malignant biliary obstruction: a systematic review and meta-analysis. World J Gastroenterol 2015;21(47):13374–85.
49. Tringali A, Giannetti A, Adler DG. Endoscopic management of gastric outlet obstruction disease. Ann Gastroenterol 2019;32(4):330–7.
50. Liu CL, Lo CM, Lai EC, et al. Endoscopic retrograde cholangiopancreatography and endoscopic endoprosthesis insertion in patients with Klatskin tumors. Arch Surg 1998;133(3):293–6.
51. Vienne A, Hobeika E, Gouya H, et al. Prediction of drainage effectiveness during endoscopic stenting of malignant hilar strictures: the role of liver volume assessment. Gastrointest Endosc 2010;72(4):728–35.

52. Park J-S, Jeong S, Kobayashi M, et al. Safety, efficacy, and removability of a fully covered multi-hole metal stent in a swine model of hilar biliary stricture: a feasibility study. Endosc Int Open 2019;7(4):E498–503.

53. Dave M, Elmunzer BJ, Dwamena BA, et al. Primary sclerosing cholangitis: meta-analysis of diagnostic performance of MR cholangiopancreatography. Radiology 2010;256(2):387–96.

54. Lindor KD, Kowdley KV, Harrison EM. ACG clinical guideline: primary sclerosing cholangitis. Am J Gastroenterol 2015;110(5):646–59. Available at: https://journals.lww.com/ajg/Fulltext/2015/05000/ACG_Clinical_Guideline__Primary_Sclerosing.10.aspx.

55. Fricker ZP, Lichtenstein DR. Primary sclerosing cholangitis: a concise review of diagnosis and management. Dig Dis Sci 2019;64(3):632–42.

56. Ponsioen CY, Arnelo U, Bergquist A, et al. No superiority of stents vs balloon dilatation for dominant strictures in patients with primary sclerosing cholangitis. Gastroenterology 2018;155(3):752–9.e5.

57. Aabakken L, Karlsen TH, Albert J, et al. Role of endoscopy in primary sclerosing cholangitis: European society of gastrointestinal endoscopy (ESGE) and European association for the study of the liver (EASL) clinical guideline. Endoscopy 2017;49(06):588–608.

58. Kimura Y, Takada T, Kawarada Y, et al. Definitions, pathophysiology, and epidemiology of acute cholangitis and cholecystitis: Tokyo guidelines. J Hepatobiliary Pancreat Surg 2007;14(1):15–26.

59. Lan Cheong Wah D, Christophi C, Muralidharan V. Acute cholangitis: current concepts. ANZ J Surg 2017;87(7–8):554–9.

60. Kiriyama S, Kozaka K, Takada T, et al. Tokyo guidelines 2018: diagnostic criteria and severity grading of acute cholangitis (with videos). J Hepatobiliary Pancreat Sci 2018;25(1):17–30.

61. Poincloux L, Rouquette O, Buc E, et al. Endoscopic ultrasound-guided biliary drainage after failed ERCP: cumulative experience of 101 procedures at a single center. Endoscopy 2015;47(9):794–801.

62. Khashab MA, Messallam AA, Penas I, et al. International multicenter comparative trial of transluminal EUS-guided biliary drainage via hepatogastrostomy vs. choledochoduodenostomy approaches. Endosc Int Open 2016;4(2):E175–81.

63. Ogura T, Takenaka M, Shiomi H, et al. Long-term outcomes of EUS-guided transluminal stent deployment for benign biliary disease: Multicenter clinical experience (with videos). Endosc Ultrasound 2019;8(6):398–403.

64. James TW, Fan YC, Baron TH. EUS-guided hepaticoenterostomy as a portal to allow definitive antegrade treatment of benign biliary diseases in patients with surgically altered anatomy. Gastrointest Endosc 2018;88(3):547–54.

65. Cotton PB, Elta GH, Carter CR, et al. Rome IV. Gallbladder and Sphincter of Oddi Disorders. Gastroenterology 2016. https://doi.org/10.1053/j.gastro.2016.02.033.

66. Geenen JE, Hogan WJ, Dodds WJ, et al. The efficacy of endoscopic sphincterotomy after cholecystectomy in patients with sphincter-of-Oddi dysfunction. N Engl J Med 1989;320(2):82–7.

67. Toouli J, Roberts-Thomson IC, Kellow J, et al. Manometry based randomised trial of endoscopic sphincterotomy for sphincter of Oddi dysfunction. Gut 2000;46(1):98–102.

68. Eversman D, Fogel EL, Rusche M, et al. Frequency of abnormal pancreatic and biliary sphincter manometry compared with clinical suspicion of sphincter of Oddi dysfunction. Gastrointest Endosc 1999;50(5):637–41.

69. Suarez AL, Pauls Q, Durkalski-Mauldin V, et al. Sphincter of Oddi manometry: reproducibility of measurements and effect of sphincterotomy in the EPISOD study. J Neurogastroenterol Motil 2016;22(3):477–82.
70. Seifert E, Schulte F, Stolte M. Adenoma and carcinoma of the duodenum and papilla of Vater: a clinicopathologic study. Am J Gastroenterol 1992;87(1):37–42.
71. Ito K, Fujita N, Noda Y, et al. Diagnosis of Ampullary Cancer. Digestive Surgery 2010;27(2):115–8. https://doi.org/10.1159/000286607.
72. Ridtitid W, Tan D, Schmidt SE, et al. Endoscopic papillectomy: risk factors for incomplete resection and recurrence during long-term follow-up. Gastrointest Endosc 2014;79(2):289–96.
73. Chini P, Draganov PV. Diagnosis and management of ampullary adenoma: the expanding role of endoscopy. World J Gastrointest Endosc 2011;3(12):241–7.
74. Chathadi KV, Khashab MA, Acosta RD, et al. The role of endoscopy in ampullary and duodenal adenomas. Gastrointest Endosc 2015;82(5):773–81.
75. Espinel J, Pinedo E, Ojeda V, et al. Endoscopic management of adenomatous ampullary lesions. World J Methodol 2015;5(3):127–35.
76. Harewood GC, Pochron NL, Gostout CJ. Prospective, randomized, controlled trial of prophylactic pancreatic stent placement for endoscopic snare excision of the duodenal ampulla. Gastrointest Endosc 2005;62(3):367–70.
77. Kim SH, Moon JH, Choi HJ, et al. Usefulness of pancreatic duct wire-guided endoscopic papillectomy for ampullary adenoma for preventing post-procedure pancreatitis. Endoscopy 2013;45(10):838–41.
78. Loperfido S, Angelini G, Benedetti G, et al. Major early complications from diagnostic and therapeutic ERCP: a prospective multicenter study. Gastrointest Endosc 1998;48(1):1–10.
79. Freeman ML, Nelson DB, Sherman S, et al. Complications of endoscopic biliary sphincterotomy. N Engl J Med 1996;335(13):909–18.
80. Wang P, Li Z-S, Liu F, et al. Risk factors for ERCP-related complications: a prospective multicenter study. Am J Gastroenterol 2009;104(1):31–40.
81. Williams EJ, Taylor S, Fairclough P, et al. Risk factors for complication following ERCP; results of a large-scale, prospective multicenter study. Endoscopy 2007;39(9):793–801.
82. Dumonceau J-M, Kapral C, Aabakken L, et al. ERCP-related adverse events: European society of gastrointestinal endoscopy (ESGE) guideline. Endoscopy 2020;52(2):127–49.
83. Chandrasekhara V, Khashab MA, Muthusamy VR, et al. Adverse events associated with ERCP. Gastrointest Endosc 2017;85(1):32–47.
84. Khashab MA, Chithadi KV, Acosta RD, et al. Antibiotic prophylaxis for GI endoscopy. Gastrointest Endosc 2015;81(1):81–9.
85. Balan GG, Sfarti CV, Chiriac SA, et al. Duodenoscope-associated infections: a review. Eur J Clin Microbiol Infect Dis 2019;38(12):2205–13.
86. Jenssen C, Alvarez-Sanchez MV, Napoleon B, et al. Diagnostic endoscopic ultrasonography: assessment of safety and prevention of complications. World J Gastroenterol 2012;18(34):4659–76.
87. Jacobson BC, Adler DG, Davila RE, et al. ASGE guideline: complications of EUS. Gastrointest Endosc 2005;61(1):8–12.
88. Saumoy M, Kahaleh M. Safety and Complications of interventional endoscopic ultrasound. Clin Endosc 2018;51(3):235–8.
89. Khan MA, Akbar A, Baron TH, et al. Endoscopic ultrasound-guided biliary drainage: a systematic review and meta-analysis. Dig Dis Sci 2016;61(3):684–703.

Principles of Intramural Surgery

Christine Tat, MD[a], Juan S. Barajas-Gamboa, MD[a], Matthew Kroh, MD[b],*

KEYWORDS

- Intramural surgery • Endoscopic surgery • Third space endoscopy

KEY POINTS

- Intramural surgery is an emerging minimally invasive surgical technique that is based on flexible endoscopy. The technique utilizes the submucosal plane to separate the mucosal layer from the underlying muscle, thereby minimizing the risk of full-thickness perforation and gastrointestinal leakage.
- Currently, there are 5 main applications of intramural surgery: peroral endoscopic myotomy for achalasia, peroral pyloromyotomy for gastroparesis, submucosal tunneling endoscopic resection of subepithelial tumors, flexible endoscopic diverticulotomy for Zenker diverticulum, and peroral endoscopic tunneling for restoration of the esophagus.
- There are 4 key steps: initial submucosal bleb injection and mucosal incision for entry point, creation of submucosal tunnel, myotomy or resection of lesion, and closure of the mucosal entry point.

INTRODUCTION

As the field of surgery evolves, minimally invasive surgery has expanded into many different forms. Although laparoscopic surgery is the most commonly considered of the minimally invasive surgical techniques, other modifications include the use of tele-robotics and increasingly complex procedures performed by flexible endoscopy. One of these forms is intramural surgery. Intramural surgery employs advanced flexible endoscopic techniques to accomplish surgical goals. Gastrointestinal endoscopy has existed for more than 60 years, but, in the past decade, novel procedures have been introduced, partly based on techniques and tools used for endoscopic mucosal resection (EMR) and endoscopic submucosal dissection (ESD).[1] Intramural surgery has emerged as a continuation of these techniques.

In the literature, intramural surgery is known interchangeably as third-space endoscopy. The first space refers to the true gastrointestinal lumen. The second space

[a] Digestive Disease Institute, Cleveland Clinic Abu Dhabi, PO Box 112412, Abu Dhabi, United Arab Emirates; [b] Digestive Disease Institute, Cleveland Clinic Abu Dhabi, Cleveland Clinic Lerner College of Medicine, PO Box 112412, Abu Dhabi, United Arab Emirates
* Corresponding author.
E-mail addresses: KrohM@ClevelandClinicAbuDhabi.ae; KrohM@ccf.org

describes the peritoneal or thoracic cavities, and thus the third space is in reference to the intramural or submucosal space.[2] The submucosal space is the plane between the mucosa and the muscularis propria comprised of loose areolar tissue. Recognition of this intermediate plane as a working space presents a different application for advanced flexible endoscopic techniques.

Natural orifice transluminal endoscopic surgery (NOTES) received significant attention and research protocols approximately a decade ago.[3] In its true sense, this used flexible endoscopy to perform surgeries without leaving any external scars, although often under the surveillance or assistance of laparoscopy. Most commonly, the operative field was established through the stomach or vagina. There was considerable concern, however, regarding leakage from the gastrotomy or enterotomy site as well as the limited clinical improvements on existing techniques. Laparoscopic surgery was well established as a minimally invasive technique, supported by literature that demonstrated safe and effective results with short hospital length of stay and reduced pain. The external scars were relatively small with minimal complications, although trocar site pain and hernia commonly are reported. Consequently, NOTES has had limited clinical applications.

Nevertheless, NOTES provided the fundamental concept necessary to develop intramural surgery. In 2007, Sumiyama and colleagues[4] were the first to describe submucosal endoscopy with mucosal flap safety valve. They showed technical feasibility and safety with both ex vivo organ tissues and in vivo pig study. First, with endoscopic guidance, a submucosal tunnel was created using carbon dioxide (CO_2) insufflation and balloon dissection. Then, a full-thickness gastric muscle resection was performed. In their last step, the mucosal flap was sealed. The closure of the mucosal flap layer was and remains critical in protecting against peritoneal spillage. Following that study, Pasricha and colleagues[5] demonstrated feasibility and safety of submucosal endoscopic esophageal myotomy in porcine model. Soon after, Inoue and colleagues[6] published the first results of peroral endoscopic myotomy (POEM) for achalasia in humans. There were 17 patients in the study. All patients had significant improvement in their dysphagia symptom score (mean 10–1.3; $P = .0003$) and there were no serious complications.

APPLICATIONS OF INTRAMURAL SURGERY

Currently, POEM is the most studied procedure in the area of intramural surgery. Since the establishment of safety, feasibility, and efficacy of POEM, including data on 5-year and longer outcomes, intramural surgery has expanded to include several other procedures.[7] These include submucosal tunneling endoscopic resection (STER), peroral pyloromyotomy (POP), flexible endoscopic diverticulotomy (FED) for Zenker diverticulum, and, most recently a new application, peroral endoscopic tunneling for restoration of the esophagus (POETRE).[8]

STER removes subepithelial gastrointestinal tumors originating from the muscularis propria. The most commonly reported locations for resection are esophagus and stomach. Although most of these tumors are benign, some harbor malignant potential. En bloc resection rates via this technique range from 83.3% to 100% in the foregut.[9–11]

In patients with refractory gastroparesis, POP, also known as gastric-POEM, provides an alternative to traditional open or laparoscopic pyloromyotomy. After establishing the submucosal tunnel, the pyloric muscle is divided to the duodenum. Early studies show that POP is technically feasible, safe, and effective in the short term with limited accrued data on long-term efficacy and comparison to laparoscopic pyloroplasty.[12]

Recently, FED has been described as a treatment of Zenker diverticulum. Traditional open surgical approach to Zenker diverticulum was through a left neck incision with subsequent cricopharyngeal myotomy with and without diverticulectomy. Previously, the main alternative to the open surgical approach was a method by rigid endoscopy and a stapled diverticuloplasty to the true lumen of the esophagus. Rigid endoscopy, however, has limitations. This technique requires general anesthesia and neck hyperextension. There was a relatively high rate of inability to complete the procedure secondary to small diverticular size.[13] In a review by Leong and colleagues,[14] out of 585 cases, 45 (7.7%) of cases were terminated prematurely. The most common reason was due to small pouch, accounting for 42% of incomplete cases. Subsequently, FED was developed as an additional technique for treatment of Zenker diverticulum. This approach involves submucosal tunneling to divide the septum between the esophageal and diverticular lumen. The cricopharyngeal muscle is contained in this septum and thus divided as well.[15]

In 2017, Wagh[16] published the first study detailing POETRE as a procedure used to treat complete esophageal obstruction. Complete esophageal occlusion is rare but occurs most frequently in patients after chemoradiation for head and neck malignancies. This technique utilizes submucosal tunneling for re-establishing the esophageal lumen after iatrogenic obliteration. The submucosal tunnel is created using combination of antegrade and retrograde (ie, by gastrostomy tube tract) endoscopy.

PREPARATION AND EQUIPMENT

The foundation of intramural surgery lies in flexible endoscopy. Therefore, it is key to first have a solid understanding of endoscopic surgical tools. In this section, the general equipment and most frequently used endoscopic tools are introduced.

Endoscope

A standard endoscope used for diagnostic endoscopy is a front-viewing gastroscope and it has a 2.8-mm working channel (GIF-HQ190, Olympus, Tokyo, Japan). It has an outer diameter of 9.2 mm and includes an integrated water channel.[8] This endoscope can be used for most of the intramural surgery-related procedures. Alternatively, other endoscopes have instrument channels that range in from 1.2 mm to 6.0 mm in size.[15] Different-sized working channels can accommodate a variety of instruments. Therapeutic endoscopes may have channel sizes as large as 6.0 mm for the purpose of foreign body removal or blood evacuation. Also, water jet capability generally is included with a standard endoscope. This function is vital to most intramural surgical procedures. The water jet infusion helps with clearing the operative field, especially in the setting of bleeding or accumulated tissue debris.

Electrosurgical Knives

There are several electrosurgical knives that are commonly used for intramural surgery[8]:

- Triangle Tip (TT) Knife (KD-640L, Olympus)
- TT Knife J (KD-645L, Olympus)
- HybridKnife (20,150–060, Erbe Marietta, Georgia, USA)
- HookKnife (KD-620LR, Olympus)
- And less commonly, ESD knives also may be used, including ITknife nano (KD-612L/U, Olympus).

For most intramural surgery procedures, the authors' group prefers to use the TT knife (KD-640L, Olympus).

Transparent Cap

Most procedures utilize a transparent endoscopic cap that is fitted over the head of the gastroscope.[12] The size and shape of the cap vary depending on manufacturer and indication. These are similar to those used in other applications, including EMR, ESD, and radiofrequency ablation. A beveled silicon-based cap can help guide the endoscope through tissues, elevating tissue planes, and therefore minimizing smudge to the gastroscope camera. The authors prefer to tape the cap to the endoscope head in order to prevent unintentional detachment of the cap from the endoscope.

Submucosal Injection Solutions

Either methylene blue or indigo carmine dye can be used to inject the submucosal space. The submucosal space preferentially absorbs these dyes; therefore, they are helpful for identifying the plane of interest.[8] This allows for differentiation of the submucosal plane from the mucosa and the muscular layers. The authors prefer to use a premixed injection solution composed of 20 mL of 1% methylene blue dye and 500 mL of 0.9% sodium chloride. Additionally, 1 mL of 1:1000 epinephrine may be added for its hemostatic effects, although some endoscopists avoid epinephrine due risk of cholinergic side effects.[17]

Other Relevant Equipment and Accessories

- Electrosurgical generator (VIO 300 D, Erbe)
- Carr-Locke injection needle (23 gauge, 4 mm; US Endoscopy Mentor, Ohio)
- Multi-3V Plus (B-V232P-A, Olympus)
- Hemostatic clips (Resolution 360 Clip, Boston Scientific Malborough, Massachusetts)
- Coagulation forceps (FD-410LR, Olympus)
- Roth Net retriever (US Endoscopy)

PROCEDURE
Preprocedure

Prior to the procedure, a patient should have a detailed work-up to confirm diagnosis. The specific work-up depends on the disease process, stage, and type of procedure. Preoperatively, all patients are kept nothing by mouth. They may be placed on a liquid diet for days preceding the procedure to allow for adequate clearance of food from the lumen of the gastrointestinal tract. This varies depending on surgeon's preference and the procedure type.

Intramural surgery may be performed either in the endoscopy suite or the operating room. General endotracheal intubation typically is used because the procedures tend to be longer in duration, and this allows for best control of the airway and minimizes aspiration risk. Patients can be placed either in a supine or the left lateral decubitus position. Each position has distinct advantages and disadvantages. For example, the left lateral decubitus position can increase the difficulty of POEM procedure in patients with end-stage sigmoid achalasia.[17] Whereas the supine position may lead to poor visualization due to fluid pooling with a posterior myotomy during POEM. At the authors' institution, the supine position is preferred for POEM and left lateral decubitus for POP, STER, and Zenker diverticulotomy. The abdomen is exposed in order observe for signs of significant capnoperitoneum and subsequent access for decompression, if needed.

After the patient is positioned, the patient receives general anesthesia with tracheal intubation in order to minimize aspiration risk. The patient receives preoperative intravenous antibiotics. Prophylactic antibiotics should cover gram-negative bacteria, anaerobic bacteria, and fungus for POEM procedure and may be tailored based on the type and location of procedure performed.[12] The authors use 400 mg of ciprofloxacin, 500 mg of metronidazole, and 200 mg of fluconazole prior to mucosal incision during POEM.

Procedural Steps

At the beginning of any procedure, a diagnostic endoscopy is performed. This is important to assess the baseline anatomy in order to plan the remaining procedure accordingly. For example, location and size should be noted for subepithelial tumors planned for resection. Subepithelial tumors that are greater than 3.5 cm in size less likely are less likely to be removed successfully. The large tumor size limits the extent of the submucosal tunnel. Additionally, the ideal location for tumor resection is along the greater curvature of the distal gastric body and commonly esophageal lesions are more easily accessible.[9] Tumors originating from the proximal fundus or lesser curvature pose more challenges in developing the submucosal tunnel because the location necessitates operating in the retroflexed position or abrupt angulation secondary to esophagogastric (EG) junction.

With achalasia, it is important to examine the esophagus for dilation, peristalsis (or lack of peristalsis) and degree of tightness at the lower esophageal sphincter. Landmarks, including distance of the EG junction from the incisors, and mucosal findings, including significant esophagitis or overlying fungal infections, also may be identified. In both achalasia and gastroparesis, there may be significant residual food and debris that warrant evacuation at the onset of the case.

CO_2 is the insufflating gas of choice. CO_2 has the advantage of rapid diffusion and absorption in tissues compared with room air. Upon absorption into tissues, CO_2 travels by blood flow to the lungs and is eliminated by expiration. Given its favorable properties, it has lower rates of clinically apparent subcutaneous emphysema, mediastinal emphysema, pneumothorax, and capnoperitoneum.[9]

In laparoscopy, CO_2 can be used with high flow rates because the maximum pressure is set at an upper limit and it can be titrated to reduce the hemodynamic changes associated with capnoperitoneum. Endoscopy lacks the capacity, however, to set an upper pressure limit. Thus, extraluminal extravasation of CO_2 can produce significant pneumoperitoneum, pneumomediastinum, and pneumothorax. Increased end-tidal CO_2, increased ventilator peak pressures, and signs of abdominal compartment syndrome may result. It is important to actively communicate with the anesthesiologist regarding hemodynamic changes throughout the case. Increases in any of these parameters should prompt evaluation of the abdomen and lung fields.

Initial submucosal bleb injection with mucosal flap incision

Once a thorough diagnostic endoscopy is complete, the procedure begins by selection of the site for initial submucosal injection and mucosal entry point. Importantly, this mucosal incision should be of appropriate distance away from the planned myotomy site. Distance between the mucosal entry point and the myotomy ensures that there is not be a full-thickness injury and thus reduce the risk of mediastinal or peritoneal leakage. As originally described by Sumiyama and colleagues,[4] this mucosal entry point serves as an essential "mucosal flap safety valve."

The exact location of the initial submucosal injection and mucosal entry point depends on the procedure and the planned length of myotomy or space needed for lesion resection. For example, in POEM, the mucosal incision ranges from 10 cm to 15 cm proximal to the EG junction,[17] whereas for POP, the mucosal entry point is approximately 5 cm from the pylorus.[18] The entry point for STER should be at 5 cm proximal to the subepithelial tumor.[10] The site for initial incision for FED for Zenker diverticulum is at 3 cm proximal to the septum or overlying the septum in preparation for muscle division.[19] For POETRE, the mucosal incision is at 5 cm proximal to the blind end of the esophagus for antegrade tunneling and 5 cm distal to the obstruction for retrograde tunneling.[16]

After selection of the entry point, a submucosal bleb is raised by injecting the submucosal solution with a 25-gauge 4-mm needle. As discussed previously, the authors' submucosal injection solution of choice is a mixture composed of 20 mL of 1% methylene blue dye, 1 mL of 1:1000 epinephrine, and 500 mL of 0.9% sodium chloride, typically not utilizing 1 mL of 1:1000 epinephrine. The dye stains the mucosa and muscularis propria differentially and allows for easier identification of the submucosa, which typically appears dark blue. When the injection is in the correct plane, a sizable weal develops. The bleb should increase in size proportionate to the amount of crystalloid mixture injected. If this weal does not appear, the needle tip likely is in the muscularis propria and should be withdrawn slowly back into the submucosal space.

A mucosal incision then is created over the submucosal bleb (**Fig. 1**). Electrosurgical knives and power settings vary depending on endoscopist's preference and procedure. The authors prefer to use the TT knife (KD-640L, Olympus) with the following settings: cut—Endo Cut Q effect 2 and coag—Spray Coag Effect 2 at 50 W. The TT knife has the ability to cut in any direction without inconveniently rotating the knife. The power settings allow for ease of cut combined with control of mild bleeding. The incision itself generally is 1 cm to 2 cm in length and it can be either transverse or longitudinal. A longitudinal incision may be beneficial in facilitating closure at the end of the case. After the initial incision, the TT knife can be used to place downward pressure on the lip of the mucosa. This separates the mucosa from the underlying submucosa. Entry into the submucosal space is evident when flimsy areolar tissue is encountered.

Creation of submucosal tunnel

The second step of the procedure is creation of the submucosal tunnel (**Fig. 2**). The submucosal space can be navigated successfully with a combination of CO_2 insufflation and careful dissection, in addition to injection of additional dye as needed. This

A

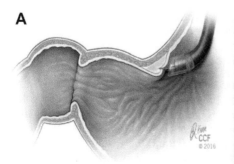

B

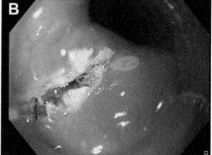

Fig. 1. (*A*) Initial submucosal bleb injection with mucosal flap incision. (*B*) Endoscopic image of submucosal bleb injection with mucosal flap incision during POEM. ([*A*] Reprinted with permission, Cleveland Clinic Center for Medical Art & Photography ©2020. All Rights Reserved.)

A

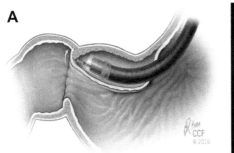

B

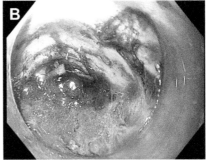

Fig. 2. (*A*) Creation of submucosal tunnel. (*B*) Endoscopic image of submucosal tunnel during POEM. ([*A*] Reprinted with permission, Cleveland Clinic Center for Medical Art & Photography ©2020. All Rights Reserved.)

space is composed of flimsy areolar tissue and blood vessels, which are more pronounced in the stomach than on the esophageal side. The plane can be dissected with the TT knife and electrocautery. Use of short bursts of energy is sufficient to break the loose areolar tissues, which also limits thermal injury to the overlying mucosa. Any moderate to large size blood vessels should be controlled with hemostatic techniques. Coagulation settings can be adjusted to amount of bleeding and vessel size. Larger vessels may need to be individually grasped by forceps with application of appropriate coagulation.

Creation of the submucosal tunnel is greatly facilitated by the transparent cap and endoscope unit. The transparent cap is attached to the working end of the endoscope. This cap has several functions. First, it provides an approximate 5 mm to 7 mm working space in front of the endoscope, allowing the camera lens to not be in constant contact with tissue. When the camera lens is smudged and unable to be cleaned with the integrated irrigation system, the endoscope is removed from the patient and a cotton swab tip is inserted through the cap to clean the endoscope's camera lens. This allows for removal of larger segments of accumulated tissue and adherent blood. Second, the beveled end permits ease of dissection into the submucosal space creating tissue retraction. The cap guides the endoscope through the tunnel and toward the myotomy site facilitating separation of the tissue layers with gentle pressure.

Progression of the procedure and dissection of the entire submucosal tunnel typically requires repeated submucosal injections commensurate with distance needed for the procedure. Different devices allow for injection ranging from standard injection needles to combined knife-injection devices. The authors prefer to use a standard biliary extraction balloon inserted through the scope and advanced just beyond the transparent cap. The balloon is inflated in order to prevent backflow of the premixed solution. Multiple injections assist in differentiating the mucosa from the muscularis propria and thus minimize the chances of inadvertent injury to the mucosa. Fluid dissection also promotes tissue layer separation. It is important to be mindful of the mucosa because adequate distance between the mucosa incision and myotomy needs to be maintained in order to prevent a full-thickness injury. It is helpful to occasionally remove the endoscope from the tunnel and re-examine the true lumen for mucosal perforations and distal progression of the dissection to the target tissue, as needed. Depending on the severity and location, accidental injury to the mucosa can be repaired with clips or commonly may not be clinically significant and left as is. Major full-thickness injury with devitalization of tissue may require conversion to laparoscopy or an open procedure, although this is rare.

During dissection of the submucosal tunnel, it is also helpful to maintain orientation of the endoscope and to be cognizant of the scope's position relative to that of the mucosa and muscularis propria. Occasionally, inattentiveness to the endoscope's position can lead to creation of a spiral tunnel, which also increases the risk of mucosal injury.[20]

Myotomy

The third step of the procedure is the myotomy or lesion excision (**Fig. 3**). The site of myotomy differs depending on specified procedure. The myotomy also can be performed with the same TT knife used throughout the case. POEM requires a 2-cm to 4-cm submucosal tunnel to the myotomy site. Multiple techniques can be useful to identify the distal extent of planned myotomy. Anatomic landmarks from the intramural view include identification of the thickened lower esophageal sphincter with concomitant narrowing, identification of the more disorganized cardiac sling muscle fibers of the stomach, larger perforating veins through the submucosa of the stomach than in the esophagus, an opening of the space with decreased limitation on the gastric side, identification of blue dye in the cardia by at least 2 cm to 3 cm from an intraluminal view, and distance from the incisors (although this may be inaccurate secondary to bowing of the scope) as well as placement of second narrow-caliber scope in the true lumen to see the extent of dissection by the primary operating scope. Fluoroscopy can be useful in guiding the submucosal passage toward the myotomy site.[17] In addition to these possible techniques, the authors also prefer to place a

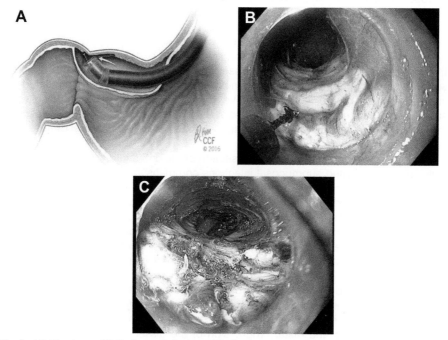

Fig. 3. (*A*) Myotomy. (*B*) Endoscopic image of before myotomy during POEM. (*C*) Endoscopic image of after myotomy during POEM. ([*A*] Reprinted with permission, Cleveland Clinic Center for Medical Art & Photography ©2020. All Rights Reserved.)

radio-opaque hemostatic clip endoscopically on the gastric cardia at a position that corresponds with the distal end of the underlying myotomy at the beginning of the procedure. When the endoscope and the radio-opaque clip are in the same position on fluoroscopy, the distal myotomy site has been reached. This location is taken into consideration with the other findings, listed previously, to ensure adequate myotomy length during POEM.

At the myotomy, the circular muscle layer of the muscularis propria is divided, with intended preservation of the longitudinal muscle fibers. Some centers prefer, however, to perform a full-thickness myotomy, including both circular and longitudinal muscular layers. The length of myotomy is 7 cm to 10 cm on the esophagus with 2 cm to 3 cm on the stomach, although this may altered based on anatomy and the disease being treated. The authors prefer posterior myotomy because this allows for a quicker and more easily accomplished myotomy. Alternatively, the myotomy also can be performed on the anterior, or less commonly lateral positions. Alternate myotomy locations may be used after previous surgical or endoscopic myotomy to avoid scar and reoperative fields.

In cases of POP, the tunnel is carried out to approximately 4 cm to 6 cm between the mucosal incision and the myotomy site. The pylorus is easily identified endoscopically and the distal myotomy on the duodenum is minimal. The myotomy divides the pylorus completely onto the duodenum and also 1 cm to 2 cm of the gastric antrum that is immediately adjacent to the pylorus. Gastric antral myotomy is limited to prevent destruction of the antral motor complex. The authors favor creating the submucosal tunnel and myotomy along the lesser curvature of the stomach through a horizontal mucosal incision. In the authors' experience, the greater curvature approach leads to more retroflexion of the endoscope and thus difficulty of the case.

FED of Zenker diverticulum involves a 3-cm submucosal tunnel followed by a division of the septum between the esophagus and the diverticulum. The cricopharyngeus muscle is enclosed in the septum and therefore it is divided.

For subepithelial tumors, the submucosal tunnel starts 3 cm to 5 cm proximal to the lesion but also should extend distal to the lesion in order to secure sufficient working space for resection and complete identification of the target lesion before resection. The distal side of the tumor often is the more difficult side. The myotomy extent is determined by the need for a circumferential enucleation of the tumor.

POETRE involves a 5-cm submucosal tunnel distal and proximal to the site of obstruction.[16] In POETRE, there is no myotomy. Instead, when both endoscopes converge at the site of obstruction, the antegrade endoscope travels from the submucosal space into and through the fibrotic portion until it reaches the true lumen of the retrograde endoscope. Use of fluoroscopy is key in this step. Fluoroscopy helps maintain the orientation of both endoscopes along the long axis of esophagus and therefore guides the dissection through the fibrotic region toward the true lumen. This portion of the case is blind and, therefore, has the highest risk of full-thickness perforation. Upon entry into the true lumen, esophageal continuity is restored, and a guide wire is passed through the recanalized track. Then, an esophageal stent is deployed over the guide wire. This esophageal stent keeps the recanalized track patent.

Mucosal flap closure

Finally, the last step involves closure of the mucosal flap. In general, a vertical orientation facilitates closure. In the authors' practice, they prefer to close the mucosa with hemostatic clips. The first clip is placed in the most distal position. This clip is the most difficult to place but it helps to align the 2 edges of the mucosa with 1 portion of the clip residing in the true lumen and the other in the submucosal space. This assures that the

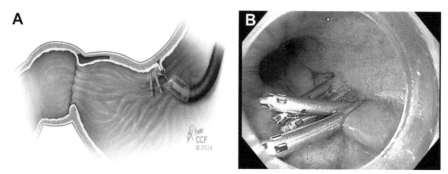

Fig. 4. (*A*) Mucosal flap closure. (*B*) Endoscopic image of mucosal flap closure. ([*A*] Reprinted with permission, Cleveland Clinic Center for Medical Art & Photography ©2020. All Rights Reserved.)

clip is in the apex of the incision and allows for alignment of the mucosal edges. The rest of the clips are placed sequentially toward the most proximal site for closure (**Fig. 4**). Careful attention should be paid to the most proximal clip to ensure sealing and prevent submucosal passage of fluid or contrast study bolus. Endoloops may be helpful in providing additional support if the tissues are severely inflamed and macerated. Alternatively, the mucosal flap can be closed with endoscopic sutures (OverStitch, Apollo Endosurgery, Austin, Texas), over-the-scope clips (OTSC Clip, Ovesco Endoscopy AG, Tuebingen, Germany), or fully covered metal stents.[17] These devices may be limited based on regional or institutional availability, or the working area may be limited by the luminal space of the organ.

At the completion of the procedure, the patient's abdomen should be observed for capnoperitoneum, which can lead to abdominal compartment syndrome.[21] If during or after the procedure the patient has hemodynamic compromise in the setting of distension, the abdomen should be decompressed. This can be performed by placing a 20-gauge needle angiocatheter in the abdomen to evacuate the CO_2. Similarly, hemodynamic compromise in the setting of diminished breath sounds, tracheal deviation, or other signs of pneumothorax should prompt immediate needle decompression of the involved chest.

Postprocedure

After the procedure, patients may be admitted to the hospital and kept nothing by mouth, based on the procedure performed and the experience of the team. It usually is not necessary to check an upright chest radiograph immediately after the procedure. In the authors' practice, however, they obtain this chest radiograph as a baseline. Small pneumothorax or pneumomediastinum without clinical signs is likely to resolve spontaneously. If a patient clinically deteriorates, however, a follow-up upright chest radiograph showing worsening pneumothorax or increasing free intraperitoneal gas may prompt intervention.

After POEM, the authors routinely obtain an upper gastrointestinal contrast study with water-soluble contrast on postoperative day 1. This study evaluates for leak or obstruction. One reason for early partial obstruction is significant tissue edema and this may be more pronounced at the EG junction. This often resolves spontaneously with time, and a postprocedure day 1 study may not accurately reflect the extent and long-term success of myotomy. If the upper gastrointestinal contrast study shows no concerning issues, the patient is initiated on a liquid diet.

Length of stay depends on the procedure but usually is approximately 1 day. Some patients are discharged on the same day, and this has been shown to be safe for patients undergoing procedures at higher volume centers.[22] Patients are discharged home with a liquid diet for 1 week to 2 weeks. Patients are placed on proton pump inhibitors and/or sucralfate therapy at discharge in order to prevent ulceration at the mucosotomy.

Complications

Overall, intramural surgery has a low rate of complications, compared with open or laparoscopic procedures. A majority of the complications are minor and not life threatening. In a multicenter study that included 1826 patients, Haito-Chavez and colleagues[23] showed that only 156 adverse events occurred. Of those, 116 (6.4%) were mild, 31 (1.7%) were moderate, and only 9 (0.5%) were severe. Complications in intramural surgery include pneumoperitoneum, pneumothorax, pneumomediastinum, hemorrhage, and perforation.[17]

Clinically significant pneumoperitoneum can be decompressed with 20-gauge needle in the abdomen, and pneumothorax should be decompressed with needle thoracostomy—with or without subsequent tube placement based on the clinical scenario. In a systematic review and pooled analysis by Patel and colleagues,[24] pneumoperitoneum occurred in 30.6% of cases but only 8% required decompression. The study also noted that pneumothorax occurred in 11% of the cases but only 2.7% required decompression.

As with any invasive procedure, hemorrhage always is a potential complication. Still, most hemorrhage is minor and self-limited. Delayed bleeding is rare. A large retrospective analysis of POEM by Zhang and colleagues[25] included 1680 patients with only 3 (0.2%) cases of delayed bleeding.

Clinically significant hemorrhage occurs in only 1.1% of patients in the pooled analysis by Patel and colleagues[24] for POEM. Significant hemorrhage warrants emergent repeat endoscopy. Hemostatic clips, electrocautery with grasping devices, and other hemostatic techniques can be applied as well. Rarely, hemorrhage necessitates laparoscopic or open surgical intervention. A study by Rodriguez and colleagues[26] included 100 POP procedures with only 4 patients with gastrointestinal bleeding. Of the 4 patients, 2 had unknown sources and the other 2 had mucosal ulcers on endoscopy. None required traditional surgical intervention.

In an analysis of 1826 POEM patients by Haito-Chavez and colleagues,[23] the most common adverse event was inadvertent mucosotomy (n = 51; 2.8%). Of these, 46 were managed endoscopically with endoclips (n = 40), over-the-scope clip (n = 2), and endoscopic suturing (n = 4). Only 1 patient with a large mucosal tear required surgical repair. The most potentially devastating complication is a postprocedural esophageal leak, but this constituted only 0.7% of the adverse events. A majority were treated endoscopically (n = 10) and only 3 patients required surgery. Thus, similar to other adverse events in intramural surgery, most do not require surgical intervention.

DISCUSSION

Intramural surgery is a safe and effective endoscopic surgical technique that offers many applications. Although NOTES is not performed commonly, in many ways this technique has allowed for the progression to intramural surgery. Advanced endoscopic procedure, such as EMR, ESD, and full-thickness resection, utilize similar techniques and tools that now are used in intramural surgery. Intramural surgery expands on the fundamental principles of flexible endoscopy. Synonymous with third-space endoscopy, intramural surgery relies on the third space or the submucosal space as its main operative pathway.

In the era of minimally invasive surgery, intramural surgery offers an expanding new clinical area. The success of POEM has launched growing interest in this movement. The number of applications is increasing. The evolution of intramural surgery has generated opportunities to treat conditions that previously had limited solutions. Recanalization of esophageal occlusion through POETRE is the latest innovative use of intramural surgery.

SUMMARY

Intramural surgery is an emerging minimally invasive surgical technique that is based on flexible endoscopy. The technique utilizes the submucosal plane or third space to separate the mucosal flap from the myotomy or target lesion, thereby minimizing the risk of full-thickness perforation and gastrointestinal leakage. POEM is the first successful application of intramural surgery, but other procedures include POP, STER, FED, and POETRE. Further exploration in this field will propel the field into new horizons.

CLINICS CARE POINTS

- Intramural surgery is an advanced endoscopic technique that utilizes the submucosal space.
- The mucosal entry point is at a distance from the myotomy, limiting the risk of full-thickness perforation.
- The submucosal injection should create a bleb. Otherwise, the needle may be in the muscularis propria and it should be withdrawn back into the submucosal space.
- The transparent cap attached to the end of the endoscope provides a short working space in front of the endoscope. This minimizes smudge on the lens of the endoscope.
- The location and length of myotomy depends on the specific application of intramural surgery (ie, POEM vs POP).
- At the end of the procedure, the abdomen should be observed for capnoperitoneum and abdominal compartment syndrome. Abdomen may need to be decompressed with a 20-guage needle.

DISCLOSURE

M. Kroh has no conflict of interest relevant to this publication. He is a consultant for Medtronic and Ethicon. The remaining authors have no conflicts of interest relevant to this publication and nothing to disclose.

REFERENCES

1. Maydeo A, Dhir V. Third-space endoscopy: stretching the limits. Gastrointest Endosc 2017;85(4):728–9.
2. Khashab MA, Pasricha PJ. Conquering the third space: challenges and opportunities for diagnostic and therapeutic endoscopy. Gastrointest Endosc 2013;77(1):146–8.
3. Strong AT, Rodriguez J, Kroh M, et al. Intramural Surgery: A New Vista in Minimally Invasive Therapy. J Am Coll Surg 2017;225(2):339–42.

 4. Sumiyama K, Gostout CJ, Rajan E, et al. Submucosal endoscopy with mucosal flap safety valve. Gastrointest Endosc 2007;65(4):688–94.
 5. Pasricha PJ, Hawari R, Ahmed I, et al. Submucosal endoscopic esophageal myotomy: a novel experimental approach for the treatment of achalasia. Endoscopy 2007;39(9):761–4.
 6. Inoue H, Minami H, Kobayashi Y, et al. Peroral endoscopic myotomy (POEM) for esophageal achalasia. Endoscopy 2010;42(4):265–71.
 7. Teitelbaum EN, Dunst CM, Reavis KM, et al. Clinical outcomes five years after POEM for treatment of primary esophageal motility disorders. Surg Endosc 2018;32(1):421–7.
 8. Nabi Z, Nageshwar Reddy D, Ramchandani M. Recent Advances in Third-Space Endoscopy. Gastroenterol Hepatol (N Y) 2018;14(4):224–32.
 9. Liu BR, Song JT. Submucosal Tunneling Endoscopic Resection (STER) and Other Novel Applications of Submucosal Tunneling in Humans. Gastrointest Endosc Clin N Am 2016;26(2):271–82.
10. Xu MD, Cai MY, Zhou PH, et al. Submucosal tunneling endoscopic resection: a new technique for treating upper GI submucosal tumors originating from the muscularis propria layer (with videos). Gastrointest Endosc 2012;75(1):195–9.
11. Gong W, Xiong Y, Zhi F, et al. Preliminary experience of endoscopic submucosal tunnel dissection for upper gastrointestinal submucosal tumors. Endoscopy 2012;44(3):231–5.
12. Allemang MT, Strong AT, Haskins IN, et al. How I Do It: Per-Oral Pyloromyotomy (POP). J Gastrointest Surg 2017;21(11):1963–8.
13. Ishaq S, Sultan H, Siau K, et al. New and emerging techniques for endoscopic treatment of Zenker's diverticulum: State-of-the-art review. Dig Endosc 2018; 30(4):449–60.
14. Leong SC, Wilkie MD, Webb CJ. Endoscopic stapling of Zenker's diverticulum: establishing national baselines for auditing clinical outcomes in the United Kingdom. Eur Arch Otorhinolaryngol 2012;269(8):1877–84.
15. Barajas-Gamboa J, Corcelles R, Kroh M. Endoscopic Intramural Surgery Part II: Muscular Division. Dig Dis Interv 2018;02(04):368–74.
16. Wagh MS, Draganov PV. Per-oral endoscopic tunneling for restoration of the esophagus: a novel endoscopic submucosal dissection technique for therapy of complete esophageal obstruction. Gastrointest Endosc 2017;85(4):722–7.
17. Grimes KL, Inoue H. Per Oral Endoscopic Myotomy for Achalasia: A Detailed Description of the Technique and Review of the Literature. Thorac Surg Clin 2016;26(2):147–62.
18. Li L, Spandorfer R, Qu C, et al. Gastric per-oral endoscopic myotomy for refractory gastroparesis: a detailed description of the procedure, our experience, and review of the literature. Surg Endosc 2018;32(8):3421–31.
19. Hernández Mondragón OV, Solórzano Pineda MO, Blancas Valencia JM. Zenker's diverticulum: Submucosal tunneling endoscopic septum division (Z-POEM). Dig Endosc 2018;30(1):124.
20. Ponsky JL, Marks JM, Pauli EM. How I do it: per-oral endoscopic myotomy (POEM). J Gastrointest Surg 2012;16(6):1251–5.
21. Tao J, Patel V, Mekaroonkamol P, et al. Technical Aspects of Peroral Endoscopic Pyloromyotomy. Gastrointest Endosc Clin N Am 2019;29(1):117–26.
22. Landreneau JP, Strong AT, Ponsky JL, et al. Enhanced recovery outcomes following per-oral pyloromyotomy (POP): a comparison of safety and cost with same-day discharge versus inpatient recovery. Surg Endosc 2019. https://doi.org/10.1007/s00464-019-07085-2.

23. Haito-Chavez Y, Inoue H, Beard KW, et al. Comprehensive Analysis of Adverse Events Associated With Per Oral Endoscopic Myotomy in 1826 Patients: An International Multicenter Study. Am J Gastroenterol 2017;112(8):1267–76.

24. Patel K, Abbassi-Ghadi N, Markar S, et al. Peroral endoscopic myotomy for the treatment of esophageal achalasia: systematic review and pooled analysis. Dis Esophagus 2016;29(7):807–19.

25. Zhang XC, Li QL, Xu MD, et al. Major perioperative adverse events of peroral endoscopic myotomy: a systematic 5-year analysis. Endoscopy 2016;48(11):967–78.

26. Rodriguez J, Strong AT, Haskins IN, et al. Per-oral Pyloromyotomy (POP) for Medically Refractory Gastroparesis: Short Term Results From the First 100 Patients at a High Volume Center. Ann Surg 2018;268(3):421–30.

Peroral Esophageal Myotomy

Sabrina Drexel, MD[a],*, Sami Kishawi, MD[b], Jeffrey Marks, MD[b]

KEYWORDS

- Achalasia • POEM • Peroral endoscopic myotomy • Esophageal myotomy

KEY POINTS

- Achalasia is the second most common esophageal motility disorder treated surgically.
- A complete workup including barium swallow, esophageal manometry, and upper endoscopy is necessary before surgical intervention.
- Peroral endoscopic myotomy (POEM) is a newer technique used to treat achalasia endoscopically, instead of treating with traditional laparoscopic approaches.
- POEM is a safe, effective treatment of achalasia, but postoperative gastroesophageal reflux disease remains an important consideration.

INTRODUCTION

First described in 1674 by Sir Thomas Willis, achalasia is a neurodegenerative motility disorder of the esophagus defined by loss of peristalsis and impaired relaxation of the lower esophageal sphincter (LES).[1–3] It is the most common esophageal motility disorder and the second most common esophageal pathology requiring surgery, after antireflux surgery LES laxity. The incidence of achalasia is approximately 1.6 per 100,000 people and is most prevalent in the third through seventh decades of life.[4] Its cause is presently unknown, and index of suspicion must be high. Untreated achalasia may progress to megaesophagus and poses an estimated 28-fold increased risk of esophageal cancer, typically squamous cell carcinoma.[5]

The primary symptom of achalasia is progressive dysphagia to solids and liquids. Additional symptoms include gastroesophageal reflux, cough, and chest pain. Weight loss is not uncommon among patients with achalasia, particularly those with higher grades of disease, as enteral contents go undigested.

[a] Northwest Minimally Invasive Surgery, 2222 Northwest Lovejoy Street, Suite 322, Portland, OR 97210, USA; [b] Department of Surgery, University Hospitals Cleveland Medical Center, 11100 Euclid Avenue, Cleveland, OH 44106-5047, USA
* Corresponding author. Northwest Minimally Invasive Surgery, LLC, 2222 Northwest Lovejoy Street, Suite 322, Portland, OR 97210.
E-mail address: Dr.sabrinadrexel@gmail.com
Twitter: @SabrinaDrexelMD (S.D.)

Surg Clin N Am 100 (2020) 1183–1192
https://doi.org/10.1016/j.suc.2020.08.004
0039-6109/20/© 2020 Elsevier Inc. All rights reserved.

Initially, patients often perform diet modification including soft foods or liquid diet. Oftentimes, patients have been symptomatic for many months before receiving a diagnosis of achalasia. Medical therapy can include calcium channel blockers, nitrate, and antireflux medications; however, interventional therapies are the mainstay of treatment. Some patients can initially be treated with endoscopic therapies, including balloon dilation of the LES or botulin toxin injection. However, these are often temporizing measures, and symptoms usually return after several weeks to several months.

Traditionally, surgical management of achalasia has been through a Heller myotomy, oftentimes with fundoplication, now most commonly done through a laparoscopic approach.[2] Peroral endoscopic myotomy (POEM), on the other hand, uses endoscopic techniques to avoid thoracic or abdominal incisions to achieve the same goal: relaxation of the LES to allow passage of enteral contents.

The first POEM was performed in 2008 in Japan and was formally described in 2010 by Inoue and colleagues[6] in a case series of 17 patients. Since then, POEM has grown in popularity and is now being performed worldwide for the treatment of achalasia and other esophageal motility disorders.

DIAGNOSIS

The diagnosis of achalasia is based on various modalities. The 3 most common investigative studies used to confirm the diagnosis of achalasia are timed barium swallow, esophageal manometry, and endoscopy (**Fig. 1**).

Briefly, a barium swallow study involves ingestion of contrast. This study helps define the anatomy of the distal esophagus, specifically at the gastroesophageal junction. Achalasia is demonstrated as a narrowing at the LES with limited passage of contrast beyond the gastroesophageal junction (see **Fig. 1**A). Variations include dilation, megaesophagus, or sigmoid esophagus just proximal to the LES, which often indicate long-standing achalasia. These are important variations to note, as they can affect surgical approach, discussed in a later section. The barium swallow study is typically the first diagnostic study to identify and evaluate esophageal anatomic abnormalities and to rule out mechanical obstructions.

Manometry is another essential study used in the diagnosis of achalasia and is widely considered the gold standard. Manometry specifically measures muscular function through pressure transducers traversing the upper esophageal sphincter, body of the esophagus, and LES. Achalasia demonstrates elevated resting LES pressure, failure of LES relaxation, and lack of peristalsis in the distal two-thirds of the esophagus (**Fig. 2**B).

Esophagogastroduodenoscopy (EGD) provides direct visualization of the esophagus and is an important adjunctive diagnostic tool to rule out other causes of LES obstruction, termed pseudoachalasia. Pseudoachalasia is most commonly caused by malignancy—specifically gastric carcinoma, lung carcinoma, or lymphoma—and mimics the clinical presentation of achalasia in roughly 2% to 4% of patients with suspected idiopathic achalasia.[7] Typical EGD findings for achalasia include retained food particles, mucosal irritation or inflammation most prominent near the LES, and distal esophageal dilation, especially evident in chronic disease (**Fig. 2**C).

Additional information can be provided by an endoluminal functional lumen imaging probe (EndoFLIP), a novel tool that measures cross-sectional area, pressure, and distensibility to assess esophageal anatomic abnormality in real time.[8] This diagnostic tool uses impedance planimetry through a balloon-tipped catheter that takes the shape of esophagus to calculate and define esophageal geometry specifically at the LES. It can be used as a diagnostic tool immediately before a POEM procedure and

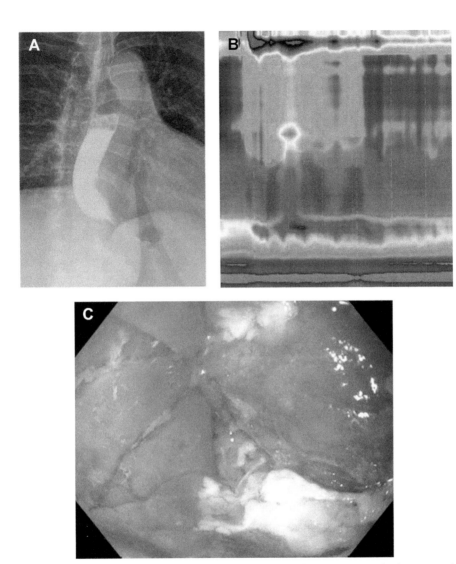

Fig. 1. Classic barium swallow findings of distal esophageal narrowing at the lower esophageal junction (*A*). Manometry composite swallow shows elevated mean LES pressure with lack of esophageal body peristalsis (*B*). Lower third of esophagus on upper endoscopy with food debris, mucosal inflammation, and LES narrowing (*C*).

then immediately after the myotomy to assess how the LES geometry and diameter has changed.[9] EndoFLIP has been shown to reliably evaluate the LES junction, but its usefulness in clinical practice in still evolving.

PREOPERATIVE PLANNING

Many patients with achalasia will have retained food and secretions in their esophagus at the time of the procedure; therefore, patients require general anesthesia. A detailed history and physical examination is a prerequisite. If necessary, the patient should be seen by anesthesia before the procedure and complete cardiopulmonary workup as

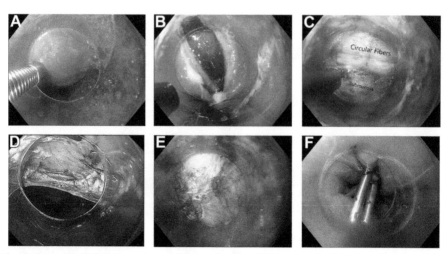

Fig. 2. Steps to POEM procedure. After performing EGD, a cap is placed on the tip of the gastroscope. The esophagus is injected using a sclerotherapy needle to form a submucosal wheal (*A*). A 3 cm mucosotomy is created (*B*). A submucosal tunnel is created past the lower esophageal sphincter and onto the stomach (*C, D*). The circular fibers are divided (*E*). The mucosotomy is closed with TTS clips (*F*). TTS, through-the-scope.

appropriate. Up to 43% of patients have had prior interventions, including botulin injections, pneumatic dilations, or prior myotomy; it is essential to ascertain this medical history, as prior therapies make POEM more challenging due to scarring and fibrosis at the LES.[10]

Patients should be maintained on a clear liquid diet for 48 hours before their POEM. We prescribe oral fluconazole and nystatin preoperatively to reduce infection due to the incidence of candidiasis in these patients.

PATIENT POSITIONING

There is no evidence to support supine versus left lateral positioning. The authors choose to leave patients supine and tuck the left arm to allow for more working space for the endoscopist. Patients are administered general anesthesia, and the endotracheal tube is positioned to the right in the patient's mouth. We then rotate the operation room table away from the anesthesia team at about a 45° angle, to allow for the surgical endoscopist to stand at the head of the bed. The patient is given a single dose of cefazolin for surgical prophylaxis. The abdomen is exposed in case the patient develops pneumoperitoneum and requires decompression during the procedure.

PROCEDURAL APPROACH

The equipment needed to perform a POEM is listed in **Box 1**. The procedure is started with a diagnostic EGD. No bite block is used, as we place an overtube at the time of EGD. After ruling out any cause for pseudoachalasia, the gastroscope is removed and fitted with a distal cap. The distance from the mouth to the gastroesophageal junction is measured, and then the gastroscope is retracted by about 14 cm. The goal is to create a long enough submucosal tunnel to allow for 5 to 7 cm of esophageal and 2 to 3 cm of gastric myotomy. The site of proposed mucosotomy is then chosen, and a submucosal wheal is raised in this area using a sclerotherapy needle (**Fig. 2**A). We

---

Box 1
List of supplies for peroral endoscopic myotomy

1. Erbe machine for electrocautery

2. Diagnostic gastroscope (GIF-190)

3. Overtube (if desired)

4. Cap for gastroscope

5. Sclerotherapy needle

6. Endoscopy knife (triangle knife)

7. Biliary injection catheter

8. Endoscopic TTS clips

9. Methylene blue, epinephrine

Abbreviation: TTS, through-the-scope.

---

use a mixture of methylene blue, epinephrine, and saline (500 mL 5% dextrose with 125 mg methylene blue and 2.5 mg of 1:1000 epinephrine), but other institutions may use isosulfan blue or indigo carmine with or without epinephrine. The blue staining helps to delineate the submucosa from the circular muscle fibers (see **Fig. 2**C). A 2 to 3 cm longitudinal mucosotomy is created with an endoscopic knife (we preferably use the triangle tip knife). The gastroscope is inserted into the mucosotomy, and a submucosal tunnel is created using the electrosurgical knife (**Fig. 2**D). The width of the submucosal tunnel is about one-third the circumference of the esophagus. Care is taken to ensure the submucosal remains parallel to the esophageal lumen, as it is easy to create a corkscrew shaped tunnel, which then leads to difficulty defining important landmarks. Additional methylene blue is injected as needed with a blunt biliary injection catheter to improve visualization of the junction between submucosa and muscle. The blunt injection catheter is used over the sclerotherapy needle to prevent vessel or mucosal injury once within the submucosal tunnel.

Once the submucosal tunnel has been created onto the stomach, the myotomy is performed. We verify dissection onto the stomach by obtaining a retroflex view in the stomach showing the methylene blue dye extending onto the gastric wall (**Fig. 3**). Other endoscopists use a dual endoscope technique to assess the distal extent of the submucosal dissection plane, whereas others rely on intraoperative fluoroscopy to confirm dissection beyond the LES onto the gastric wall.

Once we are confident we have extended the submucosal tunnel past the gastroesophageal junction, we begin the myotomy. We prefer to only cut the circular esophageal fibers, starting 3 cm below the inferior aspect of the mucosotomy, to allow for a mucosal covering over a nonmyotomized area of the esophagus. Full-thickness myotomy is commonly performed as well, and to date there are no data supporting one technique over the other. All circular fibers are cut in a vertical fashion using the triangular knife for the length of the submucosal tunnel (**Fig. 2**E). The gastroscope is then inserted back into the stomach, noting whether the LES is more patent than prior passes of the gastroscope. The mucosotomy is then closed with through-the-scope clips (**Fig. 2**F). The stomach is desufflated, and the gastroscope and overtube are removed.

Debate exists over whether an anterior versus posterior myotomy is preferred. One randomized trial showed higher intraoperative mucosal injuries with the anterior myotomy but higher rates of postoperative esophageal acid exposure in the posterior

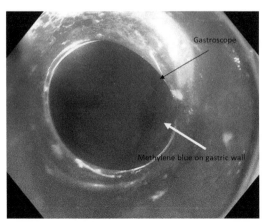

Fig. 3. Retroflex view of gastroesophageal junction showing dissection plane onto stomach wall.

group.[11] They concluded the approaches were equivalent. Other randomized studies have not shown any difference in acid exposure or intraoperative complications.[12,13] We prefer to perform an anterior myotomy, unless the patient has had a prior myotomy (surgical or endoscopic), at which time we will preferentially perform a posterior myotomy.

Selective circular myotomy versus full-thickness myotomy has also been debated. A laparoscopic myotomy intentionally creates a full-thickness myotomy, as access to the circular fibers requires cutting the longitudinal fibers first from the outside. Full-thickness myotomy is not necessary to treat achalasia or other esophageal motility disorders; however, full-thickness myotomy often occurs during POEM when the longitudinal layer is thin and separates with transection of the circular fibers. These intermittent full-thickness transections do not seem to have any significant clinical relevance.[14] Some centers intentionally perform a full-thickness myotomy during POEM, and there does not seem to be any significant difference other than shorter operative times in the full-thickness group.[15]

POSTOPERATIVE CARE

Patients are admitted overnight postoperatively; although in certain centers, patients are discharged on the same day. They are started on clear liquids the evening of surgery. Many experience chest discomfort, similar to other foregut procedures. Pain is controlled with multimodal analgesia, including acetaminophen, nonsteroidal antiinflammatory drugs, and opioids if needed.

Most patients are discharged home on postoperative day one on a full-liquid diet. They are kept on full liquids for 1 week, then advanced to a soft diet for 1 week. All patients are prescribed a proton pump inhibitor (PPI) for 6 months after POEM. At that time, their PPI is discontinued and a 24-hour pH study is conducted to assess for acid reflux.

MANAGEMENT OF COMPLICATIONS
Intraoperative Concerns

Aspiration on induction remains a major concern for patients with achalasia. We recommend rapid sequence induction for all patients. Any patient with suspected aspiration may benefit from intraoperative bronchoscopy before extubation.

Other anesthetic concerns include elevated peak airway pressures and high end-tidal CO_2.[16] Close communication between the endoscopist and the anesthetist is required. If the patient has elevated peak airway pressures, the stomach should be suctioned of insufflated CO_2 and the abdomen assessed for continued distention and suspicion for pneumoperitoneum. If necessary, the peritoneal cavity can be decompressed with a 14-gauge angiocatheter. This will typically promptly resolve elevated airway pressures and difficulty with ventilation. Hyperventilation and an increase in tidal volume can usually resolve the hypercapnia.[17,18] Subcutaneous emphysema and mediastinal emphysema can also occur as a result of the POEM, which can be observed in the postoperative period.

Bleeding in the submucosal tunnel can be difficult to control, as working space is limited. Prevention of bleeding by identifying vessels during creation of the submucosal tunnel can maintain a clear view. If bleeding is encountered, pulsed irrigation and gentle suction can be used. Gentle manual pressure with either the knife, injection catheter, or the distal cap can usually tamponade a vessel. Coagulation forceps can be used if necessary.[19] However, take caution using electrocautery on the mucosal flap, as this can lead to thermal injury and full-thickness perforation.

Postoperative Concerns

Full-thickness perforation of the esophageal wall often occurs during the myotomy. However, if there is any concern about the integrity of the mucosal closure, an esophagram can be obtained on postoperative day 1. An esophageal leak can initially be treated with NPO status and time. Rarely, the patient needs to be left NPO with distal enteral feeding.

Another postoperative concern is failure for symptoms to resolve, which could be due to an incomplete myotomy. These patients need a complete repeat workup with EGD, barium UGI, and esophageal manometry. These studies will confirm persistent elevated pressures at the LES. Patients with prior surgical or endoscopic myotomy can safely be treated with a repeat POEM.[20,21]

OUTCOMES

Overall, POEM is a safe and durable treatment of achalasia. Technical success rates of POEM are as high as 100%,[22] with clinical success rates routinely greater than 90%.[23,24] It has been shown to have similar outcomes to laparoscopic Heller myotomy,[25–27] with less operative time and shorter hospital stay. Return to activities of daily living has also been shown to be significantly faster in patients who undergo POEM over laparoscopic myotomy.[28] There are similar rates of relief from dysphagia between the 2 groups, and POEM provides a significant quality of life improvement at 1 year.[29] In addition, POEM patients use significantly less narcotics than patients who undergo laparoscopic myotomy, both during their hospitalization and at the time of discharge.[30]

Gastroesophageal reflux disease (GERD) after POEM remains a concern, as a partial fundoplication is typically performed with surgical myotomy. Some evidence shows similar esophageal acid exposure after Heller myotomy versus POEM,[31] whereas others continue to demonstrate increased esophageal acid exposure after POEM, without an increase in patient-reported GERD symptoms.[32] Reflux esophagitis seems to be higher in the short term for patients undergoing POEM.[33] Several researchers have demonstrated similar postoperative PPI use after POEM and laparoscopic myotomy,[34] and others did not find any difference in GERD-related quality of life outcomes between the 2 groups.[35] The possibility of acid reflux after the procedure should be discussed with the patient during the consent process, and we recommend 6 months of PPI therapy postoperatively.

POEM has been used to treat other esophageal motility disorders with promising results, including diffuse esophageal spasm, nutcracker esophagus, and jackhammer esophagus. These diseases require a longer myotomy to treat, which is not achievable via a laparoscopic approach. One study showed significant improvements in Eckardt scores and chest pain, with an overall clinical response rate of 93%.[36] Repeat manometry in these patients showed resolution of initial abnormalities. About one-fourth of POEMs performed worldwide are now for esophageal motility disorders other than achalasia.[37] The endoscopic technique of POEM has also been applied to esophageal and gastric tumor resection, known as peroral endoscopic submucosal tumor resection.

Debate still exists around several concepts regarding POEM, including length and location of myotomy, selective circular versus full-thickness myotomy, treatment of GERD after POEM, and use of newer diagnostic adjuncts such as EndoFLIP. These exciting minimally invasive endoscopic therapies will continue to evolve and enhance patient care with shorter hospitalizations, less pain, and excellent clinical outcomes.

SUMMARY

POEM has been accepted as an endoscopic alternative to laparoscopic myotomy for the treatment of achalasia. It remains a safe and effective procedure, even in patients with a history of prior myotomy. Awareness of anesthetic challenges and postoperative complications remains paramount for the safe practice of endoscopic surgery.

CLINICS CARE POINTS

- POEM has become the standard treatment of achalasia at many centers around the world.
- Close communication with anesthesia regarding airway pressures and end-tidal CO2 remain a crucial aspect of the procedure for patient safety.
- Always use CO_2 and not air for insufflation.
- Leave the abdomen exposed and periodically check for pneumoperitoneum.
- The anterior versus posterior approaches seem to be equivalent at this time.
- Patients can safely undergo POEM after prior laparoscopic or endoscopy myotomy.

DISCLOSURE

The authors have nothing to disclose.

REFERENCES

1. Boeckxstaens GE, Zaninotto G, Richter JE. Achalasia. Lancet 2014;383(9911): 83–93.

2. Tuason J, Inoue H. Current status of achalasia management: a review on diagnosis and treatment. J Gastroenterol 2017;52:401–6.

3. Stavropoulos SN, Friedel D, Modayil R, et al. Diagnosis and management of esophageal achalasia. BMJ 2016;354:i2785.

4. Ahmed Y, Othman MO. Peroral endoscopic myotomy (POEM) for achalasia. J Thorac Dis 2019;11(Suppl 12):S1618–28.

5. Leeuwenburgh I, Scholten P, Alderliesten J, et al. Long-term esophageal cancer risk in patients with primary achalasia: a prospective study. Am J Gastroenterol 2010;105(10):2144–9.
6. Inoue H, Minami H, Kobayashi Y, et al. Peroral endoscopic myotomy (POEM) for esophageal achalasia. Endoscopy 2010;42(4):265–71.
7. Kahrilas PJ, Kishk SM, Helm JF, et al. Comparison of pseudoachalasia and achalasia. Am J Med 1987;82(3):439–46.
8. Massey BT. EndoFLIP Assessment of Achalasia Therapy: Interpreting the Distensibility Data Is a Bit of a Stretch. Gastroenterology 2013;144(4):e17–8.
9. Familiari P, Gigante G, Marchese M, et al. EndoFLIP system for the intraoperative evaluation of peroral endoscopic myotomy. United Eur Gastroenterol J 2014;2(2):77–83.
10. Stavropoulos SN, Modayil RJ, Friedel D, et al. The International Per Oral Endoscopic Myotomy Survey (IPOEMS): a snapshot of the global POEM experience. Surg Endosc 2013;27:3322–38.
11. Ramchandani M, Nabi Z, Reddy DN, et al. Outcomes of anterior myotomy versus posterior myotomy during POEM: a randomized pilot study. Endosc Int Open 2018;6(2):E190–8.
12. Khashab MA, Sanaei O, Rivory J, et al. Peroral endoscopic myotomy: anterior versusposterior approach: a randomized single-blinded clinical trial. Gastrointest Endosc 2019;91(2):288–97.e7.
13. Tan Y, Lv L, Wang X, et al. Efficacy of anterior versus posterior per-oral endoscopic myotomy for treating achalasia: a randomized, prospective study. Gastrointest Endosc 2018;88(1):46–54.
14. Inoue H, Tianle KM, Ikeda H, et al. Peroral endoscopic myotomy for esophageal achalasia: technique, indication, and outcomes. Thorac Surg Clin 2011;21:519–25.
15. Li QL, Chen WF, Zhou PH, et al. Peroral endoscopic myotomy for the treatment of achalasia: a clinical comparative study of endoscopic full-thickness and circular muscle myotomy. J Am Coll Surg 2013;217:442–51.
16. Nishihara Y, Yoshida T, Ooi M, et al. Anesthetic management and associated complications of peroral endoscopic myotomy: A case series. World J Gastrointest Endosc 2018;10(9):193–9.
17. Wang X, Tan Y, Zhang J, et al. Risk factors for gas-related complications of peroral endoscopic myotomy in achalasia. Neth J Med 2015;73:76–81.
18. Ren Z, Zhong Y, Zhou P, et al. Perioperative management and treatment for complications during and after peroral endoscopic myotomy (POEM) for esophageal achalasia (EA) (data from 119 cases). Surg Endosc 2012;26:3267–72.
19. Bechara R, Onimaru M, Ikeda H, et al. Per-oral endoscopic myotomy, 1000 cases later: pearls, pitfalls, and practical considerations. Gastrointest Endosc 2016;84(2):330–8.
20. Orenstein SB, Raigani S, Wu YV, et al. Peroral endoscopic myotomy (POEM) leads to similar results in patients with and without prior endoscopic or surgical therapy. Surg Endosc 2015;29:1064–70.
21. Ngamruengphong S, Inoue H, Ujiki MB, et al. Efficacy and Safety of Peroral Endoscopic Myotomy for Treatment of Achalasia After Failed Heller Myotomy. Clin Gastroenterol Hepatol 2017;15(10):1531–7.e3.
22. Inoue H, Sato H, Ikeda H, et al. Per-Oral Endoscopic Myotomy: A Series of 500 Patients. J Am Coll Surg 2015;221(2):256–64.
23. Ponds FA, Fockens P, Lei A, et al. Effect of Peroral Endoscopic Myotomy vs Pneumatic Dilation on Symptom Severity and Treatment Outcomes Among Treatment-

Naive Patients With Achalasia: A Randomized Clinical Trial. JAMA 2019;322(2): 134–44.

24. Teitelbaum EN, Soper NJ, Santos BF, et al. Symptomatic and physiologic outcomes one year after peroral esophageal myotomy (POEM) for treatment of achalasia. Surg Endosc 2014;28(12):3359–65.

25. Talukdar R, Inoue H, Nageshwar Reddy D. Efficacy of peroral endoscopic myotomy (POEM) in the treatment of achalasia: a systematic review and meta-analysis. Surg Endosc 2015;29:3030–46.

26. Patel K, Abbassi-Ghadi N, Markar S, et al. Peroral endoscopic myotomy for the treatment of esophageal achalasia: systematic review and pooled analysis. Dis Esophagus 2016;29:807–19.

27. Marano L, Pallabazzer G, Solito B, et al. Surgery or Peroral Esophageal Myotomy for Achalasia: A Systematic Review and Meta-Analysis. Medicine (Baltimore) 2016;95:e3001.

28. Ujiki MB, Yetasook AK, Zapf M, et al. Peroral endoscopic myotomy: A short-term comparison with the standard laparoscopic approach. Surgery 2013;154(4): 893–7 [discussion: 897–900].

29. Ward MA, Gitelis M, Patel L, et al. Outcomes in patients with over 1-year follow-up after peroral endoscopic myotomy (POEM). Surg Endosc 2017;31(4):1550–7.

30. Docimo S Jr, Mathew A, Shope AJ, et al. Reduced postoperative pain scores and narcotic use favor per-oral endoscopic myotomy over laparoscopic Heller myotomy. Surg Endosc 2017;31(2):795–800.

31. Bhayani NH, Kurian AA, Dunst CM, et al. A comparative study on comprehensive, objective outcomes of laparoscopic Heller myotomy with per-oral endoscopic myotomy (POEM) for achalasia. Ann Surg 2014;259(6):1098–103.

32. Sanaka MR, Thota PN, Parikh MP, et al. Peroral endoscopic myotomy leads to higher rates of abnormal lesophageal acid exposure than laparoscopic Heller myotomy in achalasia. Surg Endosc 2019;33(7):2284–92.

33. Werner YB, Hakanson B, Martinek J, et al. Endoscopic or Surgical Myotomy in Patients with Idiopathic Achalasia. N Engl J Med 2019;381(23):2219–29.

34. Schneider AM, Louie BE, Warren HF, et al. A Matched Comparison of Per Oral Endoscopic Myotomy to Laparoscopic Heller Myotomy in the Treatment of Achalasia. J Gastrointest Surg 2016;20(11):1789–96.

35. Chan SM, Wu JC, Teoh AY, et al. Comparison of early outcomes and quality of life after laparoscopic Heller's cardiomyotomy to peroral endoscopic myotomy for treatment of achalasia. Dig Endosc 2016;28(1):27–32.

36. Khashab MA, Messallam AA, Onimaru M, et al. International multicenter experience with peroral endoscopic myotomy for thetreatment of spastic esophageal disorders refractory to medical therapy (with video). Gastrointest Endosc 2015; 81(5):1170–7.

37. Minami H, Inoue H, Haji A, et al. Per-oral endoscopic myotomy: emerging indications and evolving techniques. Dig Endosc 2015;27:175–81.

Peroral Pyloromyotomy

Megan Lundgren, MD*, John H. Rodriguez, MD

KEYWORDS

- Peroral pyloromyotomy • POP • G-POEM • Gastroparesis
- Delayed gastric emptying

KEY POINTS

- A diagnosis of gastroparesis must be confirmed before any consideration of gastric emptying procedure.
- A multidisciplinary approach to the management of medically refractory gastroparesis, as well as for patient selection for peroral pyloromyotomy, is ideal and should include gastroenterologists, surgical, nutritional, psychological, and pain management experts.
- Short-term results of peroral pyloromyotomy for medically refractory gastroparesis are promising. Long-term study of peroral pyloromyotomy outcomes is ongoing.

 Video content accompanies this article at http://www.surgical.theclinics.com.

INTRODUCTION
History of Endoluminal Surgery for Gastroparesis

Endoluminal surgery is continuously advancing. The development of the endoscopic pyloromyotomy for gastroparesis is the result of a rich history in endoscopic surgery. Endoscopy started within the lumen of the bowel, and subsequently procedures were extended into the peritoneal cavity, traversing the bowel wall. More recently endoluminal surgery extended into the submucosal space. This intramural surgery requires dissection and expansion of the tissue layer between the mucosa and the muscularis propria.[1]

During the development of natural orifice transluminal endoscopic surgery, a mucosal flap valve was created using dissection of the submucosal space to offset leakage. Ultimately, the application of intramural surgery in patients with achalasia by Dr Inoue resulted in the POEM procedure, described by Inoue and colleagues[2] in 2008. Following this, the endoscopic pyloromyotomy was described in a pig model by Kawai and colleagues. The aim of their study was to determine if a complete endoscopic pyloromyotomy could be completed, with an initial goal of potentially treated

General Surgery, Digestive Disease Institute, Cleveland Clinic, 9500 Euclid Avenue Desk A100, Cleveland, OH 44195, USA
* Corresponding author.
E-mail address: Megan.pratt.lundgren@gmail.com
Twitter: @meganlundgrenMD (M.L.); @johnrodriguezMD (J.H.R.)

Surg Clin N Am 100 (2020) 1193–1200
https://doi.org/10.1016/j.suc.2020.08.015
0039-6109/20/© 2020 Elsevier Inc. All rights reserved.

surgical.theclinics.com

infantile hypertrophic pyloric stenosis. The investigators found that using the saline lift technique used by Inoue for the POEM the submucosal space could be successfully dissected, and the circular and longitudinal muscle fibers at the pylorus can be endoscopically delineated, allowing for a precise, and safe, myotomy. The success of their myotomy was measured with histopathological analysis as well as manometry. The investigators closed their discussion with the proposal that this technique could be used not only for infantile hypertrophic pyloric stenosis but also for postsurgical delayed gastric emptying.[3]

Peroral endoscopic myotomy continued to be developed from the time of Kawai's report, and in 2013 the first human model was reported by Kashab and colleagues. The most frequent indications for the procedure include idiopathic, diabetic, and postsurgical gastroparesis. Gastroparesis is discussed in more detail in the following section.

NATURE OF THE PROBLEM AND DIAGNOSIS
Gastroparesis

Gastroparesis is a combination of delayed gastric emptying, absence of mechanical gastric outlet obstruction, and documented slow gastric emptying. Patients present with early satiety, postprandial fullness, nausea, vomiting, bloating, and epigastric abdominal pain. Gastroparesis results from a derangement of extrinsic neuronal control, dysfunction of the interstitial cells of Cajal and intrinsic nerves, and some element of dysfunction of smooth muscle. Proper function of the stomach entails the breakdown of foodstuff within its lumen, using shear forces. Shear forces are created by contraction of the stomach wall, whereas the pylorus is closed. This is the culmination of extrinsic vagal innervation, intrinsic cholinergic innervation, and transmission of signals through the interstitial cells of Cajal to the smooth muscle of the stomach, including the pylorus. Women are affected most commonly, and the overall prevalence of gastroparesis is 24 per 100,000 persons. This is an important and significant disease, as it decreases the quality of life of the affected patients and also decreases their overall survival.

Postsurgical gastroparesis occurs with injury to the vagus nerve during other operations—at risk with fundoplication, esophagectomy, gastrectomy, heller myotomy, etc.

Idiopathic gastroparesis is the most common cause of gastroparesis—these patients are under the umbrella of many potential causes inclusive of immunologic, neurologic, connective tissue disorders, metabolic disorders, and dysautonomia from causes other than diabetes.[4]

The cause of gastroparesis in diabetic patients is not fully understood; however, diabetic patients with other neuropathies are more likely to have diabetic gastroparesis.[5]

As demonstrated here, gastroparesis is a complex, multifactorial problem.

Diagnosis

Typically, when a patient presents with one or more of the symptoms of gastroparesis, endoscopy is first performed to rule out ulcers or obstructions. Once these conditions are ruled out, the gold standard for diagnosis of gastroparesis is the 4-hour solid-phase gastric emptying study. A gastric emptying study is the ingestion of a radiolabeled solid meal (typically scrambled eggs, bread, and water) with subsequent measuring of radioactivity in the stomach at intervals postingestion. Normal gastric emptying is defined as 37% to 90% retention at 1 hour, 30% to 60% at 2 hours, and 0% to 10% at 4 hours. If there is greater that 60%

retention of radioactivity at 2 hours or greater than 10% retention at 4 hours this is considered to be delayed gastric emptying. The percent retention at 4 hours is used to define severity of delayed emptying: 10% to 20% mildly delayed, 20% to 35% moderately delayed, and greater than 35% as severely delayed gastric emptying. An important adjunct to the gastric emptying study in the workup for gastroparesis is the transit study, using a wireless motility capsule. If a patient has a global motility disorder, diagnosed using the transit study times through the small bowel and colon, management is altered. If an endoscopy has not already been performed, it should be routinely obtained to rule out obstruction or ulcer. If a patient has had prior foregut surgery, it can be useful to obtain an upper gastrointestinal contrast study to rule out recurrences, for instance, of hiatal hernias and another anatomic issue that could be complicating symptoms congruent with gastroparesis. Laboratory studies can be obtained, as metabolic derangements are common in patients with gastroparesis related to frequent emesis, dehydration, and comorbid conditions.[6] A gastroparesis cardinal symptom index can be performed for a subjective measure of gastroparesis symptoms, displayed in **Table 1**.

ANATOMY AND PHYSIOLOGY

In regard to peroral endoscopic pyloromyotomy, the anatomy of the pylorus itself, as well as its nervous and blood supply, is important to review. In addition, awareness of the structures surrounding the pylorus is significant.

The pylorus is a sphincter, an underlying muscular ring. It is a high-pressure zone at rest. Proximal and distal pyloric loops are described, but difficult to identify endoscopically, and work in a coordinated fashion. The pylorus is different structurally from the adjacent tracts, the antrum and the duodenum; however, the proximal pylorus is coordinated with gastric contractions, and this coordination results in closure of the lumen of the pylorus, which prevents early passage of foodstuff from the antrum to the duodenum. The gastroduodenal artery is the main supply of blood to the pylorus; however, there is also supply from the right gastric artery. The pylorus, similar to the remainder of the stomach, is lined by mucosa, with underlying muscularis mucosae and submucosa containing pyloric glands, a circular muscle, and longitudinal muscle layer. The gastric electrical pacemaker, is located in the greater curvature of the

Table 1 Gastroparesis cardinal symptom index		
Symptom Subscale	**Symptoms**	**Scale (None to Very Severe)**
Nausea/Vomiting	Nausea	0–5
	Retching	0–5
	Vomiting	0–5
Fullness/Early satiety	Fullness	0–5
	Inability to finish meal	0–5
	Fullness after a meal	0–5
	Loss of appetite	0–5
Bloating/Distention	Bloating	0–5
	Visibly larger belly	0–5

stomach. At rest, there are slow waves emitted from the pacemaker to the pylorus 3 cycles per minute, as well as migrating motor complexes marked by electrical spikes. These complexes help to clear gastric content through the pylorus after it has been properly sheared and digested to chyme. After a meal, the antrum undergoes repetitive, shearing contractions against a closed pylorus.[7]

PREOPERATIVE PLANNING

Before performance of peroral pyloromyotomy the diagnosis must be confirmed using the American society of gastroenterology guidelines, confirming symptoms of gastroparesis, without gastric obstruction or ulcer and delayed emptying demonstrated on gastric emptying study. The gastroparesis cardinal symptom index can be used to assess preprocedural symptomatology; this can be used as a postprocedural comparison. Multidisciplinary clinics for gastroparesis including gastroenterologists, surgical, nutritional, psychological, and pain management experts allow for ease of appropriate patient selection for this procedure. Attempted conservative treatments such as dietary changes, glycemic control, antiemetic, and prokinetic medications should be documented. At times, the patients have required a jejunal feeding tube access or central access for parenteral nutrition for severe malnutrition before surgical consultation for an emptying procedure. Patients should ideally undergo informed consent inclusive of a discussion of a laparoscopic pyloroplasty versus endoscopic pyloromyotomy. The details of both procedures and the need for general endotracheal anesthesia should be discussed with the patient.

Patients with gastroparesis are at high risk for aspiration during induction of anesthesia. Therefore, the preoperative plan should include a full-liquid diet 2 days before the procedure, a clear-liquid diet the day before, and the patient should be directed to remain nothing per os the midnight before the procedure.

If the patient has a previously placed gastric electrical stimulator, this should be turned off the morning of the procedure.[8]

The risks of the procedure, primarily postprocedure gastrointestinal bleeding and risk of full-thickness perforation should be discussed with the patient.

PREPARATION AND POSITIONING
Positioning

The patient is placed supine on the operating room table. The arms can be left out. Intravenous access is obtained by the anesthesia team. The patient undergoes general orotracheal intubation. The surgical endoscopist should create a platform of steps/foot stools to the left of the patient. This will enable the surgical endoscopist a more comfortable working height than vertical motion of the operating table will allow.[8]

PROCEDURAL APPROACH

As with any procedure, the appropriate equipment availability should be confirmed before procedure start. For peroral pyloromyotomy this will include the following:

1. Standard diagnostic endoscope
2. Overcap
3. Electrosurgical endoscopic knife
4. Electrosurgical unit
5. Injection needle with retractable tip
6. Endoscopic clips (at least 3)

1. Step 1—submucosal injection: an injection needle is used to deliver a submucosal injection of a solution containing blue dye. The site is chosen based on the anatomy of the stomach. The authors prefer a site along the lesser curve 3 to 5 cm proximal to the pylorus. The shape of the stomach will determine the site. In patients with a J-shaped stomach, this maneuver may need to be performed in a semiretroflexed position. The site of initial injection must be distal to the incisura angularis. The goal of this step is to form a bleb that will separate the mucosa from the muscular layers of the stomach to avoid a full-thickness perforation at the site of the initial incision. The solution consists of methylene blue diluted in normal saline. Premixed gel solutions are commercially available and tend to dissipate slower in the submucosal plane.

2. Step 2—mucosal incision: once the bleb is formed, a transverse incision is made using an endoscopic knife connected to an energy source with cut current. The incision should be large enough to accommodate the diameter of the endoscope being used. The mucosa of the stomach can be of variable thickness. It is important to ensure complete mucosa incision before extending the incision laterally. In many cases, the submucosa will be adhered to the mucosa and will not allow for mucosal separation after initial incision. The beveled cap can be used to place tension and simultaneously use the electrosurgical knife with spray coagulation to divide these fibers. The endoscope is then completely inserted into the submucosal plane to develop the tunnel.

3. Step 3—tunneling: once the endoscope is inserted into the submucosal plane, tunneling toward the pylorus is performed. The critical step is achieving proper orientation in the submucosal plane before proceeding with distal dissection. The blue dye will stain the submucosal plane, whereas the mucosa and muscularis will not uptake dye. Once the muscle fibers are identified, dissection is continued distally at the junction of the muscularis and submucosa. It is critical to avoid any mucosal injuries during this dissection. The orientation of the muscle fibers in the antrum follow a cone shape, with the apex being the pyloric sphincter. The tunnel dissection ends just distal to the pylorus. The mucosa of the duodenum becomes perpendicular to the tunnel just distal to the pylorus. Therefore, further dissection is unnecessary and likely to result in mucosal injury.

4. Step 4—division of the pylorus: after the tunnel is completed, the pylorus should be clearly visualized. The pylorus can then be divided using the electrosurgical knife. This step can be achieved in several ways based on individual preference. Using cut current will result in clean division of the muscle fibers with minimal charring of the tissue. The downside is a higher potential for bleeding if small vessels are encountered during division of the pylorus. Coagulation current is highly effective as well but can result in more charring of the muscle fibers. This can make visualization somewhat difficult. Complete division is achieved once the circular fibers that compose the pyloric sphincter are completely divided. One can usually visualize a subtle change in the orientation of the muscle fibers that compose the gastric wall. In some cases, build up of blue dye can be seen dissecting between the pylorus and gastric wall.

5. Step 5—closure of the mucosotomy: once division of the pylorus is completed, the endoscope is withdrawn from the tunnel and the pylorus visualized from the lumen of the stomach. In most cases, widening of the pylorus with a somewhat oval-shaped opening can be immediately seen. Hemostasis within the tunnel is ensured, and closure of the mucosotomy is performed. Hemostatic clips are a great and simple tool to reapproximate the mucosal edges. The authors prefer to start at a corner and proceed from one end to the next.

Illustrative figures demonstrating the procedure can be reviewed in **Fig. 1** and each step can be reviewed in Video 1.

RECOVERY AND REHABILITATION

After an uncomplicated peroral pyloromyotomy, the patients can be discharged to home after time in the postanesthesia recovery unit. For patients with significant co-morbid conditions an overnight stay is not unreasonable to monitor for complications related to anesthesia; this is up to the discretion of the surgeon and anesthesia team.

The most common symptom resulting immediately after the procedure is nausea, new or increased from preprocedure symptoms. Management should be aggressive, as this can result in electrolyte derangements, dehydration, and readmission. Patients can also experience distention related to the carbon dioxide pneumoperitoneum, and reassurance should be given. In rare cases, tense capnoperitoneum must be decompressed with a 14-gauge Angio catheter or Veress needle.

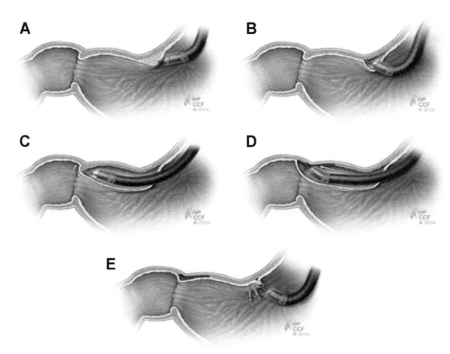

Fig. 1. (*A*) Step 1 of the per oral pyloromyotomy—injection of methylene blue to create a submucosal wheal about 3 cm oral to the pylorus. (*B*) Step 2 of the per oral pyloromyotomy—mucosal incision: a transverse incision is made using an endoscopic knife connected to an energy source with cut current in the mucosa over the bleb. (*C*) Step 3 of the per oral pyloromyotomy—tunneling, once the endoscope is inserted into the submucosal plane, tunneling toward the pylorus is performed. (*D*) Step 4 of the per oral pyloromyotomy—division of the pylorus: after the tunnel is completed, the pylorus is clearly visualized and can then be divided using the electrosurgical knife. (*E*) Step 5 of the per oral pyloromyotomy—closure of the mucosotomy with endoscopic clips. Reprinted with permission, Cleveland Clinic Center for Medical Art & Photography ©2020. All Rights Reserved.

MANAGEMENT

The results of the endoscopic pyloromyotomy are not expected to be immediate, secondary to edema related to the procedure, and this should be discussed with the patient before and after the procedure. The patients are discharged home with full-liquid dietary instructions and told to follow-up in 2 weeks for advancement to mechanical soft diet. At around 4 weeks postoperatively, the patients are typically able to resume a regular diet. Every patient is prescribed 4 weeks of a proton pump inhibitor and a mucosal protective medication. Diabetic patients are closely followed for glycemic control.

Some surgical endoscopists prefer to perform an upper gastrointestinal contrast study on postoperative day 1 before resumption of a liquid diet and before discharge. At the 4-week visit, a gastroparesis cardinal symptom index is performed. In addition, a follow-up gastric emptying study is obtained at this time, to assess for improvement compared with preoperative measurements.

OUTCOMES

In 2018 results from the author's institution were published on the outcomes of the first 100 patients. In this group of patients, after 90 days the body mass index (BMI) was not significantly increased in the underweight patients; however, for the patients overweight by BMI, at 90 days the BMI had decreased (33.7 vs 32.9, $P = .04$). The gastroparesis cardinal symptom indexes improved significantly. In the 63% of patients who had a follow-up gastric emptying study, 78% of those patients had significant improvement in gastric emptying, with 57% of those achieving normal gastric emptying. Complications included 1 return to the operating room for laparoscopic decompression of capnoperitoneum; 4 episodes of gastrointestinal bleeding, 2 of which were associated with ulcers at the tunnel location; and 2 patients requiring prolong rehydration via intravenous access. There were no full-thickness perforations. There was one dearth within 90 days determined to be of cardiac cause.[9]

SUMMARY

Peroral pyloromyotomy, an innovative intramural endoscopic procedure, is a successful management option for appropriately selected patients who suffer from medically refractory gastroparesis. Gastroparesis is a debilitating disorder of the gastrointestinal tract, which significantly decreases quality of life and overall survival. This article describes the history and background, the indications for, the diagnosis of, and the preparation, technique, and short-term outcomes of peroral pyloromyotomy. Further study is required to determine the long-term outcomes of this endoluminal technique.

CLINICS CARE POINTS

- A diagnosis of gastroparesis must be confirmed before any consideration of gastric emptying procedure.
- A multidisciplinary approach to the management of medically refractory gastroparesis, as well as for patient selection for peroral pyloromyotomy, is ideal and should include gastroenterologists, surgical, nutritional, psychological, and pain management experts.
- Long-term study of peroral pyloromyotomy outcomes is ongoing.

DISCLOSURE

M. Lundgren has nothing to disclose. J. Rodriguez has consulting relationships relevant to this topic, including Cook, Gore, Medtronic, Boston Scientific, and Pacira Pharmaceutical.

SUPPLEMENTARY DATA

Supplementary data related to this article can be found online at https://doi.org/10.1016/j.suc.2020.08.015.

REFERENCES

1. Khashab MA, Pasricha PJ. Conquering the third space: challenges and opportunities for diagnostic and therapeutic endoscopy. Gastrointest Endosc 2013;77(1): 146–8.
2. Inoue H, Minami H, Kobayashi Y, et al. Peroral endoscopic myotomy (POEM) for esophageal achalasia. Endoscopy 2010;42(04):265–71.
3. Kawai M, Peretta S, Burckhardt O, et al. Endoscopic pyloromyotomy: a new concept of minimally invasive surgery for pyloric stenosis. Endoscopy 2012; 44(02):169–73.
4. Ibele A, Gould J. Gastroparesis: a comprehensive approach to evaluation and management. 1st edition. Springer; 2020. https://doi.org/10.1007/978-3-030-28929-4.
5. Vijayvargiya P, Camilleri M. Gastroparesis. In: Lacy BE, DiBaise JK, Pimentel M, et al, editors. Essential medical disorders of the stomach and small intestine. A clinical casebook. Cham (Germany): Springer; 2019. p. 23–50.
6. Cline M, Rouphael C. Diagnostic Evaluation of Gastroparesis. In: Ibele A, Gould J, editors. Gastroparesis. Cham (Germany): Springer; 2020. https://doi.org/10.1007/978-3-030-28929-4_3. Available at:.
7. Landa ST, Dumon KR, Dempsey DT. Anatomy and physiology of the stomach and pylorus. In: Grams J, Perry K, Tavakkoli A, editors. The SAGES manual of foregut surgery. Cham (Germany): Springer; 2019. https://doi.org/10.1007/978-3-319-96122-4_3. Available at:.
8. Allemang MT, Strong AT, Haskins IN, et al. How I do it: per-oral pyloromyotomy (POP). J Gastrointest Surg 2017;21:1963–8. https://doi.org/10.1007/s11605-017-3510-2. Available at:.
9. Rodriguez J, Strong AT, Haskins IN, et al. Per-oral Pyloromyotomy (POP) for medically refractory gastroparesis. Ann Surg 2018;268(3):421–30.

Submucosal Tunneling Endoscopic Resection

Vaibhav Wadhwa, MD, Francisco X. Franco, MD, Tolga Erim, DO*

KEYWORDS

- Submucosal tunnel endoscopic resection • Extraluminal tumors
- Video-assisted thoracoscopic surgery • Video-assisted thoracoscopic enucleation
- Submucosal tumors • Submucosal lesions • Subepithelial lesions
- Muscularis propria

KEY POINTS

- Poor compliance, higher cost, and multiple endoscopic ultrasound follow-ups for submucosal tumors (SMTs) are the reasons why most patients prefer an excisional rather than a monitoring approach.
- Submucosal tunneling endoscopic resection (STER) is mainly recommended for upper gastrointestinal submucosal tumors (GISTs) originating from the muscularis propria layer.
- Regardless of the location, current guidelines recommend en bloc resection of GISTs larger than 2 cm for their well-known malignant potential as well as resistance to chemotherapy and radiation therapy.
- Tumors greater than 3.5 cm presenting an irregular tortuous shape present a higher challenge even for experienced endoscopists.
- Medical centers with expertise in endoscopic resection techniques should be the only ones performing STER procedure for SMTs to achieve maximum success rate including the management of any potential complications.

 Video content accompanies this article at http://www.surgical.theclinics.com.

INTRODUCTION

Because of the advancement in endoscopic equipment and improved radiology technique as well as the increased use of endoscopy routinely in the clinical practice, the detection rate of submucosal tumors (SMTs) has increased.[1–4] Upper gastrointestinal SMTs (GISTs) include a wide variety of neoplastic (malignant and benign) and

---

Funding: No funding source.
Department of Gastroenterology and Hepatology, Digestive Disease Institute, Cleveland Clinic Florida, 2950 Cleveland Clinic Boulevard, Weston, FL 33331, USA
* Corresponding author. Department of Gastroenterology, Cleveland Clinic Florida, Weston, FL 33331.
E-mail address: erimt@ccf.org

nonneoplastic lesions growing underneath the mucosa (intramural), such as the following GIST from multipotential mesenchymal stem cells originating mostly from muscularis propria (MP) layer, pancreatic rests (aberrant pancreas), lipomas, neuroendocrine tumors from enterochromaffin cells; schwannomas, which are benign nerve sheath tumors usually of the soft tissue; cysts; varices; and leiomyomas to mention most of them, the latter being more prevalent than others.[2]

These lesions are usually incidental findings and asymptomatic, sometimes requiring multiple endoscopic procedures to be characterized.[5] SMTs less than 3 cm are mostly benign in nature; however, mesenchymal neoplasms such as GISTs can become malignant at smaller sizes. Needle biopsy has the highest accuracy in these cases but due to the fact that sampling errors occur when obtaining the specimen, it makes it difficult to completely rule out the malignant potential of GISTs.[1,2] When dealing with this type of scenario, the options are limited to conventional endoscopic surveillance, endoscopic ultrasound (EUS), or resection of the tumor when the patient is asymptomatic. EUS is helpful due to its ability to clearly delineate the esophageal or gastric layers, making it possible to differentiate the structural origin of the lesions for accurate characterization and eventual treatment planning.[5] On the other hand, EUS is unable to absolutely distinguish GISTs from other hypoechoic lesions from the fourth layer, such as leiomyomas (benign). Thus, EUS-guided fine-needle aspiration or biopsy (EUS-FNA/FNB), even though it has relatively poor diagnostic yield on lesions less than 2 cm, is an important test for accurate detection of subepithelial lesions.[6]

An important factor to consider is the stress and anxiety that an uncertain diagnosis creates in patients as they are followed-up over a long period of time. In fact, studies report that compliance with surveillance is less than 50% for EUS for SMTs.[7]

For tumor resection the authors count on a handful of options, including open surgery, laparoscopic, video- assisted thoracoscopic surgery (VATS), and endoscopic procedures such as endoscopic muscularis excavation, endoscopic full-thickness resection, and endoscopic submucosal dissection (ESD), which have been relegated to a second choice due to higher risk of postoperative complications such as perforation, massive bleeding, and incomplete resection.[2,8,9]

A relatively more recent endoscopic procedure called submucosal tunneling endoscopic resection (STER) has been available for approximately 8 years, and it is considered a feasible minimally invasive procedure mainly recommended for resection of upper GISTs originating from the MP layer. STER was inspired by peroral endoscopic myotomy (POEM) and ESD as a technique and has proved to be more successful due to a much lower perforation risk by avoiding injury of the mucosal layer, attaining a better wound healing, and minimal risk of infection.[10]

Background

It all began back in 1955 with the first description of rectal and sigmoid polypectomy as an EMR start point for early GI neoplasia. Multiple EMR techniques were used as the years passed by, such as EMR with submucosal injections (1973), finally landing on the first ESD described for en bloc gastric cancer resection for larger lesions.[4,11] Newer devices, improved techniques, and better electrosurgical devices allowed near-maximum hemostatic control and proper management of complications such as perforations.[12] In 2004, the new concept of natural orifice transluminal endoscopic surgery emerged, originally proposed for peritoneoscopy through the stomach into the abdominal cavity.[13] In 2007 Sumiyama and colleagues[14] described a procedure performed in animals as a safe access to the mediastinal cavity avoiding the mucosal injury and achieving a single side closure. This gave origin to the idea of Pasricha and colleagues[15] to perform POEM in pigs, leading to the idea of Inoue and colleagues[16] to perform the first POEM procedure in humans in Japan to treat achalasia, additionally reporting the first case series of 17 patients.

Following the basic principles of the POEM procedure, an innovative tunneling technique approaching the third space (submucosa) for tumors en bloc resection, especially those arising from MP layer in esophagus, cardia, and stomach, was first reported by Inoue and colleagues[17] from Yokohama[11] and by Xu and colleagues[18] from Shanghai in 2012. The main characteristic of this technique is the creation of a submucosal tunnel serving as a working space to introduce the endoscope and resect the tumor.[19,20]

The concept of submucosal endoscopy with mucosal flap safety valve has enabled endoscopists to securely use submucosal space. All third-space endoscopy procedures use a similar technique—a submucosal tunnel is created, and then a myotomy is performed or a subepithelial tumor is dissected away from the initial site of the mucosal incision. The other potential indications for third-space endoscopy include refractory gastroparesis, Zenker diverticulum, and restoration of completely obstructed esophageal lumen.[4]

Basic Principles

The submucosa contains loose connective tissue that attaches the mucosa to the MP layer. Separation of this weak attachment can be carried out by injection of normal saline or similar solutions, creating a space for tunneling of the submucosa without damaging the mucosa or the MP layer. Normal saline injection is considered the most cost-effective method to divide the layers (this can be performed in any part of the GI tract). Enough quantity of normal saline has to be injected in order to properly lift the mucosa to create a tunnel leading to the target lesion and safely dissect it and extract it by using an electrocautery knife (**Fig. 1**).

SUBMUCOSAL TUNNELING ENDOSCOPIC RESECTION TECHNIQUE

Preoperative confirmation of the presence, layer of origin, size, and risk of malignancy of the SMT is essential (Video 1). Computed tomography and MRI can be helpful in differentiation of large lesions; however, EUS ± FNA/FNB is invariably used to provide

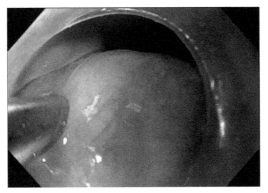

Fig. 1. Submucosal injection of dilute methylene blue and normal saline solution showing lifting of the esophageal mucosa. This demonstrated adequacy of lift is critical for tunnel creation.

the highest level of detail of the lesion as well as to help distinguish the tumor from extrinsic compression from adjacent structures or hemangiomas/varices.[21,22]

The required devices and accessories that are similar for all third-space endoscopic procedures are as follows: a high-definition endoscope, an electrosurgical generator capable of providing customization of current settings, transparent caps, and carbon dioxide (CO_2) insufflator. The accessories include coagulations forceps, hot biopsy forceps, a variety of endoscopic electrosurgical procedures, endoscopic flushing pumps, and endoclips.[23] The patient is positioned supine or left-lateral decubitus, under general anesthesia, and properly intubated to secure the airway.[24] Endoscopic tunneling procedures should only be carried out with CO_2 insufflation, never with room air, given high risk of pneumothorax and pneumoperitoneum.

Tumor identification: the tumor is precisely localized under direct vision endoscopically, assisted with EUS (see **Fig. 1**). A plastic cap attached to the endoscope is helpful in visualization of the lesion, as it can push away folds and keep the lumen open.[19] What determines the feasibility of the procedure includes the size and location of the lesion, along with the shape of it, tumors greater than 3.5 cm presenting and irregular tortuous shape present a higher challenge even for experienced endoscopists. The hardest to localize are SMTs close to the cardia especially near the gastric fundus due to their unfixed position.[25]

Substance injection: the submucosal injection is performed 3 to 5 cm from the SMT and 2 to 3 cm if rectal or gastric SMTs. The typical solution is a combination of dilute methylene blue or indigo carmine with normal saline.[26] The dye used in the injectate helps to highlight the submucosal space, that is, when in doubt, blue is safe to dissect because the mucosa and muscle will not take up the dilute dye. Epinephrine may be used in a dilute manner as part of the solution; however, this is not absolutely necessary. The investigator does not use epinephrine routinely (see **Fig. 1**).

Tunneling: a longitudinal incision in the mucosal layer of 1.5 to 2 cm is considered enough to obtain a tunnel entry; the dissection begins along the borders about 0.5 cm on each side of the first incision; this allows quicker entry into the submucosal layer (Image 2). An inverse "T" incision allows easier tumor extraction, especially in larger lesions. Once entry is established, the tunnel is extended using a side to side dissection of the submucosal fibers with the electrocautery knife, always avoiding injury of the flap by keeping the dissecting plane as near as possible to the MP layer.[27,28]

Tumor dissection, resection, and closing: the tumor is dissected with the ultimate goal of not causing damage to the capsule, which is crucial for patient prognosis (Image 3). Usually it is dissected at the MP layer; unless the tumor is originating from the deep MP layer or showing a tight connection with the MP or serosa, then a full-thickness resection should be attempted.[4]

Smaller SMTs ($\leq$2 cm) are clearly not as big a challenge as the bigger tumors in the GI tract. If the lesion is too large to be retrieved through the entry incision and preoperative evaluation points to a benign tumor, a snare might be used following the enucleation to cut the tumor into as many pieces needed to take it out. An extra-mucosal window near the tumor area is always a second option in case of large tumors.[29] Once resection is completed the tunnel is lavaged with normal saline, and hemostasis of any oozing vessels with coagulation forceps should be accomplished. Finally, the mucosal incision is closed with endoclips or an endoscopic suture device.[1,18,19,30,31]

SUBMUCOSAL TUNNELING FOR THE ESOPHAGUS

In the esophagus, SMTs less than 3 cm are deemed as benign in general terms[32]; nonetheless, some of them have a malignant potential (especially GISTs growing from MP layer)[33] and are candidates for surgical extraction. Enucleation obtained by thoracotomy used to be the conventional approach, indicated for symptomatic patients with tumors greater than 2 cm and the need for a pathologic diagnosis to exclude malignancy. This procedure is a highly invasive procedure with increased risk of postoperative complications. Thoracoscopic approach came to minimize these issues with fewer and less severe complications and higher rates of success.[34]

The most common benign esophageal tumors are leiomyomas accounting for 70% to 80% of all SMTs. However, SMTs only represent 1% or less of all tumors in the esophagus.[35] Current standard of care dictates resection of GISTs larger than 2 cm given their malignancy potential, regardless of anatomic location. STER has been increasingly used as an alternative for patients with different types of SMTs, and it has gone through an evolution over time that has expanded its utilization to larger lesions.

The creation of a mucosal flap and tunnel in STER eliminates absence of a serosal layer in the esophagus from becoming a barrier to SMT resection. The major limiting factor becomes the size of the lesion. Lesions larger than 3.5 cm can be significantly more difficult to remove due to more extensive dissection that needs to be performed to enucleate the lesion. Another disadvantage for large lesions is that they often need to be cut into smaller pieces to allow retrieval through the tunnel[36,37]; STER has been performed on SMTs greater than 3.5 cm, up to 7 cm.[29,30,38] There is experience demonstrating that the main difference between STER technique on SMTs less than 3.5 cm and greater than 3.5 cm is increasing operation time for the bigger tumors, with no significant distinction in efficacy and complications rate.[27] Others recommend that for tumors larger than 4 cm originating deeper in the MP layer, thoracoscopic enucleation should be performed because it is hard to remove this type of tumors en bloc, especially considering larger lesions may be associated with increased risk of perforation, fistula, and secondary infection[24,39] (**Figs. 2–5**).

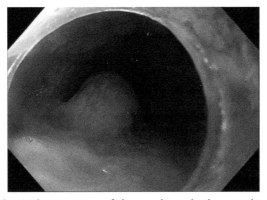

Fig. 2. Endoscopic luminal appearance of the esophageal submucosal tumor.

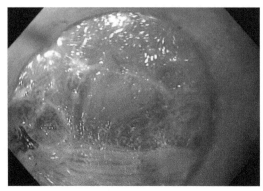

Fig. 3. Initial appearance of the submucosal tumor in the tunnel.

SUBMUCOSAL TUNNELING FOR THE STOMACH

STER in the stomach has several limitations related to anatomic characteristics (a large lumen, flaccid walls, an unfixed position, and thick mucosa), which makes rendering the generation of a submucosal tunnel significantly more challenging compared with doing so in the esophagus. Still, STER has been performed throughout the stomach, particularly on SMTs close to the cardia including the fundus, the lesser curvature of the gastric corpus, and in the greater curvature of the gastric antrum.[40,41]

If en bloc resection without piecemeal retrieval is desired, the diameter of the tumor should be 3.5 cm or smaller. The tunnel is not likely to be able to accommodate a larger lesion for single piece retrieval.[42]

STER has been studied and well defined in the removal of gastrointestinal lesions in most locations.

A fairly large review of STER for esophageal and gastric SMTs showed significant curative resection rates.[1] This included a total of 736 upper GISTs from 703 patients, with the following curative resection rates—esophageal SMTs 100% (208/208); esophagogastric junction 100% (78/78); and gastric 100% (115/115)—and en-bloc resection rates—esophageal 98.6% (205/208); esophagogastric junction 96.2% (75/78); and gastric 97.9% (95/97). There were no reports of local recurrence or distant metastasis in any of the studies with mean follow-up ranging from 1 to 36 months.[1]

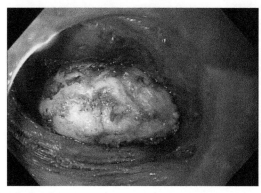

Fig. 4. Tumor is dissected out.

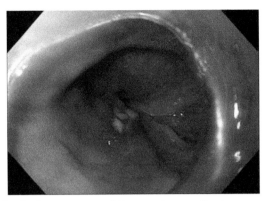

Fig. 5. Endoscopic luminal appearance of the esophagus after tumor removal.

The largest systematic review and meta-analysis on STER for upper-GISTs included 28 studies (20 retrospective and 8 prospective) comprising total 1041 patients and 1085 lesions.[43] Nearly all but one of the studies were conducted in China. The reported pooled complete resection rate was 97.5% (95% confidence interval [CI], 96.0%–98.5%), and the pooled en bloc resection rate was 94.6% (95% CI, 91.5%–96.7%). The highest reported adverse events were subcutaneous emphysema and/or pneumomediastinum of up to 14.8% (95% CI, 10.5%–20.5%), and perforation was estimated to be about 5.6% (95% CI, 3.7%–8.2%).[43]

STER can be highly challenging in the fundus; however, there has been some evidence that has reported complete resection in this area. Lu and colleagues[40] described 18 patients with 19 gastric fundus SMTs were able to undergo en bloc resection with mean size of 2.1 cm in diameter. Another study by the same group described 45 patients who underwent STER (47 tumors resected) in the cardia, fundus, or antrum with complete curative resection and no local recurrence noted on a median follow-up of 11 months.[26]

Long-term outcomes for patients with upper GISTs, originating from the MP layer, who underwent STER have been reported in one Chinese retrospective study of 180 patients (7 in the upper esophagus, 66 in the middle esophagus, 51 in the lower esophagus, 43 in esophagogastric junction, and 13 in the stomach). Most of the lesions were leiomyomas (146/180) and GISTs (28/180) with schwannomas (4/180), calcifying fibrous tumors (2/180) making up the rest. The en bloc resection rate was 90.6% and the curative resection rate being 100% with median resection time being 45 minutes (range, 15–200 mins). Piecemeal resection rate was related to size of tumor and irregularity of shape. The reported complication rate was 8.3% (pneumothorax in 10/180, major bleeding in 2/180, mucosal injury in 2/180, and esophageal-pleural fistula in 1/180). Most of the patients (177/180) were followed-up with no local recurrence or evidence of metastasis with a median follow-up of 36 months.[44]

Complications of STER include bleeding, mucosal laceration, and gas-related complications (including subcutaneous emphysema, mediastinal emphysema, pneumothorax, and pneumoperitoneum), with gas-related complications being the most common and reported in most studies. These complications tend to occur when the patient undergoes a full-thickness resection and after removal of the esophagogastric junction SMTs. Bleeding and mucosal perforations are less common but can be managed endoscopically most of the time. Large lacerations have been reported in some cases, which required esophageal stent placement.[24,45] Most gas-related complications seem to resolve on their own and do not require any intervention.[46] The risk factors of these complications include full-thickness MP resection, resection of multiple SMTs, and esophagogastric junction location. Rare complications such as large pneumothorax, thoracic effusion requiring drainage, etc. can also occur and will require intervention.[46]

It is imperative to establish that medical centers with expertise in endoscopic resection techniques should be the only ones performing STER procedure for SMTs in order to get the maximum success rate, including the management of any potential complication[25] (**Figs. 6–10**).

SUBMUCOSAL TUNNELING ENDOSCOPIC RESECTION VERSUS VIDEO-ASSISTED THORACOSCOPIC SURGERY/VIDEO-ASSISTED THORACOSCOPIC ESOPHAGECTOMY

The current surgical standard of care for the resection of esophageal SMTs is video-assisted thoracoscopic surgery (VATS) or video-assisted thoracoscopic enucleation, particularly for tumors greater than 2 cm arising from the MP. Both VATS and STER are minimally invasive techniques that have highest efficacy with low complication rates; however, STER has advantages over VATS when comparing procedure time, length of hospital stay, and cost.[28] Also, postprocedure chest pain was lower when compared with that of thoracoscopic enucleation group.[34]

A Chinese study of 166 patients with large symptomatic SMTs in the esophagus and esophagogastric junction who underwent either STER or VATS showed no statistical difference in en bloc resection, with all tumors receiving complete resection. No local recurrence was seen on follow-up in both groups. The major complication with STER was pneumothorax or pleural effusion, and for VATS group it was esophageal–pleural fistula. However, with irregularly shaped lesions, STER was technically more difficult with en bloc resection, and more complications were related to these lesions.[47]

The only randomized controlled trial comparing VATS and STER enrolled 66 patients with esophageal SMT originating from MP. Of the patients who underwent VATS or STER, en bloc resection rate was 100% for VATS and 83.3% (26/30) for STER, but this was not statistically significant. On follow-up, no local recurrence was recorded. STER, even with piecemeal resection, had 100% curative resection with no local recurrence. Complications were similar in the 2 groups. Compared with VATS, STER had decreased procedure time and cost. The investigators

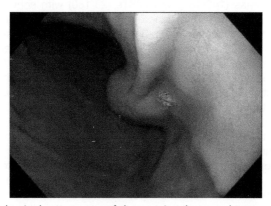

Fig. 6. Endoscopic luminal appearance of the gastric submucosal tumor.

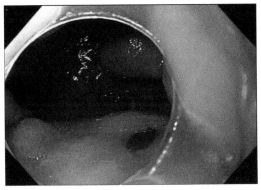

Fig. 7. Submucosal injection before creating tunnel; note the orientation with regard to the submucosal tumor.

concluded that STER may be beneficial over VATS for esophageal SMTs with less than 2 cm diameter.[48]

SUBMUCOSAL TUNNELING ENDOSCOPIC RESECTION-ET

GISTs can have extraluminal growth patterns or even occur outside of the GI tract (EGISTs), although there is a possibility that EGISTs get detached from its MP layer where they grew initially due to the extensive extraluminal growth.[49,50]

GISTs are well known to be resistant to chemotherapy and radiotherapy; therefore, complete en bloc resection is essential to avoid recurrence and complications of non-metastatic tumors. Because of the success of STER in patients with submucosal endoscopic tumor resection (SET) and SMTs arising from the MP, STER has been studied for application in SETs showing exophytic growth (STER-ET). STER-ET in expert hands can be a successful alternative to laparoscopic excisional methods by significantly lowering morbidity, and it can also make it easier to approach lesions behind the stomach or near the esophagogastric junction, which are always problematic.[51,52]

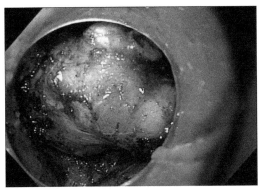

Fig. 8. Tumor is dissected out.

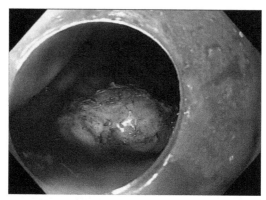

Fig. 9. Tumor is retrieved out of the tunnel.

There are very limited data on this technique. In a prospective trial by Cai and colleagues, use of STER was evaluated for GI SETs with extraluminal growth. These lesions were at the level of cardia or proximal lesser curvature of the stomach. Of the 8 patients who underwent STER-ET, en bloc curative resection rate was 100%; however, one of the tumors was too large to be removed through the SM channel and had to be excised into 2 pieces to facilitate removal. There were no major adverse events or complications observed postoperatively. The major barrier encountered using this technique was the success rate of en bloc resection related to the tumor size, which preoperatively is considered one of the factors that determine the feasibility of this approach.[52]

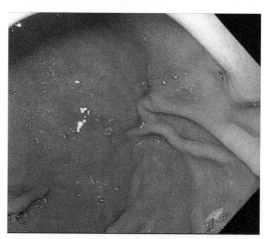

Fig. 10. Endoscopic luminal appearance of the stomach at site of tumor resection at 22-month follow-up.

SUMMARY

Minimally invasive endoscopic resection procedures continue to evolve, with STER being a durable option for en bloc resection of SMTs. Whether STER can be effectively used for larger (>3.5 cm) lesions remains to be seen. STER-ET is a novel approach for removal of extraluminal tumors, but data are currently limited to support its use. Further studies are needed to evaluate outcomes of efficacy, en bloc resection rate, recurrence, complications, and potential tumor seeding for various lesion types, sizes, locations, and different patient populations.[53]

CLINICS CARE POINTS

Pearls

- STER was inspired by ESD as a technique that proves to be more successful due to a much lower perforation risk by avoiding deliberate injury of the mucosal layer accomplishing a better wound healing and minimal risk of infection.
- In addition to being minimally invasive, en bloc endoscopic resection has the advantage of precise histopathological diagnosis of depth of invasion, differentiation, and possible involvement of either vessels or lymphatics.
- Because of the reduced area of the tunnel the recommended diameter of the tumor should be up to 3.5 cm in order to ensure a total capsule resection (en bloc).
- In the gastric region, STER is intended to be performed on SMTs close to the cardia including the fundus, the lesser curvature of the gastric corpus, and in the greater curvature of the gastric antrum.

Pitfalls

- From the esophageal anatomy point of view, there is only a thin membrane outside the MP, and STER is a complicated procedure; therefore, a 3.5 cm maximum tumor size is what most of the studies recommend for this procedure, giving the endoscopist enough room to maneuver.
- Studies recommend that, for tumors larger than 4 cm originating deeper in the MP layer, thoracoscopic enucleation should be performed, as it is hard to remove this type of tumors en bloc, also considering those are associated to increased risk of perforation, fistula, and secondary infection
- STER in the stomach has its limitations related to anatomic characteristics (a large lumen, increased flexibility, an unfixed position, and thick mucosa), which makes it different from esophageal procedure, rendering the generation of a submucosal tunnel more challenging compared with doing so in the esophagus; therefore not all gastric SMTs are suitable for STER.

DISCLOSURE

The authors have no conflicts of interest.

SUPPLEMENTARY DATA

Supplementary data related to this article can be found online at https://doi.org/10.1016/j.suc.2020.08.016.

REFERENCES

1. Jain D, Desai A, Mahmood E, et al. Submucosal tunneling endoscopic resection of upper gastrointestinal tract tumors arising from muscularis propria. Ann Gastroenterol 2017;30(3):262–72.

2. Song S, Wang X, Zhang S, et al. Efficacy and complications of submucosal tunneling endoscopic resection for upper gastrointestinal submucosal tumors and exploration for influencing factors. Z Gastroenterol 2018;56(4):365–73.
3. Chen T-H, Hsu C-M, Chu Y-Y, et al. Association of endoscopic ultrasonographic parameters and gastrointestinal stromal tumors (GISTs): can endoscopic ultrasonography be used to screen gastric GISTs for potential malignancy? Scand J Gastroenterol 2016;51(3):374–7.
4. Wadhwa V, Gupta K, Erim T. Endoscopic intramural surgery part 1: resectional therapies. Dig Dis Interv 2018;02(04):359–67.
5. Papanikolaou IS, Triantafyllou K, Kourikou A, et al. Endoscopic ultrasonography for gastric submucosal lesions. World J Gastrointest Endosc 2011;3(5):86–94.
6. Franco MC, Schulz RT, Maluf-Filho F. Opinion: How to manage subepithelial lesions of the upper gastrointestinal tract? World J Gastrointest Endosc 2015; 7(18):1262–7.
7. Kushnir VM, Keswani RN, Hollander TG, et al. Compliance with surveillance recommendations for foregut subepithelial tumors is poor: results of a prospective multicenter study. Gastrointest Endosc 2015;81(6):1378–84.
8. Shi Q, Zhong Y-S, Yao L-q, et al. Endoscopic submucosal dissection for treatment of esophageal submucosal tumors originating from the muscularis propria layer. Gastrointest Endosc 2011;74(6):1194–200.
9. Białek A, Wiechowska-Kozłowska A, Pertkiewicz J, et al. Endoscopic submucosal dissection for the treatment of neoplastic lesions in the gastrointestinal tract. World J Gastroenterol 2013;19(12):1953–61.
10. Duan T-Y, Tan Y-Y, Wang X-H, et al. A comparison of submucosal tunneling endoscopic resection and endoscopic full-thickness resection for gastric fundus submucosal tumors. Rev Esp Enferm Dig 2018;110(3):160–5.
11. Chiu PWY, Inoue H, Rösch T. From POEM to POET: applications and perspectives for submucosal tunnel endoscopy. Endoscopy 2016;48(12):1134–42.
12. Committee AT, Maple JT, Abu Dayyeh BK, et al. Endoscopic submucosal dissection. Gastrointest Endosc 2015;81(6):1311–25.
13. Kalloo AN, Singh VK, Jagannath SB, et al. Flexible transgastric peritoneoscopy: a novel approach to diagnostic and therapeutic interventions in the peritoneal cavity. Gastrointest Endosc 2004;60(1):114–7.
14. Sumiyama K, Gostout CJ, Rajan E, et al. Transesophageal mediastinoscopy by submucosal endoscopy with mucosal flap safety valve technique. Gastrointest Endosc 2007;65(4):679–83.
15. Pasricha PJ, Hawari R, Ahmed I, et al. Submucosal endoscopic esophageal myotomy: a novel experimental approach for the treatment of achalasia. Endoscopy 2007;39(09):761–4.
16. Inoue H, Minami H, Kobayashi Y, et al. Peroral endoscopic myotomy (POEM) for esophageal achalasia. Endoscopy 2010;42(04):265–71.
17. Inoue H, Ikeda H, Hosoya T, et al. Submucosal endoscopic tumor resection for subepithelial tumors in the esophagus and cardia. Endoscopy 2012;44(3): 225–30.
18. Xu M-D, Cai M-Y, Zhou P-H, et al. Submucosal tunneling endoscopic resection: a new technique for treating upper GI submucosal tumors originating from the muscularis propria layer (with videos). Gastrointest Endosc 2012;75(1):195–9.
19. Chen H, Li B, Li L, et al. Current status of endoscopic resection of gastric subepithelial tumors. Am J Gastroenterol 2019;114(5):718–25.
20. Werner YB, Rösch T. POEM and submucosal tunneling. Curr Treat Options Gastroenterol 2016;14(2):163–77.

21. Nishida T, Kawai N, Yamaguchi S, et al. Submucosal tumors: comprehensive guide for the diagnosis and therapy of gastrointestinal submucosal tumors. Dig Endosc 2013;25(5):479–89.

22. Chu Y, Qiao X, Gao X, et al. Combined EUS and CT for evaluating gastrointestinal submucosal tumors before endoscopic resection. Eur J Gastroenterol Hepatol 2014;26(8):933–6.

23. Nabi Z, Nageshwar Reddy D, Ramchandani M. Recent advances in third-space endoscopy. Gastroenterol Hepatol (N Y) 2018;14(4):224–32.

24. Tan Y, Huo J, Liu D. Current status of submucosal tunneling endoscopic resection for gastrointestinal submucosal tumors originating from the muscularis propria layer. Oncol Lett 2017;14(5):5085–90.

25. Li Q-L, Chen W-F, Zhang C, et al. Clinical impact of submucosal tunneling endoscopic resection for the treatment of gastric submucosal tumors originating from the muscularis propria layer (with video). Surg Endosc 2015;29(12):3640–6.

26. Lu J, Jiao T, Li Y, et al. Heading toward the right direction—solution package for endoscopic submucosal tunneling resection in the stomach. PLOS ONE 2015; 10(3):e0119870.

27. Wang H, Tan Y, Zhou Y, et al. Submucosal tunneling endoscopic resection for upper gastrointestinal submucosal tumors originating from the muscularis propria layer. Eur J Gastroenterol Hepatol 2015;27(7):776–80.

28. Tan Y, Lv L, Duan T, et al. Comparison between submucosal tunneling endoscopic resection and video-assisted thoracoscopic surgery for large esophageal leiomyoma originating from the muscularis propria layer. Surg Endosc 2016; 30(7):3121–7.

29. Ng JJ, Chiu PWY, Shabbir A, et al. Removal of a large, 40-mm, submucosal leiomyoma using submucosal tunneling endoscopic resection and extraction of specimen using a distal mucosal incision. Endoscopy 2015;47(Suppl 1 UCTN): E232–3.

30. Tan Y, Zhu H, Lv L, et al. Enlarging an accidental mucosotomy to facilitate tumor extraction during submucosal tunneling endoscopic resection for a giant esophageal leiomyoma. Gastrointest Endosc 2016;83(1):248–9.

31. Du Z, Ding W, Chen T. Suitability and efficacy of submucosal tunneling endoscopic resection for the treatment of giant leiomyoma in the middle and lower esophagus. Dis Esophagus 2019;32(12):doz059.

32. Demetri GD, von Mehren M, Antonescu CR, et al. NCCN task force report: update on the management of patients with gastrointestinal stromal tumors. J Natl Compr Canc Netw 2010;8:S1–44. Suppl 2(0 2).

33. Joensuu H, Hohenberger P, Corless CL. Gastrointestinal stromal tumour. Lancet 2013;382(9896):973–83.

34. Li Q-Y, Meng Y, Xu Y-Y, et al. Comparison of endoscopic submucosal tunneling dissection and thoracoscopic enucleation for the treatment of esophageal submucosal tumors. Gastrointest Endosc 2017;86(3):485–91.

35. Seremetis MG, Lyons WS, deGuzman VC, et al. Leiomyomata of the esophagus. An analysis of 838 cases. Cancer 1976;38(5):2166–77.

36. Ye L-P, Zhang Y, Mao X-L, et al. Submucosal tunnelling endoscopic resection for the treatment of esophageal submucosal tumours originating from the muscularis propria layer: an analysis of 15 cases. Dig Liver Dis 2013;45(2):119–23.

37. Liu B-R, Song J-T, Kong L-J, et al. Tunneling endoscopic muscularis dissection for subepithelial tumors originating from the muscularis propria of the esophagus and gastric cardia. Surg Endosc 2013;27(11):4354–9.

38. Liu H, Wei L-L, Zhang Y-Z, et al. Submucosal tunnelling endoscopic resection (STER) for the treatment of a case of huge esophageal tumor arising in the muscularis propria: a case report and review of literature. Int J Clin Exp Med 2015; 8(9):15846–51.

39. Tan Y, Liu D. En bloc submucosal tunneling endoscopic resection for a giant esophageal leiomyoma. Gastrointest Endosc 2015;82(2):399.

40. Lu J, Zheng M, Jiao T, et al. Transcardiac tunneling technique for endoscopic submucosal dissection of gastric fundus tumors arising from the muscularis propria. Endoscopy 2014;46(10):888–92.

41. Li B, Liu J, Lu Y, et al. Submucosal tunneling endoscopic resection for tumors of the esophagogastric junction. Minim Invasive Ther Allied Technol 2016;25(3): 141–7.

42. Wang X-Y, Xu M-D, Yao L-Q, et al. Submucosal tunneling endoscopic resection for submucosal tumors of the esophagogastric junction originating from the muscularis propria layer: a feasibility study (with videos). Surg Endosc 2014;28(6): 1971–7.

43. Lv X-H, Wang C-H, Xie Y. Efficacy and safety of submucosal tunneling endoscopic resection for upper gastrointestinal submucosal tumors: a systematic review and meta-analysis. Surg Endosc 2017;31(1):49–63.

44. Chen T, Zhou P-H, Chu Y, et al. Long-term outcomes of submucosal tunneling endoscopic resection for upper gastrointestinal submucosal tumors. Ann Surg 2017;265(2):363–9.

45. Du C, Linghu E. Submucosal tunneling endoscopic resection for the treatment of gastrointestinal submucosal tumors originating from the muscularis propria layer. J Gastrointest Surg 2017;21(12):2100–9.

46. Chen T, Zhang C, Yao L-Q, et al. Management of the complications of submucosal tunneling endoscopic resection for upper gastrointestinal submucosal tumors. Endoscopy 2016;48(2):149–55.

47. Chen T, Lin Z-W, Zhang Y-Q, et al. Submucosal tunneling endoscopic resection vs thoracoscopic enucleation for large submucosal tumors in the esophagus and the esophagogastric junction. J Am Coll Surg 2017;225(6):806–16.

48. Chai N, Du C, Gao Y, et al. Comparison between submucosal tunneling endoscopic resection and video-assisted thoracoscopic enucleation for esophageal submucosal tumors originating from the muscularis propria layer: a randomized controlled trial. Surg Endosc 2018;32(7):3364–72.

49. Reith JD, Goldblum JR, Lyles RH, et al. Extragastrointestinal (soft tissue) stromal tumors: an analysis of 48 cases with emphasis on histologic predictors of outcome. Mod Pathol 2000;13(5):577–85.

50. Agaimy A, Wünsch PH. Gastrointestinal stromal tumours: a regular origin in the muscularis propria, but an extremely diverse gross presentation. A review of 200 cases to critically re-evaluate the concept of so-called extra-gastrointestinal stromal tumours. Langenbecks Arch Surg 2006;391(4):322–9.

51. Gupta M, Sheppard BC, Corless CL, et al. Outcome following surgical therapy for gastrointestinal stromal tumors. J Gastrointest Surg 2006;10(8):1099–105.

52. Cai M-Y, Zhu B-Q, Xu M-D, et al. Submucosal tunnel endoscopic resection for extraluminal tumors: a novel endoscopic method for en bloc resection of predominant extraluminal growing subepithelial tumors or extra-gastrointestinal tumors (with videos). Gastrointest Endosc 2018;88(1):160–7.

53. Committee AT, Aslanian HR, Sethi A, et al. ASGE guideline for endoscopic full-thickness resection and submucosal tunnel endoscopic resection. VideoGIE 2019;4(8):343–50.

Per Oral Zenker Diverticulotomy

Harry J. Wong, MD[a,b,*], Michael B. Ujiki, MD[b]

KEYWORDS

• Zenker diverticulum • Diverticulotomy • Flexible endoscopy • Submucosal tunneling
• Z-POEM • STESD

KEY POINTS

- Zenker's diverticulum (ZD) is a rare but treatable surgical disease affecting the elderly.
- Surgical interventions include open surgery, rigid endoscopic, and flexible endoscopic diverticulotomy, with increasing trend toward flexible endoscopic approach.
- Per oral endoscopic myotomy (Z-POEM) with submucosal tunneling is a new promising technique that has been shown to be safe and effective in the management of ZD.

BACKGROUND

Zenker diverticulum (ZD) is a rare esophageal disorder with prevalence of 0.01% to 0.11% and annual incidence of 2 per 100,000, mostly affecting the elderly population.[1,2] It is a pulsion-type diverticulum that originates from the pharyngoesophageal junction between the inferior constrictor and the cricopharyngeus muscles in an area of muscle weakness termed Killian triangle. Although the pharyngeal pouch is a false diverticulum of mucosa resulted from herniation of pharyngeal soft tissue, the common wall or septum between the esophageal and diverticula lumens is full thickness containing the cricopharyngeus muscle.

Because the pathogenesis of ZD involves impaired relaxation of the cricopharyngeus muscle during swallowing, the mainstay of the treatment requires a complete cricopharyngeal myotomy/septotomy the allow open flow of food from pouch into the esophageal lumen. Although multiple surgical and endoscopic interventions exist for ZD, the optimal approach is not clear because there are no prospective randomized trials to definitively demonstrate the superiority of one approach. In this article, we describe an effective method using flexible endoscopy and submucosal tunneling technique to treat ZD, also termed per oral endoscopic myotomy (Z-POEM).

[a] Department of Surgery, University of Chicago Medicine, Chicago, IL, USA; [b] Department of Surgery, NorthShore University HealthSystem, 2650 Ridge Avenue, Evanston, IL 60201, USA
* Corresponding author. 2650 Ridge Avenue, GCSI rmB665, Evanston, IL 60201.
E-mail address: Harry.Wong@uchospitals.edu

Surg Clin N Am 100 (2020) 1215–1226
https://doi.org/10.1016/j.suc.2020.08.005
0039-6109/20/© 2020 Elsevier Inc. All rights reserved.

INDICATIONS FOR REPAIR

Usually diagnosed on contrast esophagram or upper endoscopy, the presentation of ZD is characterized by a wide range of symptoms including dysphagia, regurgitation, cough, reflux, gurgling, aspiration, globus sensation, and halitosis. Most patients with ZD are often symptomatic and should undergo repair to prevent complications, such as aspiration pneumonia or nutritional failure. However, many patients progress to an advanced state with nutritional compromise without having been appropriately diagnosed or offered surgical therapy. Moreover, because ZD commonly manifest in elderly patients, intervention tends to carry higher morbidity and mortality. That being said, surgical intervention is successful in relieving symptoms in 80% to 100% of patients.[3]

HISTORY AND EVOLUTION OF INTERVENTIONS

First reported by Ludlow in 1769, surgical treatment of ZD was described around the same time as von Zenker's landmark paper in 1877.[4] Although traditionally treated with open transcervical approach with cricopharyngeal myotomy and diverticulectomy, management has trended toward endoscopic approaches over the last several decades. Endoscopic procedures focusing on dividing the esophageal diverticular septum was initially introduced in 1917 but was quickly abandoned given high surgical morbidity and mortality. With the modification of diathermic coagulation and introduction of the endoscopic stapler in the 1990s, endoscopic repair using rigid instrumentation has been increasingly adopted by many centers, proving to be a viable treatment option. Initially described in 1995, flexible endoscopic treatment of ZD has the ability to be performed under sedation with better visualization, and therefore has also been gaining popularity as a viable minimally invasive intervention.[5]

There is currently no consensus on the optimal method of intervention because most studies have been single-institutional observational studies. Systematic reviews and meta-analyses have suggested endoscopic approaches to have shorter recovery time and lower perioperative morbidity, but not enough evidence to support one approach over the other.[4,6–8] An overview of current available approaches and interventions with various instrumentations possible for ZD is shown in **Table 1**.

Table 1
Summary of interventions and instrumentations available for the treatment of Zenker diverticulum

Open Surgery	Rigid Endoscopic	Flexible Endoscopic
Cricopharyngeal myotomy	Electrocautery	Needle knife
Diverticulectomy	CO_2 laser	APC
Diverticulopexy	Endostapler	CO_2 laser
Diverticular inversion	Harmonic scalpel	Harmonic scalpel
		Hook knife
		Stag Beetle knife
		Ligasure
		Flexible rotatable bipolar forceps
		Z-POEM/STESD

Abbreviations: APC, argon plasma coagulation; STESD, submucosal tunneling endoscopic septum division.

APPROACH TO MANAGEMENT
Open Surgery

Historically, ZD was treated with an open surgical approach via a left transcervical incision, often involving diverticulectomy with cricopharyngeal myotomy added on later with the improved understanding of the pathophysiology.[9] Currently, there are different variations of the open surgical treatment, most of which include some combination of diverticulectomy, diverticulopexy, or diverticular inversion with myotomy of the cricopharyngeal muscle according to size of the diverticulum.[5,10] Based on current literature, the open approach has a good success rate (80%–100%) with overall morbidity of 10.5% and mortality of 0.6%, and risk of serious complications was low (3.3% leak/perforation, 0.2% mediastinitis, 3.3% recurrent laryngeal nerve injury, and 1.8% infection). Although open surgery is the preferred approach of some specialists for very small or large diverticula, the invasive nature and long recovery time warrants careful patient selection.[5]

Rigid Endoscopic Surgery

Initially developed to reduce postoperative morbidity, the rigid transoral endoscopic approach uses a rigid diverticuloscope to provide exposure of the common wall, with the long blade in the esophagus and short blade in the diverticulum, allowing safe division of the common wall including the cricopharyngeus. There are several methods to divide the common wall, evolving from electrocautery (Dohlman technique)[11] at first to carbon dioxide laser, and stapling devices. The rigid transoral stapling approach in particular has shown favorable results and has been accepted as a safer, less invasive, and more efficient minimally invasive therapy of choice.

Rigid endoscopic stapling procedure technique

Following induction of general anesthesia, the rigid diverticuloscope is placed in the esophagus and secured in place once optimal exposure is obtained, identifying the diverticulum. An appropriately sized endoGIA stapler is then selected and advanced through the diverticuloscope with the anvil placed into the diverticular pouch and the cartridge into the esophageal lumen. The stapler is then closed and fired, dividing the common wall and sealing the edges, effectively making the diverticulum contiguous with the posterior esophagus and dividing the cricopharyngeal muscle.[5]

Comprehensive literature reviews have reported clinical success rates upward of 90% with 4% to 7% morbidity and less than 1% mortality using the stapler approach.[10] However, the rigid endoscopic approach has many limitations. Besides the obvious need for general anesthesia, intraoperative abandonment or conversion to open has been reported to be as high as 7.7% mostly caused by inadequate neck extension or mobility and issues with small diverticular size not allowing adequate stapler engagement and firing. As shown in **Fig. 1**, current endoscopic staplers do not staple and cut all the way to the tip, which can lead to incomplete division of the septum and cricopharyngeal muscle. This is thought to be the major cause of persistent symptoms and recurrence, which has been reported to be as high as 36%.[7] However, there has been report of surgeons cutting down the blade of the anvil or applying traction sutures on the septum to achieve a more complete division.[5,12,13] More recently, there has been reports of using other dissection techniques, such as the Harmonic scalpel or Ligasure dissectors[14]; however, these techniques have not been widely adopted given consideration of potentially unsealed edges and bleeding.[5]

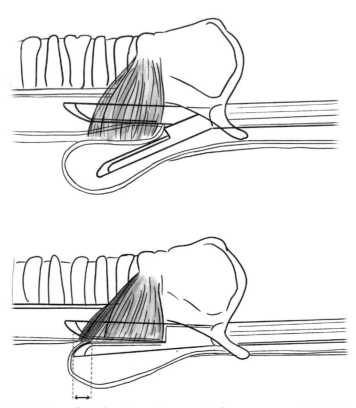

Fig. 1. Demonstration of rigid endoscopic approach for management of Zenker diverticulum, with stapler in the closed position, not all cricopharyngeal muscle fibers are divided once stapler is fired.

Flexible Endoscopic Surgery

Flexible endoscopic diverticulotomy was first introduced in 1982 with the first series reported by Mulder and colleagues.[15] Initially designed for patients who were poor surgical candidates unable to tolerate general anesthesia and those with inadequate neck extension for rigid scopes or other anatomic difficulties, the flexible endoscopic approach is becoming increasingly popular and widely accepted with multiple series demonstrating the feasibility and efficacy.[6,8,16] Along with the advancements of endoscopic techniques and instrumentation, this technique can now be performed using a variety of devices including argon plasma coagulation cautery, hook knife, needle knife, Stag Beetle knife, harmonic scalpel, and bipolar or monopolar forceps.[17]

The principle of flexible endoscopic approaches also involves the division of the common wall or septum of the diverticulum to achieve complete cricopharyngeal myotomy. The goal is to reduce the size of the diverticulum and improve pharyngeal motor function, which ultimately improves symptoms of dysphagia and regurgitation. This technique is often performed with accessory devices, such as a transparent cap loaded onto the tip of the endoscope or a soft diverticuloscope as an overtube (**Fig. 2**) that straddles the common wall between two lumens. A nasogastric tube can also be used to reference the true esophageal lumen, which may not always be apparent.

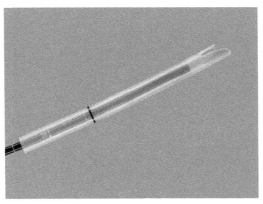

Fig. 2. Flexible diverticuloscope to be used as an overtube during flexible endoscopic Zenker diverticulotomy. (Permission for use granted by Cook Medical, Bloomington, Indiana.)

Although there are significant variations in instrumentation used, most flexible endoscopic diverticulotomies performed since its emergence involve division of the common wall using a cutting device. Once the common wall or septum between the true esophageal lumen and diverticular pouch is identified, a mucosotomy is performed over the cricopharyngeus muscle and carried down until the septum is completely divided. An Endoclip is often placed at the vertex of the incision to decrease risk of subsequent perforation. Despite the heterogeneity in recent published literature on flexible endoscopic diverticulotomy, multiple meta-analyses have demonstrated comparable outcomes to open or rigid endoscopic approaches.[6,8] A summary of clinical outcomes using recent studies on the flexible endoscopic approach is shown in **Table 2**, grouped by instrumentation type.[15,18–38]

Per Oral Endoscopic Myotomy of Zenker Diverticulum (Submucosal Tunneling Endoscopic Septum Division)

More recently, there has been emergence of a novel flexible endoscopic method using submucosal tunneling technique to achieve the cricopharyngeal myotomy. Using the same principle of the POEM for achalasia, Li and colleagues[39] first described the use of submucosal tunneling to perform Z-POEM, which is also referred to as submucosal tunneling endoscopic septum division (STESD). This technique was developed to decrease the risk of perforation encountered during the usual flexible endoscopic techniques, which has been reported as high as 6.5%.[8] The first description of the Z-POEM technique involves four major steps: (1) mucosal incision proximal to the diverticular septum, (2) submucosal tunneling, (3) septum division, and (4) mucosal closure.[39] This is slightly different than the preferred technique used by the authors at our institution where our practice involves making the mucosal incision directly over the septum. The detailed technical approach is described next.

Per oral endoscopic myotomy Zenker diverticulum/submucosal tunneling endoscopic septum division procedure technique

Once in the operating room, the patient is positioned in the supine position and induced under general anesthesia with rapid sequence intubation because the presence of ZD carries higher risk for aspiration. General anesthesia is preferred for the ease of the surgeon and comfort of the patient, although the procedure is safely performed with monitored sedation. Prophylactic antibiotics are also given. Carbon

Table 2
Summary of clinical outcomes after flexible endoscopic diverticulotomy for Zenker diverticulum based on existing published data, grouped by instrumentation and scope accessories

Reference	No. of Pts	Division Device/ Instrument	Scope Accessories	Technical Success (%)	Satisfactory Outcome (%)	Overall Morbidity (%)	Perforations (%)	Recurrence Rate (%)
Ishioka et al,[18] 1995; Hashiba et al,[19] 1999; Evrard et al,[20] 2003; Costamagna et al,[21] 2007; Vogelsang et al,[22] 2007; Case and Baron,[23] 2010; Al-Kadi et al,[24] 2010; Repici et al,[25] 2010; Huberty et al,[26] 2013; Halland et al,[27] 2016; Pescarus et al,[28] 2016; Costamagna et al,[29] 2016	546	Needle knife	Cap; soft diverticuloscope	99.3	87.2	11.4	3.7	13.0
Buttaglia et al,[30] 2015; Goelder et al,[31] 2016	83	Stag Beetle knife		100.0	88.0	10.8	3.6	2.7
Repici et al,[32] 2011; Brueckner et al,[33] 2016	78	Hook knife	Soft diverticuloscope	98.7	94.9	6.4	0.0	21.6
Costamagna et al,[21] 2007; Rabenstein et al,[34] 2007	69	APC	Cap	100.0	85.5	20.3	4.4	17.6
de la Morena Madrigal et al,[35] 2016	64	Needle knife + APC	None	93.8	91.2	40.6	1.6	21.2
Laquiere et al,[36] 2015	42	HybridKnife	Soft diverticuloscope	100.0	88.1	31.0	0.0	16.2
Christiaens et al,[37] 2007; Mulder et al,[15] 1995	37	Monopolar forceps	Cap; forcep	100.0	94.6	10.8	0.0	0.0
Manno et al,[38] 2014	19	Insulated tip knife 2	Soft diverticuloscope	100.0	100.0	0.0	0.0	10.5

Abbreviation: APC, argon plasma coagulation.
Data from Refs.[18–38]

dioxide is used exclusively for insufflation given its rapid absorption by the soft tissues to minimize any postoperative subcutaneous emphysema.

A high-definition (HQ-190) upper endoscope, loaded with an EMR cap, is used for the entirety of the procedure. First, a diagnostic upper endoscopy is performed with focus on visualization of the diverticulum and any residual food in the diverticular pouch should be cleared if done easily. Next, with the septum in the center of view (**Figs. 3**A and **4**A), the submucosa overlying the cricopharyngeus is injected with 3 to 5 mL of a mixture of saline, epinephrine, and methylene blue (or 1% indigo carmine) to create a submucosal bleb (**Fig. 3**B). This same mixture is used throughout the case to infiltrate the submucosal space. Next, a mucosotomy is performed over the midpoint of the cricopharyngeal bar with the HybridKnife (EndoCutQ 3-1-1, Erbe USA, Marietta, GA) (**Fig. 4**B). The scope is then inserted into the submucosal space, with the aid of the cap and repeated injection of the blue-dyed saline, the submucosal space is dissected in a proximal to distal direction with the HybridKnife (Forced Coag/Effect2/50W, Erbe USA) on both side of the septum down past the diverticulum and onto the circular and longitudinal fibers of the esophagus (**Figs. 3**C and **4**C). Next, a myotomy of the entire length of the cricopharyngeus is performed (**Figs. 3**D, E and **4**D, E), by cauterizing with the HybridKnife (EndoCutQ 3-1-1, Erbe USA). The scope is then withdrawn from the submucosa back into the esophagus. Once hemostasis is confirmed with no incidental mucosal entries noted, the mucosal defect is closed with Endoclips (Resolution 360 Clips, Boston Scientific, Marlborough, MA) (**Figs. 3**F and **4**F). Of note, the endoscopic Overstitch suture device (Apollo Endosurgery, Austin, TX) may be used for difficult closures. The patient is then awakened from anesthesia and taken to the recovery room. Major steps of the procedure are illustrated in **Figs. 3** and **4**.

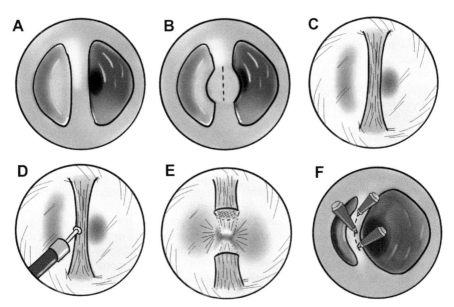

Fig. 3. Illustrated flexible endoscopic view of Z-POEM technique for ZD. (*A*) ZD on the left with the common wall/septum in the middle. (*B*) Submucosal injection and mucosal incision over the septum. (*C*) Creation of the submucosal tunnel on either side of the septum with clear exposure of the muscle fibers of cricopharyngeus. (*D*) Septum division with Hybrid-Knife. (*E*) Complete cricopharyngeal myotomy down to the esophageal wall. (*F*) Closure of mucosal entry with Endoclips.

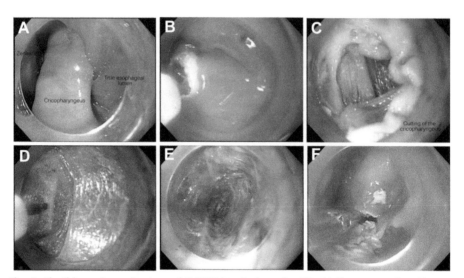

Fig. 4. Flexible endoscopic view of Z-POEM technique for ZD. (*A-F*)correspond to illustrations and descriptions in Fig 3. Flexible endoscopic view of peroral endoscopic myotomy (Z-POEM) technique for ZD. (*A*) ZD on the left with the common wall/septum in the middle. (*B*) Submucosal injection and mucosal incision over the septum. (*C*) Creation of the submucosal tunnel on either side of the septum with clear exposure of the muscle fibers of cricopharyngeus. (*D*) Septum division with HybridKnife. (*E*) Complete cricopharyngeal myotomy down to the esophageal wall. (*F*) Closure of mucosal entry with Endoclips.

After the patient has recovered from anesthesia, most are discharged to home the same day with instructions to stay on a pureed or soft diet for 2 weeks to prevent dislodgement of the Endoclips. This is different than most existing small series and case reports on this technique where patients are routinely admitted for overnight observation followed by esophagram before clearance of diet and antibiotics continued for up to 7 days postoperatively.[39–44] There is currently no evidence to suggest postoperative esophagram or prolonged antibiotic use correlate with improved clinical outcomes.

Using the Z-POEM/STESD technique has many advantages. First, submucosal tunneling allows the cricopharyngeus to be completely isolated and dissected, ensuring the complete myotomy under direct visualization up to the level of the esophageal wall. Moreover, by dissecting in the submucosal space, the integrity of the mucosal layer is preserved, decreasing the risk for perforation and secondary infection.[39,44]

Similar to all endoscopic approaches, it is thought that the flexible endoscopic approach may not be suitable for diverticula that are too large or too small. In a study by Costamagna and colleagues[29] evaluating prognostic variables for clinical success in flexible endoscopic septotomy for ZD, they found septotomy length of less than or equal to 2.5 cm and pretreatment ZD size of greater than or equal to 5 cm were independent predictors of failure to achieve symptom relief. The short septotomy length predicting failure further validates the need for complete myotomy, which is more reliably achieved with the Z-POEM approach. The problem that arises from a very large diverticulum causing persistence of recurrence of symptoms is seemingly only solved by open surgery with diverticulectomy. However, we present a possible flexible endoscopic alternative to address this issue, by performing an endoscopic diverticulopexy.

Endoscopic diverticulopexy for large diverticulum (>5 cm)

In the authors' experience, a patient with a pretreatment ZD of 6.2 cm returned after initial treatment with recurrence of dysphagia and was successfully treated with flexible endoscopic diverticulopexy. This technique requires the use of a dual-lumen scope and overstitch device with 2–0 DemeLENE suture (DemeTECH, Miami, FL). After identification of the diverticulum, the apex of the pouch is grasped with a helix device and brought into the jaws of the device. The device was then brought into the true lumen of the esophagus and another bite distal was taken on the lateral wall of the esophagus, effectively pexying the diverticular sac. Additional similar stitches should be taken until the entire diverticulum is attached to the lateral wall. The scope is then exchanged for a single-channel scope with intraoperative fluoroscopy, which is used to confirm the lumen is not obstructed. After confirming hemostasis and absence of mucosal perforation, the scope is removed.

Examining analogous literature in open surgical approaches, Vannucci and colleagues[45] described an open approach myotomy plus diverticulopexy without diverticulectomy in an observational study with 34 patients and found virtually no complications or recurrence up to 1 year postoperative. This further suggests that diverticulopexy may be the management of choice to prevent recurrence especially when a large diverticulum is present.

OUTCOMES

Numerous case series have been published regarding the use of a flexible endoscopic approach for the treatment of ZD (see **Table 2**). Although most of these studies are retrospective observational studies with heterogeneity of instrumentation, the available data demonstrate high rates of technical success and clinical response with low complications and recurrence. In a meta-analysis by Crawly and colleagues[46] comparing rigid versus flexible endoscopic repair of ZD, no difference was found in mortality, infection, or perforation. However, bleeding and recurrence were more likely after flexible endoscopic techniques (20% vs <10% and 4% vs 0%, respectively). Risk of perforation was reported to be 1% to 2% in all approaches. Only two studies have been done that directly compares rigid with flexible endoscopic approaches,[32,47] which showed no clear evidence one technique is better than the other.

In a review article by Jain and colleagues[16] reviewing 997 patients from 23 studies who underwent flexible endoscopic diverticulectomy of ZD, the authors reported composite technical success rate of 99.4% and clinical success rate of 87.9%. Although composite failure and recurrence rates were 10% and 13.6%, respectively, half of those patients in each group had success with subsequent endoscopic intervention. Perforation occurred in 5.3% with most successfully managed nonoperatively and only 0.9% requiring invasive management. There were no reported mortalities. Unlike the rigid endoscopic approach, diverticulum size did not affect the efficacy or safety of the intervention.

Given the novel nature of Z-POEM, the specific flexible endoscopic approach using submucosal tunneling described previously has not been included in existing meta-analysis and systematic reviews. With mostly case reports available, there is only one large multi-institutional study that included 75 patients by Yang and colleagues.[44] This study reported overall technical success rate of 97.3% with only two technical failures caused by inability to locate the septum and failed tunnel creation, both of which might have been ameliorated if our specific approach was taken by making the mucosotomy directly over the septum. Clinical success was observed in 92% of patients with adverse events in 6.7% and only one patient reporting symptom recurrence at 12-month follow-up. These results are certainly promising; however, given the heterogeneity in the instrumentation and techniques across different centers, large-scale prospective studies using standardized techniques with long-term follow-up are needed to define the optimal intervention in the treatment of ZD. No matter the approach, it should always be considered in the context of the patient's characteristics to achieve the best outcome.

CLINICS CARE POINTS

- ZD is a rare but treatable surgical disease.
- Three main surgical interventions exist today: open surgery, rigid endoscopy, and flexible endoscopy, mainstay of which involves a cricopharyngeal myotomy.
- Endoscopic approaches are widely accepted as the preferred approach with a trend toward flexible endoscopic approaches, although somewhat limited by patient characteristics (ie, diverticulum size <5 cm).
- There is heterogeneity in instrumentation and specific techniques when performing flexible endoscopic diverticulotomy.
- Our preferred method is per oral endoscopic myotomy with submucosal tunneling technique (Z-POEM).
- There is evidence that flexible endoscopic approach including Z-POEM is safe and effective with excellent patient outcomes.
- Careful patient selection and operative intervention tailored to patient characteristics is important when evaluating patients for operative intervention for ZD.

DISCLOSURE

Dr M.B. Ujiki is a consultant for Boston Scientific, Olympus, and Cook Medical. Dr M.B. Ujiki is also a speaker for GORE, Medtronic, and Erbe.

REFERENCES

1. Bizzotto A, Iacopini F, Landi R, et al. Zenker's diverticulum: exploring treatment options. Acta Otorhinolaryngol Ital 2013;33(4):219–29.
2. Ferreira LEVVC, Simmons DT, Baron TH. Zenker's diverticula: pathophysiology, clinical presentation, and flexible endoscopic management. Dis Esophagus 2008;21(1):1–8.
3. Sen P, Lowe DA, Farnan T. Surgical interventions for pharyngeal pouch. Cochrane Database Syst Rev 2005;(3):CD004459.
4. Howell RJ, Giliberto JP, Harmon J, et al. Open versus endoscopic surgery of Zenker's diverticula: a systematic review and meta-analysis. Dysphagia 2019;34(6):930–8.
5. Beard K, Swanström LL. Zenker's diverticulum: flexible versus rigid repair. J Thorac Dis 2017;9(2):S154–62.
6. Crawley B, Dehom S, Tamares S, et al. Adverse events after rigid and flexible endoscopic repair of Zenker's diverticula: a systematic review and meta-analysis. Otolaryngol Head Neck Surg 2019;161(3):388–400.
7. Rizzetto C, Zaninotto G, Costantini M, et al. Zenker's diverticula: feasibility of a tailored approach based on diverticulum size. J Gastrointest Surg 2008;12(12):2057–65.
8. Ishaq S, Hassan C, Antonello A, et al. Flexible endoscopic treatment for Zenker's diverticulum: a systematic review and meta-analysis. Gastrointest Endosc 2016;83(6):1076–89.e5.

9. Romanelli JR, Desilets DJ, Earle DB, editors. NOTES and endoluminal surgery. Cham (Switzerland): Springer International Publishing; 2017. https://doi.org/10.1007/978-3-319-50610-4.

10. Yuan Y, Zhao Y-F, Hu Y, et al. Surgical treatment of Zenker's diverticulum. Dig Surg 2013;30(3):207–18.

11. Dohlman G, Mattsson O. The endoscopic operation for hypopharyngeal diverticula: a roentgencinematographic study. AMA Arch Otolaryngol 1960;71:744–52.

12. Aiolfi A, Scolari F, Saino G, et al. Current status of minimally invasive endoscopic management for Zenker diverticulum. World J Gastrointest Endosc 2015;7(2):87–93.

13. Jackson AS, Aye RW. Endoscopic approaches to cricopharyngeal myotomy and pyloromyotomy. Thorac Surg Clin 2018;28(4):507–20.

14. Diez Redondo P, Núñez Rodríguez H, de Benito Sanz M, et al. Endoscopic treatment of Zenker's diverticulum with Ligasure: simple, safe and effective. Endosc Int Open 2019;7(2):E203–8.

15. Mulder CJ, den Hartog G, Robijn RJ, et al. Flexible endoscopic treatment of Zenker's diverticulum: a new approach. Endoscopy 1995;27(6):438–42.

16. Jain D, Sharma A, Shah M, et al. Efficacy and safety of flexible endoscopic management of Zenker's diverticulum. J Clin Gastroenterol 2018;52(5):369–85.

17. Ishaq S, Sultan H, Siau K, et al. New and emerging techniques for endoscopic treatment of Zenker's diverticulum: state-of-the-art review. Dig Endosc 2018; 30(4):449–60.

18. Ishioka S, Sakai P, Maluf Filho F, et al. Endoscopic incision of Zenker's diverticula. Endoscopy 1995;27(6):433–7.

19. Hashiba K, de Paula AL, da Silva JG, et al. Endoscopic treatment of Zenker's diverticulum. Gastrointest Endosc 1999;49(1):93–7.

20. Evrard S, Le Moine O, Hassid S, et al. Zenker's diverticulum: a new endoscopic treatment with a soft diverticuloscope. Gastrointest Endosc 2003;58(1):116–20.

21. Costamagna G, Iacopini F, Tringali A, et al. Flexible endoscopic Zenker's diverticulotomy: cap-assisted technique vs. diverticuloscope-assisted technique. Endoscopy 2007;39(02):146–52.

22. Vogelsang A, Preiss C, Neuhaus H, et al. Endotherapy of Zenker's diverticulum using the needle-knife technique: long-term follow-up. Endoscopy 2007;39(2):131–6.

23. Case DJ, Baron TH. Flexible endoscopic management of Zenker diverticulum: the Mayo Clinic experience. Mayo Clin Proc 2010;85(8):719–22.

24. Al-Kadi AS, Maghrabi AA, Thomson D, et al. Endoscopic treatment of Zenker diverticulum: results of a 7-year experience. J Am Coll Surg 2010;211(2):239–43.

25. Repici A, Pagano N, Romeo F, et al. Endoscopic flexible treatment of Zenker's diverticulum: a modification of the needle-knife technique. Endoscopy 2010; 42(7):532–5.

26. Huberty V, El Bacha S, Blero D, et al. Endoscopic treatment for Zenker's diverticulum: long-term results (with video). Gastrointest Endosc 2013;77(5):701–7.

27. Halland M, Grooteman KV, Baron TH. Flexible endoscopic management of Zenker's diverticulum: characteristics and outcomes of 52 cases at a tertiary referral center. Dis Esophagus 2016;29(3):273–7.

28. Pescarus R, Shlomovitz E, Sharata AM, et al. Trans-oral cricomyotomy using a flexible endoscope: technique and clinical outcomes. Surg Endosc 2016;30(5):1784–9.

29. Costamagna G, Iacopini F, Bizzotto A, et al. Prognostic variables for the clinical success of flexible endoscopic septotomy of Zenker's diverticulum. Gastrointest Endosc 2016;83(4):765–73.

30. Battaglia G, Antonello A, Realdon S, et al. Flexible endoscopic treatment for Zenker's diverticulum with the SB Knife. Preliminary results from a single-center experience. Dig Endosc 2015;27(7):728–33.
31. Goelder SK, Brueckner J, Messmann H. Endoscopic treatment of Zenker's diverticulum with the stag beetle knife (sb knife): feasibility and follow-up. Scand J Gastroenterol 2016;51(10):1155–8.
32. Repici A, Pagano N, Fumagalli U, et al. Transoral treatment of Zenker diverticulum: flexible endoscopy versus endoscopic stapling. A retrospective comparison of outcomes. Dis Esophagus 2011;24(4):235–9.
33. Brueckner J, Schneider A, Messmann H, et al. Long-term symptomatic control of Zenker diverticulum by flexible endoscopic mucomyotomy with the hook knife and predisposing factors for clinical recurrence. Scand J Gastroenterol 2016; 51(6):666–71.
34. Rabenstein T, May A, Michel J, et al. Argon plasma coagulation for flexible endoscopic Zenker's diverticulotomy. Endoscopy 2007;39(2):141–5.
35. de la Morena Madrigal EJ, Pérez Arellano E, Rodríguez García I. Flexible endoscopic treatment of Zenker's diverticulum: thirteen years' experience in Spain. Rev Esp Enferm Dig 2016;108(6):297–303.
36. Laquière A, Grandval P, Arpurt JP, et al. Interest of submucosal dissection knife for endoscopic treatment of Zenker's diverticulum. Surg Endosc 2015;29(9): 2802–10.
37. Christiaens P, De Roock W, Van Olmen A, et al. Treatment of Zenker's diverticulum through a flexible endoscope with a transparent oblique-end hood attached to the tip and a monopolar forceps. Endoscopy 2007;39(2):137–40.
38. Manno M, Manta R, Caruso A, et al. Alternative endoscopic treatment of Zenker's diverticulum: a case series (with video). Gastrointest Endosc 2014;79(1):168–70.
39. Li Q-L, Chen W-F, Zhang X-C, et al. Submucosal tunneling endoscopic septum division: a novel technique for treating Zenker's diverticulum. Gastroenterology 2016;151(6):1071–4.
40. Brewer Gutierrez OI, Ichkhanian Y, Spadaccini M, et al. Zenker's diverticulum peroral endoscopic myotomy techniques: changing paradigms. Gastroenterology 2019;156(8):2134–5.
41. Delis K, Robotis J, Sachitzi E, et al. Submucosal tunneling endoscopic septum division of a Zenker's diverticulum. Ann Gastroenterol 2018;31(5):634.
42. Hajifathalian K, Dawod Q, Saumoy M, et al. Submucosal tunneling endoscopic septum division for treatment of Zenker's diverticulum. Endoscopy 2018;50(12): E340–1.
43. Yang J, Zeng X, Yuan X, et al. An international study on the use of peroral endoscopic myotomy (POEM) in the management of esophageal diverticula: the first multicenter D-POEM experience. Endoscopy 2019;51(04):346–9.
44. Yang J, Novak S, Ujiki M, et al. An international study on the use of peroral endoscopic myotomy in the management of Zenker's diverticulum. Gastrointest Endosc 2020;91(1):163–8.
45. Vannucci J, Matricardi A, Scarnecchia E, et al. Is Myotomy Plus Diverticulopexy Suitable for Symptomatic Zenker's Diverticula? Dysphagia 2019;34(2):240–7.
46. Crawley B, Dehom S, Tamares S, et al. Adverse Events after Rigid and Flexible Endoscopic Repair of Zenker's Diverticula: A Systematic Review and Meta-analysis. Otolaryngol Head Neck Surg 2019;161(3):388–400.
47. Jones DG, Aloraini A, Gowing SD, et al. Comparing outcomes of open vs flexible and rigid trans-oral endoscopic techniques for the treatment of Zenker's diverticulum. J Am Coll Surg 2014;219(4, Supplement):e67.

Moving?

Make sure your subscription moves with you!

To notify us of your new address, find your **Clinics Account Number** (located on your mailing label above your name), and contact customer service at:

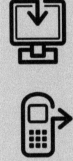

Email: journalscustomerservice-usa@elsevier.com

800-654-2452 (subscribers in the U.S. & Canada)
314-447-8871 (subscribers outside of the U.S. & Canada)

Fax number: 314-447-8029

Elsevier Health Sciences Division
Subscription Customer Service
3251 Riverport Lane
Maryland Heights, MO 63043

*To ensure uninterrupted delivery of your subscription, please notify us at least 4 weeks in advance of move.

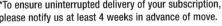